Asian Healing Traditions in Counseling and Psychotherapy

Sara Miller McCune founded SAGE Publishing in 1965 to support the dissemination of usable knowledge and educate a global community. SAGE publishes more than 1000 journals and over 800 new books each year, spanning a wide range of subject areas. Our growing selection of library products includes archives, data, case studies and video. SAGE remains majority owned by our founder and after her lifetime will become owned by a charitable trust that secures the company's continued independence.

Los Angeles | London | New Delhi | Singapore | Washington DC | Melbourne

Asian Healing Traditions in Counseling and Psychotherapy

Roy Moodley
University of Toronto

Ted Lo
University of Toronto

Na Zhu
University of Windsor

SAGE

Los Angeles | London | New Delhi
Singapore | Washington DC | Melbourne

SAGE

FOR INFORMATION:

SAGE Publications, Inc.
2455 Teller Road
Thousand Oaks, California 91320
E-mail: order@sagepub.com

SAGE Publications Ltd.
1 Oliver's Yard
55 City Road
London, EC1Y 1SP
United Kingdom

SAGE Publications India Pvt. Ltd.
B 1/I 1 Mohan Cooperative Industrial Area
Mathura Road, New Delhi 110 044
India

SAGE Publications Asia-Pacific Pte. Ltd.
3 Church Street
#10-04 Samsung Hub
Singapore 049483

Acquisitions Editor: Abbie Rickard
Editorial Assistant: Jennifer Cline
Production Editor: Andrew Olson
Copy Editor: Megan Markanich
Typesetter: Hurix Systems Pvt. Ltd.
Proofreader: Annette Van Deusen
Indexer: Judy Hunt
Cover Designer: Rose Storey
Marketing Manager: Katherine Hepburn

Printed in the United States of America.

Library of Congress Cataloging-in-Publication Data

Names: Moodley, Roy, editor. | Lo, Ted Hung-Tat, editor. | Zhu, Na, editor.

Title: Asian healing traditions in counseling and psychotherapy / [edited by] Roy Moodley, University of Toronto, Ted Lo, University of Toronto, Na Zhu, University of Windsor, Canada.

Description: Los Angeles : SAGE, [2018] | Includes bibliographical references and index.

Identifiers: LCCN 2017030914 | ISBN 9781483371436 (pbk. : alk. paper)

Subjects: LCSH: Psychotherapy–Cross-cultural studies. | Cross-cultural counseling. | Alternative medicine–Asia. | Mental healing–Asia.

Classification: LCC RC455.4.E8 .A85 2018 | DDC 362.196/89140095–dc23 LC record available at https://lccn.loc.gov/2017030914

This book is printed on acid-free paper.

FSC www.fsc.org MIX Paper from responsible sources FSC® C014174

17 18 19 20 21 10 9 8 7 6 5 4 3 2 1

Contents

Foreword

Joseph E. Trimble

Distinguished University Professor
Professor of Psychology
Western Washington University

About four decades ago, three of my close American Indian friends and I spent a few days in a traditional lodge in a remote area of South Dakota. Two Native healers, holy men, accompanied us. The healers extended us the invitation to be with them because they wanted us to hear their stories. We were there to learn about their ways of healing, along with the traditions, ceremonies, customs, and ways of their world. Through one story after another, the healers thoroughly engaged us in the deep mysteries of traditional practices we had heard about over the years, but we knew little about their deeper historical meaning. During the day, we would walk around the area by ourselves or in groups talking, reflecting, and probing deeply into the wisdom unfolding in the stories we were hearing. We prepared and cooked meals together, with family members often joining us in the chilly evenings, a small fire always burning in the center of the lodge.

On the morning of our last day with the healers, they asked us to explain how we psychologists provided "healing" for those in need. The clinical psychologist in our group, with considerable experience working in mental health settings focused on providing services for different multicultural clients, described how the client would sign up for a session, what took place in the first and subsequent sessions, how the "counseling" unfolded, and generally what would happen in each session. Another friend added a few features of the relationships between the mental health helper and the client. The healers listened intently, though often with puzzled expressions.

Following our detailed descriptions, the healers began asking the following questions: Do you personally know the clients? Why do they have an appointment with you for an hour each week? Do they always show up?

Why do you talk and talk with them and them with you? How do you know you helped or healed them? Do you ever see them again? Do you ask the spirits to help you as you talk with them? Do spirits sometimes come in the room where you're sitting? Why do you sit when the two of you talk? Why aren't others present when you talk with one another? Do you ask their ancestors to join you? Is the room where you're sitting clean and clear of evil and bad spirits? Are both of you clean and clear of anything bad that may interfere with the talking and healing? Do the clients prepare for each meeting by sweating, praying, meditating, and fasting? Do counselors prepare this way also for each meeting with the client? Why do you take notes? Does the talking occur in a sacred place? What happens to the two of them after the client is healed?

We attempted to answer each of their surprising questions. With each response, we focused more on what we were saying to them and the possibility that their questions were more profoundly meaningful and appropriate than we realized. We also knew on that day that conventional counseling and psychotherapy were a long way from including the spiritual, the sacred, or the meaning of place in the healing process and from considering the real possibility that centuries-old traditional healing practices were as powerful, if not more so, than contemporary approaches to mental health.

Recognition and acknowledgment of what was at the heart of the healers' probing questions and concerns that day wouldn't come to the evolving mental health fields until much later. In 2003, the American Psychological Association (APA) published a set of multicultural guidelines that gave attention to changes in society at large and to the emerging data about "the different needs of unique individuals and groups historically marginalized or disenfranchised within and by psychology based on their ethnic/racial heritage and social group identity or membership" (p. 377).[1] The overarching goal of the guidelines was to provide psychologists with a rationale for the urgency to address multiculturalism and diversity in education, training, research, practice, and organizational change.

Additionally, in 2009, the Association for Spiritual, Ethical, and Religious Values in Counseling endorsed a set of carefully crafted guidelines for spiritual competencies in counseling. They maintained in their report that culturally competent counselors actively give attention to the spiritual dimension of the client's life and consider the profound influence of religious, spiritual, and transpersonal beliefs, practices, and development over the life span. To this end, the practitioner is encouraged to use a client's spiritual beliefs in the pursuit of the client's therapeutic goals. Counselors are asked to carefully and thoughtfully focus on connections, similarities, and differences among religion, spirituality, and the transpersonal and to describe beliefs and practices in a cultural context. They are encouraged to articulate a client's self-exploration of personal beliefs and to explain various models of spiritual development across a client's life span. Counselors also are encouraged to demonstrate sensitivity to and acceptance of a variety of spiritual expressions from the client. And, importantly, the guidelines recommend counselors acknowledge the limits of their understanding of a client's spiritual and deeply cultural expression and demonstrate appropriate referral skills.

Fortunately, psychotherapy and counseling practices and approaches are being reshaped within the profession. There is a strong sense among practitioners and in research findings that inclusion of spirituality and collaboration with traditional healers and elders in the counseling process and intervention programs create better outcomes. Therapy offered in a manner congruent with the traditional values and spirituality of the clientele can reverse the historical trend of many immigrant populations to assimilate dominant cultural ways and worldviews exclusively to get better and healthier. With counseling and psychotherapy aligning with culture, there is now the possibility of receiving treatment supportive of one's own culture, beliefs, and spirituality. While these are exciting and promising trends, pitfalls and dangers also are associated with these endeavors. Caution is encouraged, because the development of keen sensitivity and respect is required when attempting to move into these sensitive areas. Not every client will be receptive to openly sharing his or her beliefs.

In this book, the reader will discover that Asian healers know a great deal about what works best for those who seek guidance, assistance, and healing. The relational styles of Asian healers are comparable with what we know works effectively in building and sustaining positive counseling and psychotherapeutic relationships. Effective counselors and therapists possess personal characteristics that promote positive relationships with clients, regardless of cultural background. Indeed, this is the foundation of any healing or helping process. Characteristics such as empathy, genuineness, warmth, respect, and availability are likely to be effective in any setting or ethnocultural community.

These same characteristics often exemplify the spiritual healers in numerous indigenous communities. The Inupiat Alaska Native counseling psychologist Reimer, for example, collected information from Inupiat members in an Alaska Native village concerning the characteristics they found desirable in a healer. Her respondents indicated that a healer is (a) one who is virtuous, kind, respectful, trustworthy, friendly, gentle, loving, clean, giving, and helpful; (b) one who is thoroughly strong; (c) one who works well with others by becoming familiar with people in communities; (d) one who has good communication skills; (e) one who is respected because of his or her knowledge; (f) one who is substance-free; (g) one who knows and follows the culture; and (h) one who has faith and a strong relationship with the Creator (p. 60).[2]

Asian Healing Traditions in Counseling and Psychotherapy is a seminal contribution to the evolving mental health field. The editors, Roy Moodley, Ted Lo, and Na Zhu, and their impressive array of chapter authors are to be congratulated. They are bold in addressing the legacies of Asian healing traditions and their influence on counseling and psychotherapy. The 18 chapters in the book are packed with useful material—some based on empirical findings and others based on firsthand experiences. The chapter authors invite the reader to reflect on the similarities of many Asian healing traditions with the core principles and approaches of conventional counseling and psychotherapy. The blend of their many voices, personal writing styles, and points of view add to the breadth and depth of a book that will influence the scholarly expression of Asian approaches and perspectives and help shape the direction of counseling and psychotherapy research for many years to come.

Loaded with useful tools for treatment professionals, this beautifully crafted book is especially excellent for introducing practitioners to the deeply philosophical and practical Asian approaches to healing. Anyone interested in the depth and scope of providing counseling services to culturally distinct populations should keep this book close by, as it will prove a valuable resource for assistance and inspiration for years to come. We can be optimistic that its contributions will help move the fields of counseling and psychotherapy from a Eurocentric level of understanding to one closer to eliminating cultural biases and the disregard those biases so often engender.

The challenge is clear. Science and psychology must examine their Eurocentric views, recognize its limitations, and seek to expand and transcend its assumptions, thereby restoring balance to its own original purpose, the pursuit of truth for the common good. Advances in multicultural psychology are accumulating like pieces of a multicolored quilt, giving us a much broader outlook on spirituality, culture, and psychology. The mounting number of research studies and clinical observations from those who have ventured beyond their own cultural milieu all indicate that culture in psychotherapy matters.

Scientists must seek out the wisdom holders within other cultures and meet on equal ground for the exchange of knowledge. On this point, beginning in 1987, the Dalai Lama co-initiated ongoing meetings between Buddhist scholars and top Western scientists in what is now called *Dialogues With the Dalai Lama*.[3] Similar meetings could be established among Asian elders and healers and Western scientists and educators. While this may be a challenging and daunting endeavor, it is worth the effort as a way to work toward restoring harmony among the world's people, a world in which all will benefit.

References

1. American Psychological Association. (2003). Guidelines on multicultural education, training, research, practice, and organizational change for psychologists. *American Psychologist*, *58*(5), 377–402.
2. Reimer, C. S. (1999). *Counseling the Inupiat Eskimo*. Westport, CT: Greenwood.
3. Dalai Lama. (2005). *The universe in a single atom*. New York, NY: Doubleday.

Acknowledgments

We want to express our sincere thanks and appreciation to all the authors in this book for the creative and innovative way in which they responded to our invitation to write about Asian healing traditions and its intersection with counseling and psychotherapy. These expert researchers with numerous years of practice and teaching wonderfully distilled their canon of work into the limitation of space in this book. Also, our very special thanks and gratitude go to all the clients or patients whose stories were part of the analysis. We deeply appreciate your desire and openness to engage in a holistic and integrative approach to achieve wellness, health, and mental health care.

Our deepest gratitude goes to several colleagues, friends, and family members who were very supportive during this book's development; they are Roisin Anna, Javeria Arshad, Joy Bon, Charles Chen, Zina Claude, Maya Florence, Daniel Harry, Tara Isabelle, Mama Ishii, Melissa Morton, Joe So, Anissa Talahite, and Joanne Zhu.

Our thanks go to the publication team at SAGE: Nathan Davidson, Kassie Graves, Katherine Hepburn, Megan Markanich, Carrie Montoya, Alissa Nance, Andrew Olson, Abbie Rickard, and Rose Storey.

We would also like to thank the following reviewers: Mary Olufunmilayo Adekson, St. Bonaventure University; Mary Fukuyama, University of Florida; Tonya R. Hammer, Oklahoma State University; Joanne Jodry, Monmouth University; Theresa S. Kearns-Cooper, Jackson State University; Gerard Kenny, University of the West of England; Fernand Lubuguin, University of Denver; Charmaine Sonnex, University of Northampton; Theresa Van Lith, Florida State University; Jessica Woolhiser Stallings, Emporia State University.

Introduction

The inclusion of mindfulness meditation techniques into Western therapies has clearly demonstrated that integration of Asian philosophical, religious, and healing traditions are not just a theoretical possibility but can become a major force of change in ways in which healing is understood and practiced in the West. The successful integration of mindfulness meditation into cognitive behavioral therapy (CBT) clearly demonstrates that integration of Asian healing traditions is happening at a much rapid rate than is currently acknowledged. Moreover, the mindfulness meditation scholarship generally has not been forthcoming in recognizing the traditional Asian healing roots of mindfulness meditation. No doubt, the integration of mindfulness meditation into counseling and psychotherapy, which began in the 1960s in North America through the efforts of Jon Kabat-Zinn and his mindfulness-based stress reduction (MBSR) in medicine, evolved in a significant methodology in counseling and psychotherapy.[1] In part, it has addressed the limitations and shortfalls in Western health and mental care practices, which, in turn, provided a space for conversations about the cultural and traditional healing practices of racialized and marginalized communities. Furthermore, immigrants coming to the West since the 1960s, particularly from Asia and Africa, brought with them a compendium of methods in which to heal themselves physically, mentally, emotionally, and spiritually. Indeed, many first- and second-generation immigrants today practice traditional healing alongside conventional medicine to make up for the many shortcomings of Western health and mental care practices.[2] The crisis that counseling, psychotherapy, psychology, and psychiatry are experiencing in relation to not meeting the mental health needs of a diverse multicultural society has provided a space for the inclusion of mindfulness meditation. Since mindfulness meditation now appears to be firmly rooted in Western health and mental care, other Asian healing traditions and their histories and philosophies can be explored for inclusion and integration, such as Confucianism, Taoism, and Buddhism.

While traditional, cultural, and indigenous healing practices have been used since the dawn of history, it has only recently been part of the conversation of health and mental health care in the West. Throughout the period of colonialism, cultural, indigenous, and traditional healing practices were not encouraged at best or were completely banned, outlawed, and disavowed. Notwithstanding the disruptions and oppressions of the colonial period, Asian healing traditions, like aboriginal, African, Caribbean, Hispanic, and South Asian healing traditions, have been the mainstay of health and mental health practices for wellness and well-being for the majority of people from those cultures, being practiced in various ways openly or secretly in clandestine sessions and underground and away from the public gaze or the ever seeing eye of colonial regimes. While many indigenous and traditional approaches have not changed from its earliest origins of practice, many have been modified and reconstituted to suit the sociopolitical contexts and health care needs of people from those cultures. At the same time, the lived experiences of those cultural communities also determine the growth, research, and development of the indigenous healing practices. Some of the traditional and cultural healing practices were even modified to respond to the racism and colonial oppression that people experienced—for example, voodoo healing in the Caribbean.[3] The failures of the prohibitions of traditional healing practices during the colonial hegemony are a clear sign of the strength and resilience of these practices. It also shows that these cultural healing practices are embedded in an epistemologically richly grounded past; a significant part of the evolutionary history of the community is the production of knowledge for the health and well-being of the people. In particular, Asian healing traditions can clearly trace their development to specific cultural, historical, and political periods in the Far East.

The result of gaining independence from European colonialism and the subsequent rise of nationalism led to the indigenizing psychology movement in many non-Western countries. In many cases, these movements were a direct response to oppressive colonial practices and the need to reclaim indigenous and cultural healing methods.[4] For example, in China, the Cultural Revolution saw the rise and growth of traditional Chinese medicine (TCM), with its own exclusions of some indigenous practices that it deemed superstitious. However, in more recent times, these disavowed practices are now resurfacing and are being accepted as mainstream, such as palm readings.

In the postcolonialism period and more recently through globalization and international migration, many people in the West and not just the new immigrant communities actively seek alternative and complementary treatments, such as TCM (including acupuncture, Qigong [QG]), Ayurveda, herbalism, yogic meditation, and many others for their mental and physical well-being.[5] The result of globalization and internationalization has no doubt increased the degree to which Asian healing practices are now part of a larger global or universal health and wellness practice; many are now found on the main streets in metropolitan cities in the West accessed by non Asian clients.

However, globalization has generally led to the domination of Eurocentric ideas and methods in health and mental health. This has constructed and shaped health and mental health policies and interventions across the globe. This is due, in part, to the well-established status and specialty of Western health and mental health theories and practices as the standard approach to health and well-being. But as immigration continues to characterize the Western world, it is imperative for mental health practitioners and clinicians, and those in training, to abandon their sense of self-sufficiency and actively increase their understanding of non-Western healing traditions and practices. This book, *Asian Healing Traditions in Counseling and Psychotherapy*, has been developed to address shortcomings in Western health care practices vis-à-vis the Asian communities and make a significant contribution to the already growing awareness, understanding, knowledge, and practices of the rich, centuries-old Far East Asian healing traditions amongst scholars, practitioners, researchers, and patients. *Asian Healing Traditions in Counseling and Psychotherapy* not only defines the processes involved and explains the philosophical basis for these healing practices but engages Western practitioners to seriously consider integration and collaboration toward formulating a new approach to health and mental health care.

Traditional Healing, Multiculturalism, Counseling, and Psychotherapy

Since the 1960s, the developments in multiculturalism and counseling and psychotherapy offered a tremendous potential for innovative research, theory building, and practice of multicultural (cross-cultural, intercultural, transcultural) counseling and psychotherapy. While the evolution and trajectory of U.S. multicultural counseling, psychology, and psychotherapy development attempted to parallel the sociocultural, political, and historical events within North American and European societies, it has also largely neglected to offer a critical analysis of Eurocentric approaches and methodologies. The curriculum of counseling and psychotherapy programs in Western universities are essentially ethnocentric, Eurocentric, and individualistic. Even multicultural counseling has systemically failed to address the root causes of anxiety, depression, schizophrenia, suicide deaths, and many others. The focus on cultural competencies and racial identity theories over the decades has led to a lack of research on critical issues such as oppression, domination, racism, poverty, and marginalization of ethnic minority communities. Moreover, it has also failed to theorize and engage the practice of indigenous, cultural, and traditional healing in health and mental health care.[6] Nor did it allow for an acknowledgment and focus on the traditional healing practices of Diaspora ethnic or visible minority communities: indigenous, aboriginal, First Nation, and many other indigenous communities from around the world. Indeed, on the contrary, the opposite has happened in mainstream counseling psychology and psychiatry where indigenous healing traditions have been critiqued for being unscientific, primitive, or just mumbo jumbo arising from undeveloped, unsophisticated, and nascent societies in the developing world, or in the West from the era of slavery or the colonial period.

In more recent decades, with the advent of diversity (race, gender, class, sexual orientation, disability, religion, age) taking a more prominent place in multicultural counseling, the healing traditions of non-Western cultures are also being acknowledged and accepted for their clinical and healing potential. These changes in both counseling and multicultural counseling are illustrative of the fact that counseling and psychotherapy are in dire need of change to avert the crisis that these mental health fields find themselves in: poor rates of participation by non-Western communities in psychotherapy, premature termination if they engage in therapy, and failure to adequately address the mental health needs of communities and groups that are not identified as part of the dominant culture. More importantly, there is a clear understanding that health and mental health interventions would need to be situated in local cultural contexts to solve local problems. As Good and Good said, "the meaning of illness for an individual is grounded in . . . the network of meanings an illness has in a particular culture" (p. 148).[7] It seems that indigenous and traditional healing practices are then an obvious resource for any intervention in a local context; the network of meanings for both the illness and the wellness is best mediated through practices that arise from within the same cultural contexts. Thus, in recent years, counseling and psychotherapy have become more open to the idea of locating culture more centrally in their healing project. Yet, this is not a new idea, since psychoanalysis and psychotherapy have its roots in 19th-century European culture with deeply underpinning Jewish roots through its founder, Sigmund Freud. Subsequently, each type of psychotherapy has developed out of its own cultural context and represents the dominant worldview of that time and age. For example, CBT and client-centered therapy (CCT) are uniquely North American. However, in our contemporary context, with a diverse population, each approach may find its own adherents depending on the cultural match between the therapy and the help-seekers—for example, for those with a past orientation, psychoanalysis may be meaningful, while for those with a future perspective, solution-focused therapy may be more effective.[8] Traditional healing is based on the cultural context of the specific tradition from which it arose. For example, aboriginal cultural healing practices, such as healing circles, storytelling circles, sweat lodge ceremonies, medicine wheel, and the Pimaatisiwin circle are deeply rooted in thousands of years of aboriginal cultures.[9] It is often more holistic with an emphasis on the spiritual and social aspects of an individual and his or her community. That is appealing to many who are dissatisfied with the more clinical approach in many current therapies. An integration of aspects of such traditional healing with current psychotherapies may offer a blend that is refreshing to the users and rewarding to counselors and psychotherapists. Indeed, working alongside these Western-trained practitioners are the traditional healers who are fast becoming part of the healing landscape of health services, who offer a form of medical pluralism and dual interventions by using cultural and traditional healing practices as one of many sources of healing for their health and mental health needs.[10]

The various chapters in this book are ordered in such a way to offer the reader an introduction into the complex field of Asian traditional healing and its integration into counseling, psychotherapy, and psychiatry. The earlier chapters explore the historical trajectory and the evolution of Asian healing to both contextualize its age-old roots and draw attention to the potentiality in contemporary clinical practice. Specific modalities of practices are discussed with a focus on integration into Western health and mental health approaches.

Part A: The Ancient Art of Asian Healing Traditions offers a discussion on the origins of Asian traditional healing through its exploration of Confucianism, Taoism, and Buddhism and its constructions of healing. For example, in Chapter 1: Confucianism and Healing, Kwang-Kuo Hwang explores the concept of *self-exertion* and *putting oneself in the place of another* as the core idea that arises from Confucian theory. The chapter discusses several ideas that establish a critical background to Asian healing traditions—for example: the two branches of neo-Confucianism—Cheng-Chu School of *lixne* and Lu-Wang School of *xinxue*—in the Sung–Ming dynasties; Wang Yangming's theory on the Unity of Knowledge and Practice, which was imported to Japan before the era of Meiji Restoration; and the development of Confucianism during the Cultural Revolution. Chapter 2: Taoism and Healing, by Catherine Tien-Lun Sun, on the other hand, explores how the essence of Taoism (found in the *taijitu)* illustrates the concepts of harmonious equilibrium, noninterference, mutual generation, mutual attenuation, and dynamism—for example, the human body and the universe are both conceived of being made up by the interaction and composition of *yin* and *yang*, and the five elements of metal, wood, water, fire, and earth. From this conception, the elements of traditional Chinese healing are derived. Furthermore, in Chapter 3: Buddhism and Healing, Tony Toneatto discusses how Buddhist psychology, which is primarily concerned with the alleviation of human suffering, distress, and dissatisfaction, closely resembles many clinical perspectives in clinical psychology and psychotherapy. Finally, in this section, Chapter 4: Qigong and Healing (Based on Taoist Philosophy) and Chapter 5: Ki (氣) and Healing examine the concept of *qi* or *ki* in different contexts. *Qi*, or *ki*, or sometimes referred to as the life force or energy flow, underlies many concepts in traditional healing and is explored throughout this book. Specifically, in Chapter 4, Amy L. Ai explores how the ancient art of QG, part of TCM and an energy-based health care practice and originating in Daoism (or Taoism), has the potential for clinical practice.

And Chapter 5, by Tadashi Ogawa and Mami Ishii, considers how *ki* (or *qi*) is conceptualized in a Japanese context to engage with healing and mental health.

Part B: Integrating Asian Healing Traditions Into Clinical Practices includes chapters that explore how Asian healing practices can be integrated into various clinical approaches. Specifically, in Chapter 6: Infusing Asian Healing Traditions Into Counseling Psychology, Ben C. H. Kuo and Beatriz Rodriguez-Rubio discuss the incorporation of Asian traditional healing into counseling and psychotherapy. The chapter reviews the current understanding, views, and debates on indigenous healing or helping approaches and contemporary practices and training of counseling psychology. Integration into psychotherapy is further expounded in Chapter 7: Integrating Asian Healing Traditions Into Psychotherapy by Boon-Ooi Lee, who argues that through this kind of integration psychotherapy may become more culturally relevant as worldviews embedded in psychotherapy largely reflect the Euro-American concepts of the self, human nature, well-being, and suffering. Chapter 8: Integrating Asian Healing Traditions Into Biomedicine, by Tenzin Lhundup and James H. Lake, engages the reader in an interesting conversation about the inclusion of Asian traditional healing practices into biomedicine. This chapter explores how conventional biomedicine (also known as allopathic medicine) and Asian healing traditions including TCM, Tibetan medicine, and Ayurveda, present many complex issues and opportunities in the treatment of medical and psychiatric problems. Finally, in Chapter 9: Integrating Mindfulness Meditation, Buddhism, and Therapeutic Practices, Marco Mascarin explores the relationship between Buddhism and mindfulness meditation and its integration into clinical practice. This chapter begins with the historical Buddhist traditions that gave rise to mindfulness meditation, considers several concepts of Buddhism—amongst them, the Four Noble Truths, an Eightfold Path, and right mindfulness—and articulates a strong position for strategic integration into therapeutic work.

Part C: Asian Healing Traditions and Their Contemporary Formulations considers the approaches that have been developed in the current period but has roots in culture and traditions. For example, in Chapter 10: Chinese Taoist Cognitive Psychotherapy, Yu-ping Cao, Jie Zeng, and Ya-lin Zhang discuss how Chinese Taoist cognitive psychotherapy (CTCP), a culturally grounded approach, shaped by Confucianism (e.g., social hierarchies and collective responsibility, moral development, self-cultivation, professional achievement, control over nature) and Taoism (e.g., easy enjoyment of life's pleasures, development of a flexible personality, acceptance over action, conformity to natural laws), can be a contemporary clinical approach to healing. Chapter 11: Acceptance and Commitment Therapy and Asian Thought, by Kenneth Fung and Zhuo-Hong Zhu, explores the third wave of psychotherapy, acceptance and commitment therapy (ACT) and its roots in Eastern philosophy and its integration into clinical practice. ACT consists of six interrelated processes: (1) cognitive defusion, (2) acceptance, (3) contact with the present moment, (4) self-as-context, (5) values, and (6) committed action. The chapter discusses how ACT is used to treat a variety of psychological and medical problems, neurosis, psychosis, chronic pain, and other health and mental health concerns.

In Chapter 12: Japanese Contemplative Practice of Naikan, Chikako Ozawa-de Silva and Yoshihiko Miki discuss Naikan, the introspective healing practice derived from Japanese Mahayana Buddhism, referred to as a "pre-religious practice" as it does not require any religious belief or knowledge but can lead to self-transformation through cognitive and conceptual shifts. This chapter explores how Naikan as a discursive and analytical method of structured self-reflection can lead to relief from physical and psychological discomforts. Furthermore, in Chapter 13: Morita Therapy, Charles P. Chen discusses Japanese Morita therapy as an alternative helping approach for therapeutic and counseling interventions. The chapter explores how Morita therapy supports emotional and psychological well-being as well as psychological coping and healing. Finally, in Chapter 14: Reiki Therapy, Martha P. Novoa and Emily Kedar discuss the history and origins of Reiki, its evolution and use in the West, and the future of Reiki in counseling and psychotherapy.

Part D: Asian Healing Traditions Inspire Creative Therapies explores new therapies that use Asian healing traditions and their foundation for therapeutic work. In Chapter 15: Tai Chi and Meditation, Paul Posadzki and Samantha Jacques discuss Tai Chi (TC) and meditation. This chapter considers the conceptual congruence and therapeutic benefits of both these practices. Furthermore, in Chapter 16: Hakoniwa: Japanese Sandplay Therapy, Carolyn Zerbe Enns and Makiko Kasai introduce Sandplay therapy with a Eastern paradigm that emphasizes verbal and direct expression, linear and cause–effect thinking, and a distinction between physical and mental wellbeing. This chapter discusses its relationship to Jungian and Eastern philosophy and clarifies how Japanese values and perspectives on the self and mental health are consistent with the practice of Hakoniwa. In contrast, in Chapter 17: *Oishii*: Japanese Delicious Moment Therapy, Mami Ishii and Ted Lo introduce the readers to a new and novel approach to healing and therapy. *Oishii* is a Japanese concept of "deliciousness." The holistic nature of Japanese aesthetics values the simplicity, harmony, and impermanence as seen in many traditional healing practices. This chapter explores these ideas through the four domains of wellness: (1) the body (biological), (2) the mind (psychological), (3) the spiritual (metaphysical), and (4) the social (society).

Finally, in the Conclusion: Integrating Asian Healing Traditions Into Counseling and Psychotherapy, Roy Moodley, Julie Hong, and Na Zhu offer a brief summary of some of the critical issues that were discussed. The conclusion considers issues of integration and the ways in which integration is accomplished. In bringing these ideas and thoughts together, the concluding piece endeavors to strengthen the relationship between Asian healing and Western Eurocentric clinical approaches.

REFERENCES

1. Kabat-Zinn, J. (2013). *Full catastrophe living: Using the wisdom of your body and mind to face stress, pain, and illness* (Rev. 2nd ed.). New York, NY: Bantam/Random House.
2. Moodley, R. (2011). The Toronto traditional healers project: An introduction. In R. Moodley & S. Stewart, Special issue: Integrating traditional healing practices into health promotion and education. *International Journal of Health Promotion and Education*, *49*(3), 71–136.
3. Sutherland, P., Moodley, R., & Chevannes, B. (Eds.). (2014). *Caribbean healing traditions: Implications for health and mental health*. New York, NY: Routledge.
4. Moodley, The Toronto traditional healers project.
5. Ibid.
6. Moodley, R. (2011). *Outside the sentence. Readings in critical multicultural counselling and psychotherapy*. Toronto, Canada: University of Toronto, CDCP Publications.
7. Good, B. J., & Good, M.-J. D. (1982). Towards a meaning centered analysis of popular illness categories "fright illness" and "heat illness" in Iran. In A. J. Marsella & G. M. White (Eds.), *Cultural conceptions of mental health and therapy*. Dordecht, Netherlands: Reidel.
8. Fung, K., & Lo, T. (in press). An integrative clinical approach to cultural competent psychotherapy. *Journal of Contemporary Psychotherapy*.
9. Poonwassie, A., & Charter, A. (2005). Aboriginal worldview of healing: Inclusion, bending and bridging. In R. Moodley & W. West (Eds.), *Integrating traditional healing practices into counseling and psychotherapy*. Thousand Oaks, CA: Sage.
10. Moodley, R., Gielen, U. P., & Wu, R. (Eds.). (2013). *International counseling case study handbook*. Alexandra, VA: American Counseling Association; Moodley, R., & Sutherland, P. (2009). Traditional and cultural healers and healing: Dual interventions in counselling and psychotherapy. *Counselling and Spirituality Journal*, *28*(1), 11–31.

PART A

The Ancient Art of Asian Healing Traditions

1 Confucianism and Healing

Kwang-Kuo Hwang

Four paradigmatic philosophers seem to have emerged from 600 BC to AD 200 in four places: (1) Ancient Greece, (2) the Middle East, (3) India, and (4) China. They created cultural systems common to each area without any direct transmission of ideas from one region to another. Confucianism established by pre-Qin Confucianists (Confucius, Mencius, and Xunzi) has gradually become a transcendental formal structure for sustaining the life-world of Chinese people.

This chapter explores the historical and cultural origin of Confucianism. It discusses the Chinese worldview model of equilibrium, as well as Confucian ethics for ordinary people. The chapter also considers the differences between the relative ethics of five cardinal relationships (*wu lun*) and the absolute ethics of three bonds (*san gang*). A description of illness representations and conceptualizations of health, Confucian practice of self-cultivation and its implications for psychological healing and psychotherapy will also be discussed.

Historical and Cultural Origin of Confucianism

Confucius (551–479 BC), the most respected educator in Chinese history, was born in the state of Lu (now Shandong Province) during the turmoil of the Spring and Autumn period (772–484 BC) in ancient China. His father, a mid-rank official, died when he was 3 years old. Confucius worked as a shepherd and as an accountant for a noble family. He was very interested in the rites and institutions that prevailed in a much earlier period of Chinese history during the Zhou dynasty (1122–256 BC) and devoted himself to the study of the traditional Zhou culture. During Confucius's lifetime, feudal princes were frequently trying to usurp the throne. He hoped to restore social order by advocating a return to the morality of loyalty and the ethical system of filial piety. Confucius began his career as a public teacher at the age of 22. His fame gradually increased, and it is said that he attracted 72 disciples and more than 3,000 students, which earned him a good reputation and made him well known.

In 517 BC, Duke Chao of Lu engaged in an open quarrel with three hereditary ministerial families in the state, who were continually encroaching on the authority of their feudal ruler. Confucius fled into Chi, the adjoining state, to avoid the prevailing disorder. After the rebellion was suppressed, he returned to the state of Lu at the age of 51 and obtained a position in the government. He was forced to resign after 3 months as he failed to persuade the king to destroy three castles constructed by feudal princes. From the age of 54, he toured with some of his disciples around various states for a period of 14 years, hoping that his political advocacy might be accepted by other feudal kings.

Confucius identified himself as an educator whose mandate was to rectify the world by teaching virtues. In attempting to restore the feudal social order of the early Zhou dynasty, he spent a lot of time researching and recording rites and music for ceremonies and other occasions expressing one's dedication to family, country, and state. He also edited poems and classics collected from various states, including Lu, Zhou, Sung, and Chi. He wrote a history of Lu, titled *Spring and Autumn*. In his late years, he annotated 10 supplements to the oracular text *The I Ching*, which is considered the most ancient Chinese book of philosophy and cosmology. All of these were used as teaching materials.

Interpretation of *The I Ching*

The reinterpretation of ***The I Ching*** by Confucianists has very important implications for its rationalization in ancient China. *The I Ching* was originally a divination text in ancient China. During the Spring and Autumn period (221–481 BC), Confucius and his disciples were said to have written the *Shi Yi* (十翼, *Ten Wings*) as well as a series of commentaries on *The I Ching*. The Confucianists' interpretation of *The I Ching* had transformed it into a "philosophical masterpiece" of Confucian philosophy and cosmology.[1] Meanwhile, Laozi's (or Lao Tze's; 604–531 BC) interpretation had helped the post-Warring States Taoists to develop Chinese organic sciences.[2]

The Chinese Worldview Model of Equilibrium

The works of these schools (Confucianism and Taoism) have contributed to the formation of a **Chinese worldview model of equilibrium**. Using the method of structuralism, anthropologist Li analyzed the folk religions, legends, and myths prevalent in Chinese society and constructed a Chinese worldview model of equilibrium.[3] The word *equilibrium* used in Li's model comes from the Confucian golden mean, in which the term was used to mean "to reach balance and harmony." Li proposed that the most fundamental operating rule in traditional Chinese cosmology is to seek balance and harmony between humans and nature, humans and society, and humans and ego. The most ideal and perfect states in traditional culture all aim at such a state of balance and harmony. In order to reach these ideal states, it is necessary to maintain balance and harmony within each of the three systems. The equilibrium worldview model comprises balance and harmony within each of the three systems.

Harmony With Nature

The first level of harmony is harmony with nature, which can be expressed in two aspects: (1) time and (2) space. In Chinese folk belief, harmony of temporality is manifest in the explanation of one's fortune in life in coordination with cosmic time. Four pairs of signs represent the time, date, month, and year in which a person was born. The two characters of each pair are adopted from 10 celestial stems and 12 terrestrial branches and are usually called eight characters. The eight characters that represent one's birth time may determine one's life experience or fate (*ming*). To many Chinese, fate is determined at birth. In coordination with cosmic time, an individual's life experience will take on various changes as a consequence of good or bad luck. In the traditional system of Chinese belief, fate is unchangeable, while luck can be changed with the aid of various forces. Seeking harmony with temporality is revealed in this changeable fortune.

The second aspect of maintaining balance with nature is spatial arrangement. Ideas of spatial harmony are constructed on the concepts of *yin* and *yang*, the five elements (*wu-hsin*), and the eight trigrams (*ba-gua*). The combination of these factors constitutes a belief in geomancy (*feng shui*).

Harmony Within the Individual

Maintaining harmony within the individual can be divided into two parts: (1) internal substantial harmony and (2) external formal harmony. The former explains the harmony within the human body mainly by the dynamic equilibrium between the two opposing forces of ***yin* and *yang***. Based on these concepts, a very complicated system of Chinese medicine and food has been developed. If an individual's body is basically cold, that person should consume more hot foods to keep in balance, while a person whose body is basically hot should consume more cold foods. If the body overheats, more cold food or medicine will be needed to keep the balance and vice versa. The food that people should eat changes with the weather: More hot foods should be eaten in the winter, and more cold foods should be consumed in the summer to maintain the equilibrium of *yin* and *yang* within the body. The harmony of the external form is mainly represented in the use of one's name. In the traditional Chinese theory of naming, names are not just signs or symbols; names entail a transforming force for the individual. Two aspects represent a person's name. The first is related to the five elements; the second is the number of strokes required to write one's name. Both show an individual's search for balance in external forms.

Interpersonal Harmony

Harmony existing in a person's social relationships is the steadfast goal of the Confucian value system, which itself is the ethical foundation of social order. Confucian theory of self-cultivation requires everyone to practice the doctrine of "exerting oneself" (*zhong*, 忠, literally, "loyalty") and "putting oneself in the place of the other" (*shu*, 恕, "forgiveness") in one's five cardinal relationships (*wu lun*) between father and son, sovereign and subordinate, husband and wife, older and younger brother, and friends. Since the Martial Emperor of the Han dynasty (158–87 BC) accepted Dong Zhong Shu's (179–104 BC) proposal to dismiss the hundred schools by revering Confucianism solely, the three bonds (*san gang*) had been frequently and closely linked to five cardinal ethics (*wuchang*), which delineated the absolute authority of the ruler over the minister, the father over the son, and the husband over the wife, and have had profound influence over Chinese culture in general. As the politicized Confucian ideology of control, the institution of three bonds was a deliberate attempt to utilize Confucian values for the maintenance of a specific social order. It is detrimental to human flourishing. On the contrary, the five cardinal ethics deliberated by Mencius with self-cultivation is not only compatible with but also essential to interpersonal harmony and personal growth.

Illness Representations and Conceptualizations of Health

Culture may shape not only patterns of emotional expression but also help-seeking behaviors when one experiences physical or psychological disturbances that are mediated by the concept of illness prevailing in that culture. In order to illustrate this point, a distinction should be made between the concepts of *disease* and *illness*. These ideas are underpinned by Confucianism. Disease is a pathological concept, while illness is a cultural one. In the modern concept of medicine, disease indicates infection by germs or a virus. It is a biological or pathological phenomenon that can be examined in a clinic or laboratory. Illness indicates the social recognition that one cannot appropriately carry out daily duties and that a series of acts must be taken to improve the situation. A person's illness is meaningless unless the concept of that illness is recognized in that person's culture. Disease means malfunctions of one's physique. Illness implies this but also implies a threat to the individual's social existence.[4] In her field study in a village of northern Taiwan, anthropologist Chang discovered that the peasants' illness behaviors were profoundly influenced by their concepts of illness.[5] The peasants recognized a disease by examining their own feelings and thought that an illness meant that the body felt uncomfortable and painful and that the person could not work or rest: "A feeling of hurt is an illness" (p. 125).[6] This statement points out that pain is an indicator of illness. A cold, minor cut or an incised wound is not illness. An illness means a feeling of discomfort inside the body; it makes an individual unable to assume the regularity of life.

Multiple Treatments

A disease may not be a necessary condition for seeing a medical doctor. It may depend on the extent of the seriousness of the disease. A slight disease is "feeling uncomfortable." It just requires getting more rest and taking good care of one's health. A serious disease is "feeling much discomfort, having to lie in bed and being unable to work, even move."[7] This condition causes one to see a doctor and to take medicine. Whether one sees a doctor also depends on the patient's social status. Thus, Chinese people have a specific criterion for judging the seriousness of an illness. The peasants' concepts about the cause of illness included the following:

1. Physique: congenitally weak and easily sick
2. Heredity: weak-minded with epilepsy that comes from the ancestors
3. Infection: cold, cough, or smallpox
4. Influence by external evil: god, ghost, geomantic omen, or changes of one's fortune
5. Influence by internal evil: internal heat, virtual and weak circulation

Chang further indicated that people decide the way to seek medical aid after making a self-diagnosis and conjecturing the cause of illness. If the patient believes that the disease is caused by internal factors, the person will seek help from Western or Chinese medicine for curing the discomforts of the body. If a patient feels that the disease is caused by a supernatural power, after interacting with a doctor the patient may seek help from a witch doctor. A feature of Chinese patients' medicine-seeking behavior is that they do not insist on seeing a doctor of Western medicine, Chinese medicine, or traditional therapy. They care only about the effectiveness of the treatment, leading to the multiple treatments.

Psychiatric Stigma and Shame

In Western countries, especially for the Catholics, confessions to a priest may be a part of people's lives. But there is no such practice as confession in the Chinese cultural tradition. In Buddhism, the ritual of repenting one's sins is performed within one's own mind, not before a priest. In **Confucianism**, the act of self-reflection is performed for oneself, not for others. In other words, Chinese people are not used to telling the secrets or worries in their minds to others. It is a matter of cultural reliance for a westerner to disclose personal secrets to a professional such as a counseling psychologist, but under the influence of Confucian ethics, a Chinese person tends to disclose secrets only to very close friends, if anyone at all.

Kleinman distinguished the thoughts and affects of Chinese people into two categories: (1) those that are superficial and public and that can be appropriately performed according to one's status in responding to social demands and (2) those that are hidden and private and that should be brought under control and revealed only to very few intimate persons.[8] Emotional disturbances are generally viewed as personal affairs that should be controlled by one's own will. Failure to control one's emotions is generally viewed as a sign of an immature personality. Fabrega compared psychiatric stigma in several non-Western societies and found that suffering from psychiatric disorder is a matter of extreme shame in Chinese society.[9] He reviewed the literature on Chinese law and medicine, which surprisingly indicated that the pathology of Chinese medicine contains no obvious stigma for psychiatric patients. Psychiatric stigma originates from the bureaucratic system of the Chinese Empire, which was dominated by Confucian ideology. For instance, in the Han dynasty, an insane man who killed his mother and brother was sentenced to be executed in public for his violation of Confucian ethics. Tseng said that if a patient is reporting his physical complaints repeatedly without any indication of being able to talk about a psychological disturbance, it is very likely that the patient is blocked by an intense feeling of shame or embarrassment in doing so.[10] Such a resistance might be caused by the popular belief that domestic scandals should not be publicized. Conservative Chinese may thus be unable to discuss "disgraceful affairs" within their families with a therapist.

Suppression in Communication

In their attempt to explain the formation of **somatization** orientation for Chinese people, Kleinman and Lin argued that in one's process of being socialized, a Chinese person usually has to learn to suppress feelings of unhappiness and express them by way of physical communication.[11] When suffering from psychosomatic symptoms, attention is focused on physical reactions to the stressful situation, and there is a tendency to report experience in this way. Kleinman tried to induce Chinese patients to talk about their feelings of anxiety, but patients would only say that they felt depressed, anxious, and fearful.[12] They were unable to provide concrete examples or illustrations and instead described the cause of their physical disease or the interpersonal problems directly.

Some experienced psychiatrists have also reported that Chinese patients tend to disclose their worries only to intimate friends.[13]A strong feeling of shame—and their keen sensitivity to showing only appropriate behavior in front of others—may inhibit them from disclosing their disturbances to a stranger, even one who is a psychiatrist in a system of Western medicine. This is the reason "frank and sincere communication" is regarded as the crucial technique in Chinese psychiatry, and the nature of the interpersonal relationship between the therapist and the client is viewed as the most important factor for successful psychotherapy.

Application of Confucianism Principles and Practices to Psychological Healing

Pre-Qin Confucianists advocated that from the Son of Heaven down to the mass of ordinary people, all must consider cultivation of the self as the root of everything (*Great Learning*, classic Chapter 1). The pre-Qin Confucian theory of self-cultivation consisted of four steps, namely to rectify the mind, to be sincere in thoughts, to extend knowledge to the utmost, and to investigate the world. Maintaining the tranquility and peace of mind was the first step of self-cultivation.

Rectification of the Mind

When an individual is being stirred by such emotional disturbances as terror, fond regard, sorrow and distress, it is very unlikely for him or her to maintain the state of tranquility and peace of mind. She or he tends to "look but oversee," to "hear without understanding," to "eat without taste"; it is very difficult for him or her to acquire new knowledge or solve any problem. Therefore, rectifying the mind was regarded as the first step for cultivating oneself. When an individual encounters barrier or frustration in the lifeworld due to his or her action, she or he may experience negative emotions and try to make efforts to control the external world. However, when his or her world-oriented reflection reveals that she or he is unable to overcome barriers in the external world, she or he has to seek actions that may restore the equilibrium between the actor and the external world.

The most important Confucian rule of thumb for guiding one's own conduct is this: "When you do not realize what you want, you must turn inwards and examine yourself in every aspect." That is also the criterion for distinguishing a morally superior man (*junzi*) and a mean man (*xiaojen*). When one has exerted oneself but failed in interpersonal competition, she or he must turn inward rather than grumble against heaven and blame other people. Mencius fully understood that the actor's interpretation about the source of the barrier may determine his or her usage of emotional concepts; his or her interpretation about the experience of frustration may "cover" the occurrence of a particular kind of emotional experience. Therefore, just like other pre-Qin Confucianists, he requested his disciples to be a *junzi* and suggested, "That whereby the *junzi* (morally superior man) is distinguished from other men is what he preserves in his heart; namely, benevolence and propriety."

Normative Schemata

Because the norm of reciprocity is a universal rule for interpersonal interaction, Mencius asserted this: "He who loves others is constantly loved by them. He who respects others is constantly respected by them" (*The Works of Mencius,* Li Lau, II, Chapter 28). In case a man treats others in a perverse and unreasonable manner, Mencius suggested that the *junzi* in such a case will turn round upon himself. "I must have desired benevolence. I must have desired propriety. How should this happen to me?" When an individual takes world-oriented action, she or he may make subjective and intuitive interpretation on barriers in the external world. But when one is making action-oriented reflection, she or he has to reflect on the meaning of barriers in his or her own action context and think over the most appropriate way to overcome the barrier. As such, the normative schemata of some beliefs of morality and laws that have been acquired via cultural learning may become the regulatory system for guiding the actor's reflection. Therefore, Mencius emphasized that in interpersonal interaction (treating others), affectional expression (loving others), governance of the state (ruling others), or interpersonal competition, when one has not obtained the expected return for the accomplishment of one's most appropriate behavior, one should turn inward and examine oneself in terms of such normative schemata as benevolence, wisdom, politeness, etc. (*The Works of Mencius*, Li Lou, I, Chapter 4).

The Teaching of Forbearance

Since the expression of negative emotions may destroy psychosocial homeostasis, **forbearance** became a moral response learned in socialization in Chinese culture, which emphasizes the value of harmony. During the Yuan dynasty, Wu Liang wrote a book called *Rěn Jīng* (忍經, *Classic of Forbearance*), and Hsu Ming-Kui wrote *Quàn Rěn Bǎi Zhēn* (勸忍百箴, *One*

Hundred Admonitions for Forbearance). It describes 100 episodes of *rén* (forbearance) by Zhang Gong-Yi in the Tang dynasty. Zhu Xi, a great Confucian master in the school of idealist philosophy during the Ming dynasty, wrote this in his work titled *Tóng Méng Xū Zhī* (童蒙須知, *Essential Teachings for Innocent Childhood*):

> All people as others' juniors should be generally yielding and speak in details with a gentle tone, not indulging in loud and empty talk or clamoring and teasing. Be submissive and docile so as not to spout opinions when father or a senior is lecturing or reproaching. Should seniors have unpremeditated errors in their examination or condemnation, do not refute them on the spot but forbear and keep quiet temporarily.[14]

Zhu Xi's concept of education reveals the importance of forbearance as a moral characteristic for the socialization of Confucian ethics in traditional Chinese society. Ho and Kang reviewed research on Chinese child-rearing practices and concluded that the core idea of Chinese parents for socialization of their children is to teach them how to restrain their tempers and not to fight with others.[15] In other words, the socialization process may influence the strategy a Chinese person adopts to cope with interpersonal conflicts.

Conclusion

As a virtue for self-cultivation in Confucian cultural tradition, forbearance is like a double-edged sword. On one hand, it may help an individual to get along with others harmoniously within either family or work where pre-Qin Confucian relative ethics of *wu lun* have been practiced by most group members. On the other hand, it may be detrimental to one's psychological as well as physical health in situations where the absolute ethics of three bonds (*san gang*) are enforced by the resource allocator authoritatively. Taking *self-exertion and putting oneself in the place of another* as its core ideas, Confucian theory of self-cultivation had been utilized to develop Naikan therapy and Morita therapy in Japan (Chapters 12 and 13, this volume), which were further modified into constructive living therapy in North America.[16] These therapies, which arose from Confucian principles and ideas, offer clients coping strategies to effectively engage with daily situations where an ideal outcome will result in behavioral attempts to repay the debt for what one has received from significant others and from society. In some ways, these Confucian principles can be at odds with the focus of autonomy, expression, and satisfaction of the individual in Western counseling and psychotherapy that can stand in the way of clients learning the satisfaction of serving others.[17]

DISCUSSION QUESTIONS

1. Explain the differences between Western and Asian worldviews. How can you incorporate the Chinese worldview model of equilibrium into a Western model of psychotherapy?
2. Generally, psychologists and mental health professionals appear to recognize that mainstream counseling and psychotherapy is Eurocentric. What aspects of Asian healing traditions can be incorporated into Western counseling and psychotherapy to make it more global?
3. In what ways can Confucian principles of self-cultivation be used in clinical work?
4. Do you think that Asian healing traditions such as Confucianism ideas can be applied to non-Asian clients in clinical settings effectively?

REFERENCES

1. Abraham, R. (1999). Emotional intelligence in organizations: A conceptualization [Monograph]. *Genetic, Social, and General Psychology Monographs, 125*, 209–227.
2. Needham, J. (1981). *Science and civilization in China.* Cambridge, England: Cambridge University Press.
3. Li, Y. Y. (1988). Ancestor worship and the psychological stability of family members in Taiwan. In K. Yoshimatsu & W. S. Tseng (Eds.), *Asian family mental health* (pp. 26–33). Tokyo, Japan: Psychiatric Research Institute of Tokyo; Li, Y. Y. (1992). In search of equilibrium and harmony: On the basic value orientation of traditional Chinese peasants. In C. Nakane & C. Chiao (Eds.), *Home bound: Studies in East Asian society* (pp. 127–148). Hong Kong: The Center for East Asian Cultural Studies.
4. Hwang, K. K. (2012). *Foundations of Chinese psychology: Confucian social relations.* New York, NY: Springer.
5. Chang, H. (1989). *Consciousness of darkness and democratic tradition* (in Chinese). Taipei, Taiwan: Linking Publishing.
6. Ibid.
7. Ibid.
8. Kleinman, A. (1980). *Patients and healers in the context of culture.* Los Angeles: University of California Press.
9. Fabrega, H. (1991). Psychiatric stigma in non-Western societies. *Comprehensive Psychiatry, 32*, 534–551.
10. Tseng, W. S. (1996). The Chinese psychotherapy: A cultural perspective. In W. S. Tseng (Ed.), *Chinese psychology and its therapy.* Taipei, Taiwan: Laureate. (In Chinese)
11. Kleinman, A., & Lin, T.-Y. (Eds.). (1981). *Normal and abnormal behavior in Chinese culture.* Holland, Netherlands: D. Reidel.
12. Kleinman, A. (1986). *Social origins of distress and disease: Neurasthenia, depression and pain in modern China.* New Haven, CT: Yale University Press.
13. Tseng, W. S. (1975). The nature of somatic complaints among psychiatry patients: The Chinese case. *Comprehensive Psychiatry, 16*(3), 237–245.

14. Xi, Z. (1922). *Zhuzi yulei* (classified dialogues of Master Zhu). In J. P. Bruce (Trans.), *The philosophy of human nature.* London, England: Probstain. (Original work published 1130–1200)
15. Ho, D. Y., & Kang, T. K. (1984). Intergenerational comparisons of child-rearing attitudes and practices in Hong Kong. *Developmental Psychology, 20*(6), 1004–1016.
16. Reynolds, D. K. (1995). *A handbook for constructive living.* Honolulu: University Press of Hawaii.
17. Ibid.

SUGGESTED READINGS

Hwang, K. K. (2012). *Foundations of Chinese psychology: Confucian social relations.* New York, NY: Springer.

This is the first English book that contains a series of culture-inclusive theories on Chinese psychology constructed on the presumption of relationalism.

Kleinman, A., & Lin, T. Y. (Eds.). (1981). *Normal and abnormal behavior in Chinese culture.* Holland, Netherlands: D. Reidel.

This collection of articles addresses various aspects of social behaviors and psychopathology in Chinese society.

Li, Y. Y. (1992). In search of equilibrium and harmony: On the basic value orientation of traditional Chinese peasants. In C. Nakane & C. Chiao (Eds.), *Home bound: Studies in East Asian society* (pp. 127–148). Hong Kong: The Center for East Asian Cultural Studies.

This chapter describes the Chinese worldview model of equilibrium for maintaining one's harmonious relationships with nature, society, and oneself.

Reynolds, D. K. (1995). *A handbook for constructive living.* Honolulu: University Press of Hawaii.

This is an action-based way of looking at the world that combines two Japanese psychotherapies: Naikan and Morita.

2 Taoism and Healing

Catherine Tien-Lun Sun

The healing tradition in China is more than 5,000 years old and exists side by side in Chinese heritage cultures with systems of healing founded on logical positivism and the methods of experimental science. The healing tradition in China has firm roots in **Taoism**, and this chapter purports to examine them.

The renowned sinologist Needham discerned that while Confucianism dominates Chinese social life, Taoism is equally if not more important in Chinese mental life.[1] Indeed, in Chinese heritage cultures, spirituality is predominantly experienced through two channels: (1) firstly, through a vast variety of Taoist rituals, which ensure the harmonious and balanced existence of the three worlds—the ideal this-world, the ideal other-world, and the domain of ghosts—and (2) secondly, through the broad array of medicinal and health practices directed at enhancing health and longevity.

There are two classical texts in Taoism: (1) *Tao Te Ching* contains the teachings of Laozi (or Lao-Tzu), and (2) the *Classics of Nan Hua* contains the teachings of Chuanzi. Additionally, the Taoists have their own canon in the *Dao Zang*, which contains 1,500 texts. However, unlike Buddhism where the *Dazangjing* is regarded as the benchmark for all intellectual, religious, and philosophical discourse, Taoist masters who are naturalists at heart are inclined to select only the classical texts that bear relevance to their teaching. Consequently, students trained by two masters may demonstrate significant differences in their interpretation of Tao and utilize markedly distinct techniques in the quest of longevity and immortality. Worldwide, the *Tao Te Ching* has been translated into various languages more than 300 times since the late 19th century.

One of the pioneers to bridge Western thinking with Taoism was Capra, whose *Tao of Physics* has been translated into more than 20 languages.[2]

Taoism has also been used in providing mystical interpretations of quantum physics and how it should be taught.[3] In terms of psychology and psychotherapy, the influence of Taoism has been extensive. Jung, founder of analytical psychology, wrote the preface to the German translation by Wilhelm of *Secret of the Golden Flower*, a Taoist book on meditation. It is also commonly held that Jung's treatise on synchronicity, which provides definitive confirmation for his concepts of archetypes and the collective unconscious, was inspired by his interest in Taoism.[4] Fabry was able to identify Taoist origins in Frankl's logotherapy. In fact, he saw obvious parallels between Tao and Logos. Craig, in his exposition on Tao as a system of psychotherapy, opined that Tao is the way of all beings and is dynamic in nature.[5] He further elaborated this point by likening the Tao to the existential concept of an authentic mode of living. Watts, in his many comparisons of Eastern and Western psychotherapy, declared that it is illusory to conceive ourselves to be outside Tao, as Tao is in everything and everything is Tao.[6] Thus, Watts suggested that pathology results from an egocentric management of one's body and psyche, and health emanates when one allows one's senses and feelings to be spontaneous.

Taoism has two origins, both of which are indigenous to China. The first is a blending of shamans and magicians who have existed in China since ancient times, and their practice has exerted profound and enduring impact on traditional healing, alchemy, nature worship, and demonology. The second comprises philosophers from the Warring States (approximately 476–221 BC), whose exposition on Taoism was a reaction toward the Confucian Tao of Humanity, which was deemed to be contriving and restrictive. These Taoist philosophers advocated that social harmony could not be realized in the absence of a thorough appreciation of the Tao of Nature. From these two origins, Taoism can be interpreted as a syncretic hybrid of mysticism, religion, and philosophy.

Ho deduced six meanings of Tao from this syncretic nature of Taoism.[7] The first is *daoti*, or "Tao as Reality," and views Tao as the noumenon of the universe; the second is *daoyuan*, or "Tao as Origin," and identifies Tao as the origin of the universe; the third is *daoli*, or "Tao as Principle," and refers to Tao as the law governing the processes of the universe; the fourth is *daoyong*, or "Tao as Function," and is concerned with adhering to the principles of Tao for the purpose of self-cultivation; the fifth is *daode*, or "Tao as Virtue," and points out that virtue springs from Tao and exists because of Tao; and the sixth is *daoshu*, or "Tao as Technique," and refers primarily to the use of Tao in political and military strategies.[8]

Thus, in the broadest sense, Tao is the order of nature, and it is the way the universe works. Taoism does not consider human beings to be at the center of the universe but rather as one of the numerous phenomena that has come into being through the dynamic and spontaneous interaction of cosmic forces. The Tao is perceptible through scientific and systematic observation, but it is essential that the observer remains passive and receptive.[9]

Taoist Cosmology and Worldview

Taoism configures the human body as being homologous to the universe. Thus, man is a microcosm that reflects the universe, the macrocosm, perfectly. To attain health, harmony and equilibrium must not only exist within the microcosm but between the microcosm and macrocosm.

Taoist cosmology advocates the principles of connectedness, unity, and oneness, and the *taijitu* created by the renowned scholar Zhou Dunyi from the Song dynasty (AD 1017–1073) aptly depicted these principles. According to Zhou, the circle represents Tao, or *wuji,* the Boundless Ultimate or the First Cause. *Wuji* produces the *taiji,* the "Supreme Ultimate," and in Zhou's configuration, *wuji* and *taiji* are in fact the primordial and evolving expressions of the same construct. In other words, *taiji* is the activated counterpart of *wuji*, and in this activated form, *taiji* produces *yang*. When *yang* reaches its zenith, *taiji* becomes serene, and *yin* is produced. When *yin* reaches its apex, *taiji* becomes active again to produce *yang*. In this sense, *yin* and *yang* are entrenched in each other, and through their mutual generation, **the five elements**, or *wu xin*, of metal, wood, water, fire, and earth, which are the founding matters of all phenomena, are produced. Their interaction with each other is either through inhibition or enhancement and explains all changes in Nature. *Wu xin* is employed in the explanation of tidal variations, astronomical movements, and weather conditions. They are also used to describe the physical and psychological functions of the body as well as the temperament of the host. The inhibitory and generative qualities of *wu xin* formulate the most essential principles of the Taoist system of healing.[10] The *taijitu* demonstrates that Tao, man, and all matters in the universe are in essence not only interrelated but are one and the same.

Taijitu

From the brief exposition that was just given, it is evident that Taoist cosmology refers to two realities: (1) the concrete reality of the 10,000 myriad things and (2) the abstract reality made up by the *wuji, taiji, yin* and *yang*, and the five elements. Izutsu named these two realities the Level of Multiplicity and the Level of Unity.[11] The former suggests the phenomenal level of everyday experiences and consciousness where each and every object has its own boundary and is distinguished by separateness. The latter is the level of Tao, which is boundless and infinite and is distinguished by its total lack of differentiation.

There are three worlds in Taoism. The ideal this-world is serene and impartial and can be reached through leading a simple, noncompetitive, and noncontentious life. The ideal other-world is the home of celestial beings (*hsien*). A person does not need to expire physically before he becomes a *hsien* but can achieve this state through ingesting elixirs of life, internal alchemy, and the accumulation of virtues. The third world lies in between the ideal this-world and the ideal other-world and is the domain of ghosts and demons. There is frequent travel between these three worlds—some of which are inadvertently caused while others may be intentionally cultivated. The Taoist notion of three worlds has permeated the minds of Chinese people, and we are able to witness this notion in the various spheres of everyday life, such as the pursuit of immortality, the inclusion of medicinal cuisine in the average Chinese diet, the wearing and ingestion of talisman to combat physical and psychological distress, the daily worship of deities and ancestors, and the celebration of festivals to honor ghosts and ancestors. Travel between the three worlds, if not carefully orchestrated, is likely to cause disequilibrium and lead to illness.

Life, according to the Taoist schema, is therefore a balancing act, and the best approach to attaining this is by being ***wu wei***, or "do nothing." *Wu wei* is often mistaken to be advocating inaction or inactivity. However, Needham pointed out unambiguously that *wu wei* refers to an attitude of not acting in contrary to the laws of nature.[12] Taoists believe that nature, when left alone, will take care of itself. By extension, a *wu wei* person understands the intrinsic nature of matters and allows them to work out by themselves. The Taoist expression "*wei wu wei*," or "acting without action," though seemingly oxymoronic, is interpreted as not acting against Tao or acting in accordance with Tao. It is believed that in the absence of undue interference, most matters resolve themselves in time. Thus, there is an overwhelming preference of non-action over action in Taoism.

An illustration of *wu wei* can be seen in the practice of a form of Taoist gymnastics, the *taiji* boxing. There is a set of movements involving the use of 4 taels (approximately 4 ounces) to overturn 100 catties (approximately 1,000 pounds) of weight. In these movements, the practitioner does not counter force with equal force; rather, he uses the force exerted by the opponent and directs it away from oneself. These movements look as if the attacked does not put up any resistance; rather, he gracefully pulls the attacker toward himself until the attacker loses his balance and in the process dismantles the force of the attack. The essence, of course, lies in finding the leverage point. *Wu wei* does not make a Taoist indolent; it makes him less impetuous and more strategic in dealing with the adversities in life.

As mentioned at the beginning of this chapter, while Confucianism dominates Chinese social life, Taoism directs Chinese mental life; while Confucianism is concerned with social propriety, Taoism is very much about the pursuit of personal happiness. Distinct from other Asian religions and philosophies such as Hinduism, Islam, or Buddhism, Taoism does not view life as an endless barrage of suffering and death as the ultimate liberation. Quite to the contrary, Taoists contemplate life as filled with wonders and death as a termination of these wonders. If man is indeed a microcosm that perfectly reflects nature the macrocosm, then to the Taoist mind, aging contradicts the law of rejuvenation in nature. Hence, Taoists are very intent at developing ways of self-cultivation aiming at the defiance of illness, aging, and dying. They believe that it is possible, through intentional cultivation, to possess an ageless body and to eventually attain immortality. Founded on this belief, Taoists have developed systems of internal and external alchemy. Internal alchemy comprises breathing exercises, visceral gymnastics, meditational techniques directed at activating and balancing glandular secretion, sexual practices focused on invigorating and harmonizing the *yin* and *yang* energies, medicinal cuisine, and so on. External alchemy centers on the concept of spagirism, the making of pills of immortality, and has often been commissioned by those in power.

Taoist Conceptualizations of Health and Illness

In Taoist healing, it is deemed that the universe as the macrocosm and man as the microcosm reflect each other perfectly. Alternatively stated, human life is a miniaturized version of the cosmos. Health, in Taoism, is the manifestation of a state of harmonious equilibrium between *yin* and *yang,* the five elements (metal, wood, water, fire, and earth), the six environmental conditions (dry, wet, cold, hot, wind, and flame), and the seven emotions (joy, sorrow, anger, worry, panic, anxiety, and fear). Note that there is no assigning of positive or negative value to any of these qualities, a feature which is probably in contradiction with Western conceptions. Take the example of the seven emotions: In Western parlance, we would refer to joy as having positive valence and the six other emotions as having negative valence, but in Taoism, they are all necessarily interconnected for the maintenance of harmonious equilibrium.

The Taoist conceptualizations of health and illness are contained within *The Yellow Emperor's Classic of Chinese Medicine*, or ***Huangdi Neijing***.[13] This classical text is attributed to a mythical figure, *Huangdi*, who was the first of the five earliest emperors in recorded history of China. A more popular view is that the text was believed to be compiled during the Warring States (403–221 BC).

Huangdi Neijing is generally accepted as the most authoritative text in Taoist medicine. It unequivocally stated that the law governing the intergeneration of *yin* and *yang* is at the foundation of all matters and changes. Hence, illness is attributable to the disharmony in the *yin–yang* law, and healing is not possible without being able to identify the root of the disharmony. In this sense, the Taoist approach to illness and health is not so concerned with detecting and rectifying specific pathologies but rather with the **holistic** restoration of *yin–yang* balance.

Huangdi Neijing is made up of two parts. Part 1, *Su Wen*, literally meaning "common questions," deals with the theoretical foundations, methods of diagnosis, and treatment modalities. Part 2, *Ling Shu*, translated as the "Spiritual or Miraculous Pivot," deals with the art and science of acupuncture. Each part is made up of 81 treatises. Ma noted that of the total 162 treatises, 90% refer to mental health in some form, and over 30 treatises bear psychology-related titles.[14] This distribution attests to the holistic approaches to body–mind and body–mind–nature advocated in Taoism, which is in stark contrast to Cartesian dualism upheld in Western biomedicine. The approaches illustrate that in Taoist medicine, emotional disorders are deemed to be caused by the loss of dynamic balance between *yin* and *yang* in at least one of three levels: (1) within the body and the mind, (2) between the body and the mind, or (3) between nature and the body–mind composite.

Taoism, which is indigenous to the Chinese people, and Taoist health practices, which are within easy access of the average person, have been instrumental in creating a popular health subculture. Unfortunately, as a consequence of its popularity, Taoist medicine has always carried with it an aura of amateurism, bordering on superstition, particularly in the realm of mental health. This is exemplified in the etiology and treatment of psychosis. A psychotic patient may be treated with herbal medicine and acupuncture to restore balance in accordance with some specific *yin–yang* law; at the same time, he may also be subjected to Taoist rituals of exorcism since the common cause of mental illness is often reckoned to be an unsolicited and unwanted invasion from the domain of ghosts and demons. Although there is an ostensibly holistic presentation in the combined efforts of the herbalist–acupuncturist and the exorcist who is often a part-time Taoist priest, yet in this age of scientific inquiry, the knowledge-based approach of the former is unfortunately diminished in terms of reliability and validity by the spiritually based approach of the latter.

Taoist Healing and Contemporary Practice

Consistent with Taoist cosmology and worldview, the Taoist system of healing has its unique diagnostic tools and interventions. The primary purpose of a Taoist diagnosis is to determine whether or not an imbalance has occurred, where it is located, and its overall impact on health.

The diagnostic tools employed by the Taoist practitioner and the Taoist priest are very different. The Taoist practitioner uses the four skills of *wang* (observation), *wen* (listening and smelling), *wen* (questioning), and *qie* (palpation). Observation includes looking at the whole person, from his aura and nonverbal cues, to his body posture and facial expression to discern his level of suffering, the nature of his ailment, and his attitude toward his predicament. Listening and smelling refers to listening skills and smelling the patient's breath and odors. Listening assists the practitioner to put the patient's illness into the context of his lifestyle, and smelling enables the practitioner to obtain some idea of the location of his ailment. Questioning is aimed at gathering information pertinent to understanding the patient's health condition. Palpation is the placing of the practitioner's index, middle, and ring fingers on the patient's wrist for a pulse-reading. Palpation is based on the concept that one's vital energy passes through the body through the meridian channel. Taoists believe that blockage in the meridian channel is a fundamental cause of illness, and through palpation, the practitioner is able to determine the location of the blockage.

The Taoist priest employs ritualistic practice to communicate with the world of ghosts and demons. In his configuration, illness is often reckoned to be the result of unsolicited invasions by ghosts and demons, including one's ancestors. To remedy the situation, these spirits may either be appeased through offerings or expelled through specific rituals or both.

To understand the Taoist notion of mental health and illness, it is imperative to examine the notions of *shen* (soul or spirit) and *qi* (life force). *Shen* is the spiritual capacity of the mind and is expressed both somatically and behaviorally. A person with a smart demeanor is often described as *shen qi*, meaning that he is full of spirit and life force. A person who is confused, at a loss, or not fully conscious is said to be *shen zhi bu qing*, meaning that he lacks clarity of spirit. Etymologically, the traditional form of *qi*, refers to the steam rising from rice as it cooks. In Taoism, *qi* suggests the somatic and psychological presence of the cosmic life force within our bodies. *Huangdi Neijing* specifically indicated that the movements and obstructions of *qi* reflect our emotional states as well as the synergy or the lack of it between *yin* and *yang*.

Prior to the introduction of psychiatric classifications of mental disorders in the 1980s, and based on the notions of *shen* and *qi,* mental illness in China is commonly termed *shen jing bing,* literally meaning an illness of the *shen* and *jing* (the meridians along which the *qi* flows). In other words, in the Taoist schema, which is holistic and not dualistic in nature, mental illness is caused by a destabilization of the *shen* and obstruction to the flow of *qi.* The disturbance of the *shen* and *qi* is manifested in the malfunctioning of the five internal organs of the lungs, liver, kidney, heart, and spleen or pancreas, and the concomitant and exaggerated presence of grief, anger, fear, joy, and obsession in the individual. To further elaborate this point, it should be borne in mind that the Taoist world is made up of the five elements of metal, wood, water, fire, and earth, each generating or attenuating another. The five elements correspond to the five human organs—lungs, liver, kidneys, heart, and spleen or pancreas, which are in turn the sites for grief or sadness, anger, fear, joy or overexcitement, and overthinking or obsession. Through palpation, the Taoist practitioner is able to determine where the *qi* is obstructed, and from questioning, listening, and observing, he can discern how the *shen* is destabilized.

There is a two-way relationship between the viscera and the emotions. *Huangdi Neijing* states that excessive grief can cause injury to the lungs but can also be caused by a lung ailment, excessive anger can cause injury to the liver but can also be caused by a liver infirmity, fear can cause injury to the kidneys but can also be caused by a failure in kidney functions, excessive joy or excitement is injurious to the heart but can also be caused by a heart condition, and excessive thinking and obsession injures the spleen and pancreas but can also be caused by diseases in these organs. This sort of relationship typically speaks to the acausal nature of Taoist thinking.

Bearing in mind the law of mutual generation and attenuation of the five elements, grief can be attenuated by joy and generated by obsession, anger can be attenuated by grief and generated by fear, obsession can be attenuated by anger and generated by joy, fear can be attenuated by obsession and generated by grief, and joy can be attenuated by fear and generated by anger.[15] Zhang Jingyue (AD 1563–1640), a renowned Taoist practitioner from the Ming dynasty, specifically pointed out that generation and attenuation work alongside each other to maintain balance. Generation without attenuation would lead to overstimulation, and attenuation without generation would lead to disastrous deterioration. This resonates fully with the Taoist proposition that when *yang* reaches its zenith, *yin* is produced, and when *yin* reaches its apex, *yang* is activated.

There exists a principle of Taoist healing that corresponds to the Taoist interpretation of health and illness. This principle states that when an emotion and its related organ is weak, its mother (i.e., the generating organ) needs to be enhanced; when an emotion and its related organ is overexcited, its son (i.e., the attenuating organ) must be enfeebled. If this principle is to be followed, then in the case of a bipolar disorder, the Taoist practitioner would focus on restoring balance to the spleen and pancreas. The rationale behind it is this: Depression is related to the weakened functioning of the lungs, and to reverse the situation, the mother or the spleen and pancreas needs to be enhanced; mania is related to the overexcitation of the heart, and to correct the situation, the son or the spleen and pancreas needs to be enfeebled. In short, in the treatment of bipolar disorders, there is need to stabilize the *shen* and open up the flow of *qi* in the spleen and pancreas.

In terms of bodily based approaches, herbal therapy is the most popular choice, and the leading reference is the *Compendium of Materia Medica* compiled by Li Shizhen of the Ming dynasty. A typical Taoist practitioner has immediate access to over 100 kinds of herbs, which are stored in a *baizigui*—literally translated as a chest for 100 sons. The herbs are rarely used singularly but are more often used in creative combinations. Acupuncture is another popular choice used to remove the obstruction of *qi* in the meridian channel. For those who find acupuncture needles to be too invasive, moxibustion therapy and acupressure provide other alternatives. Food therapy, which uses different tastes to counter specific emotions, is incorporated into both herbal therapy and medicinal cuisine: spicy tastes for grief, sour tastes for anger, salty tastes for fear, bitter tastes for overexcitement, and sweet tastes for obsession.

With respect to physical exercises, a number of techniques are used. The best known techniques are *taiji* boxing and *taiji* swordplay, which enhance the flow of *qi* in the body through the meridian channel. Breathing techniques, or Qigong (QG), are practiced separately or as part and parcel of the *taiji* practices. Taoist meditation aimed at balancing the secretion of the ductless glands is also believed to promote both emotional and physical health and to contribute to longevity.

Talk therapy, conducted by men of wisdom and learning, was once used to deal with irrational thinking. It is possible that talk therapy was at one time a combination of philosophical therapy and Taoist musings. In this connection, dream interpretation was used as a diagnostic tool. In recent years, Taoist cognitive therapy has gradually evolved.[16]

Other therapies include art therapy and music therapy. Art therapy, which primarily includes painting and calligraphy, has traditionally been regarded as most effective in regulating temperaments. Specifically, staying focused on the brushstrokes is claimed to stabilize the *shen* and remove blockages to the flow of *qi*. In regards to music therapy, Guo and Zhang pointed out that the five tones in traditional Chinese music are associated with the five emotions: (1) Grief can be lessened by music in the *shang* tone, (2) anger can be doused by music in the *jiao* tone, (3) fear can be lifted by music in the *yu* tone, (4) obsession can be overcome by the *gong* tone, and (5) overexcitement can be lifted by the *zheng* tone.[17]

Conclusion

The Taoist etiology of mental health and illness and its concomitant treatment modalities do not have the scientific exactitude of Western evidence-based medicine. Nonetheless, from the previously given discussion, it can be deduced that the system is based on a fully developed Taoist cosmology and worldview and has clear guidelines for the ascertaining of diagnosis, treatment modalities, and prognosis. Furthermore, above all else, it has withstood the test of time. Therefore, even if it is not scientifically on par with biomedicine, it has definite value as an alternative to Western psychotherapy and psychiatry.

In recent decades, there has been considerable effort to subject the Taoist system to scientific inquiry. *Taiji* boxing was found to improve the psychosocial status of people with cardiovascular disease risk factors.[18] Chan, Ho, and Chow were able to determine that a Taoism-based holistic model of intervention brought about positive changes in health in cancer patients, bereaved wives, and divorced women.[19] Cross-cultural studies indicated a lower incidence of psychiatric disorders in Taiwan than the United States, which provided evidence that the preventive perspective of the Taoist system had positive effects on the mental health of the Chinese people.[20] Therefore, instead of the apprehension that with globalization the Taoist system will one day be totally overwhelmed by Western biomedicine, there is reason to look forward to the development of holistic medicine worldwide under the influence of Taoism.

DISCUSSION QUESTIONS

1. The influence of Taoism on Western psychology and psychotherapy has been rather extensive. Do you agree? How would you qualify this notion?
2. The human body, in Taoism, is configured to be homologous to the universe. How would you frame your understanding of this viewpoint in the context of the *taijitu?*
3. Taoists are said to practice holistic medicine as opposed to Western medicine, which is influenced by Cartesian dualism. Between the two, where would body–mind medicine fit in?
4. Diagnostically, the Taoist practitioner uses the four skills of *wang* (observation), *wen* (listening and smelling), *wen* (questioning), and *qie* (palpation). What sort of information do you think the practitioner is trying to garner?

REFERENCES

1. Needham, J. (1972). *Science and civilization in China* (Vol. 2). Cambridge, England: Cambridge University Press. (Original work published 1956)
2. Capra, F. (2014). *The Tao of physics: An exploration of the parallels between modern physics and eastern mysticism* (5th ed.). Boston, MA: Shambhala Publications.
3. Zukav, G. (2009). *Dancing wu li masters: An overview of the new physics.* New York, NY: HarperOne.
4. Shinoda-Bolen, J. (1979). *The Tao of psychology: Synchronicity and the self.* New York, NY: HarperCollins.
5. Fabry, J. B. (1975). Logotherapy and eastern religions. *Journal of Religion and Health, 14,* 271–276; Craig, E. (2007). Tao psychotherapy: Introducing a new approach to humanistic practice. *The Humanistic Psychologist, 35*(2), 109–133.
6. Watts, A. (1961). *Psychotherapy east & west.* New York, NY: Vintage Books; Watts, A. (1975). *Tao: The watercourse way.* New York, NY: Penguin Books.
7. Ho, Y. C. (1990). The noological and mental-health views of Taoist thought: A preliminary empirical study. *Bulletin of Educational Psychology, 23,* 158–188. (In Chinese). 何英奇 (1990) 。道家思想的心靈觀與心理健康觀的初步實徵性研究。教育心理學報，23期，158–188頁
8. Ibid.
9. Sun, C. T. L. (2013). *Themes in Chinese psychology* (2nd ed.). Singapore: Cengage Learning.
10. Ibid.
11. Izutsu, T. (1968). *The absolute and perfect man in Taoism.* In *Eranos-Jahrbuch 1967: Polarität des lebens* (pp. 379–441). Zurich, Switzerland: Rhein-Verlag.
12. Needham, *Science and civilization.*
13. Ni, M. (1995). *The yellow emperor's classic of medicine.* Boston, MA: Shambhala Publications.
14. Ma, S. Y. (2005). A cursory discussion of new modes of thinking in medicine within the context of Chinese medicine, Hulu Chinese Medicine Information Net. Retrieved from http://www.hulu.com.tw/art/list.asp?unid=495 (in Chinese). 馬肇禹(2005),〈淺談中國醫學中的新醫學模式思想〉,見《胡盧中醫資訊網.

15. Guo, S., & Zhang, Z. (1986). *Traditional Chinese convalescencology.* Sichuan, China: Sichuan Science and Technology Press (in Chinese). 郭子光、張子游(1986),《中醫康復學, 四川科學技術出版社.
16. Young, D., Zhou, L., & Zhu, J.-F. (2008). Daoistic cognitive psychotherapy: Philosophical foundation and basic procedure. *World Cultural Psychiatry Research Review*, 32–36; Moss, R. C., & Perryman, K. L. (2012). East meets West: Integration of Taoism into Western therapy. *Ideas and Research You Can Use: VISTAS 2012, 1*(33).
17. Guo & Zhang, *Traditional Chinese convalescencology.*
18. Taylor-Piliae, R. E., Haskell, W. L., Waters, C. M., & Froelicher, E. S. (2006). Change in perceived psychosocial status following a 12-week Tai Chi exercise programme. *Journal of Advanced Nursing, 54*(3), 313–329.
19. Chan, C., Ho, P. S. Y., & Chow, E. (2001). A body-mind-spirit model in health: An Eastern approach. *Social Work in Health Care, 34*(3/4), 261–282.
20. Hwu, H. G., Yeh, E. K., & Chang, L. Y. (1989). Prevalence of psychiatric disorders in Taiwan defined by the Chinese diagnostic interview schedule. *Acta Psychiatrica Scandinavica, 79*, 136–147; Compton, W. M., Helzer, J. E., Hwu, H. G., Yeh, E. H., McEvoy, L., Tropp, J. E., & Spitzuagel, E. L. (1991). New methods in cross-cultural psychiatry in Taiwan and the United States. *American Journal of Psychiatry, 148*, 1697–1704.

SUGGESTED READINGS

Chan, C., Ho, P. S. Y., & Chow, E. (2001). A body-mind-spirit model in health: An eastern approach. *Social Work in Health Care, 34*(3/4), 261–282.

Cartesian dualism influenced Western medicine in that physical, emotional, and spiritual health are respectively assigned to the domains of the physician, social worker, and clergy. By contrast, Taoism and Chinese medicine hold a holistic view. The authors promote a body–mind–spirit integrated model of intervention and demonstrate that the approach was able to bring about improvement in physical and mental health as well as perceived sense of control and social support in cancer patients, bereaved wives, and divorced women.

Izutsu, T. (1968). *The absolute and perfect man in Taoism. In Eranos-Jahrbuch 1967: Polarität des lebens* (pp. 379–441). Zurich, Switzerland: Rhein-Verlag.

In making a structural comparison between Sufism and Taoism, Izutsu is able to identify and isolate the ontological concept underlying the worldview espoused in philosophical Taoism. In particular, the writings of the Taoist masters Laozi and Zhuangzi (or Zhang Zhou or Chuang-Tzu) are deemed to represent a culmination of the spiritual tradition in China.

Needham, J. (1972). *Science and civilization in China* (Vol. 2). Cambridge, England: Cambridge University Press. (Original work published 1956)

In the second of a seven-volume epic text, Needham opines that the Taoist worldview is most basic to the development of Chinese science. The idea that the Tao pervades all matters and controls all changes is at the foundation of organismic philosophy. In this, Taoism rejects the Confucian ethics-oriented interpretation of nature and substitutes it with a relativist notion in which constant change is brought about by the dynamic interplay of *yin* and *yang* as well as the five elements.

Sun, C. T. L. (2013). *Themes in Chinese psychology* (2nd ed.). Singapore: Cengage Learning.

In Chapter 2 of this book, the place of Taoism in the development of the Chinese mentality and the Chinese conception of health is juxtaposed against Confucianism and Buddhism. Then, in Chapter 11, the contribution of Taoism to the development of traditional Chinese medicine (TCM) and modern medicine is discussed.

3 Buddhism and Healing

Tony Toneatto

In his discourses with those he encountered throughout his life, Buddha declared that he was "awake"! But awake from what? The Buddha was obviously not referring to awakening from literal sleep. He was pointing to a psychological state. Having "awakened," the phenomenal world had not changed. What had altered was a subjective state. The Buddha was pointing to a radical shift in the perception of the subjective world. If the Buddha lived today, he might adopt the term *aware* to better convey what he intended to describe. What the Buddha was describing may be contrasted with the opposite of being awake or aware: darkness, ignorance, unconsciousness, or nonclarity. But exactly what was the Buddha aware of or awake from? The Buddha was referring to a discernment that dissolved the distortions of perception and cognition that obscure or veil our ability to perceive ourselves, others, and our experiences as veridically as possible.[1]

The Buddha was describing a clarity of perception and cognition that can distinguish the distorting aspects of ordinary consciousness that is the foundation of emotional suffering and illness. This clarity of perception can be termed *wisdom*. And the distortion is the outcome of the conditioned, even traumatized, inherited biases, delusions, and obscurations that prevent us from authentically encountering our perceptual world. The Buddha is describing a profound perceptual–cognitive shift that reveals the psychological basis of our emotional suffering. He clearly saw the specific ways our mind can, without the clarity that comes with discernment and wisdom, lead to modes of perception and cognition (and hence feeling and action) that produce the endless cycle of human suffering and anguish (*samsara*).[2]

This leads to an important insight about the nature of **Buddhism** that will be expanded further in this chapter. The mind and its functions are central to how we see ourselves, our world, and others. The mind maintains our suffering. The mind releases us from suffering.[3]

Historical Context

The Buddha was born approximately 2.5 millennia ago (approximately 550 BC; although others have suggested closer to 350 BC) in what is southern Nepal today as Siddhartha Gautama.[4] He was of privileged descent as his father, Suddhodana, was king of the Shakya clan. Tragically, Siddhartha's mother, Mahamaya, died days after his birth, and he was subsequently raised by his aunt and other attendants. Nevertheless, blessed as he was by virtue of his privileged birth, Siddhartha lacked nothing and had free access to every pleasure and opportunity. He had been prophesized to become either a political leader or a great sage. His father, preferring the former, ensured that Siddhartha became proficient in all of the customs and laws of his culture so that he would one day succeed him. His father kept him occupied with all manner of material goods, pleasures, and entertainments.[5] Siddhartha eventually became bored with this sensually pleasing but existentially unsatisfying existence and became curious to explore the world outside his privileged environment. So he ventured out, deliberately rebelling against his father and his upbringing. In his sojourns, Siddhartha met a very different reality. He encountered old age, disease, and death and learned that he (and everyone else, including his loved ones) would be subject to these forces. Unable to return to his previous life cloistered within the confines of his kingdom, Siddhartha made a radical, life-altering decision: to find real happiness and well-being and not the facsimile his father had offered; he had to leave the world his father had prepared for him. Biographies of the Buddha describe Siddhartha's exploits over the several ensuing years during which he encountered and was taught by Hindu mystics and yogis, all of whom were also united in their search for true, enduring happiness and health. Siddhartha, through extreme asceticism, austerities, and bodily privations, mastered the most advanced states of consciousness, meditative bliss, and absorption. Perception and sensation were blamed for suffering and our ability to transcend. If one could separate, ignore, or set aside our somatic, carnal nature from the soul, the spirit, or consciousness itself, then we could be free. Understandably, if the path of sensory indulgence, of bodily satisfaction through pleasure, had not yielded an authentic, real, stable happiness, then possibly the opposite approach might. This inherent dualism revealed the tendency of the mind to seek for the solutions outside of itself. Years of such ascetic and meditative practices, however, did not satisfy Siddhartha. They did not solve the problem of mental suffering and illness nor produce lasting healing. Thus, Siddhartha had no choice but to reject asceticism as he had done so with indulgence years before.[6]

With one-pointed determination, he sat under the pipal tree, closed his eyes, and resolved to allow his mind to become still and observed his inner world.[7] After 6 months, the limited, conditioned, societally civilized Siddhartha personality disappeared or dissolved, and the insights he had made months before were now stabilized and integrated into a coherent state of being.

He had awakened from the dream of suffering, of birth and death. He was now "the Buddha"—awakened, aware, and enlightened. An apt translation of Buddha could also be the "healed one" in the sense that the outcome of such a journey was to attain an authentic wholeness and well-being. The path to truth and wellness could be achieved only by oneself and only with dedicated effort and persistence. For several decades, the Buddha taught ceaselessly throughout the Indian continent, attracting devotees and disciples until his passing at the age of 80.[8]

Buddhism Worldview

In the centuries after the Buddha passed away, efforts were made to preserve his teachings, orally at first, but eventually written (i.e., the Pali Canon sutras). This collection of sayings of the Buddha, preserved by the Theravadins, one of the last sects that emerged following the Buddha's death, are considered the most complete set of the Buddha's spoken word. It is sometimes referred to as Southern Buddhism as it is predominant in modern-day Sri Lanka, Burma, Cambodia, Laos, and Thailand.[9] The main teachings include what are considered to be the core teachings of Buddhism such as the Three Marks of Existence, the Four Noble Truths, the Eightfold Path, dependent origination, nature of self, and nirvana. The emphasis is on personal liberation (the *arhat*), renunciation (or more accurately, discipline), mindfulness, and ethical living.[10]

By the 1st century BC, additional teachings appeared; they were believed to have been inspired or revealed by the historical Buddha (e.g., Diamond Sutra, Lotus Sutra, Heart Sutra) but hidden and preserved (e.g., in a cave, heaven, encased at the bottom of the ocean and protected by a dragon) only to be released at a later time when the need of humankind demanded it. In these writings, the Buddha is portrayed more as a transcendent, idealized superbeing, with less significance placed on the appearance of the historical Buddha (the physical manifestation of the archetypal Buddha) of the Pali Canon scriptures. Omnipresent and omniscient, the Buddha could reveal himself to anyone at any time or place. This development of the Buddhadharma is commonly labeled as the Mahayana (Great Path) or Northern Buddhism (China, Japan, Korea, Vietnam) and includes Shin Buddhism, Soto Zen and Rinzai Zen Buddhism, and Nichiren Buddhism. The main teachings include the idea of the bodhisattva, who, motivated by supreme compassion, resists final nirvana for the sake of sentient beings (in contrast to the emphasis on solitary attainment of final nirvana of the *arhat* of the Theravada). The Lotus Sutra, for example, mentions 23 celestial bodhisattvas, such as Maitreya, Manjushri, and Samantabhadra. In addition to the bodhisattvas, a vast pantheon of divine, archetypal, celestial Buddhas are described, infinite in number and teaching Dharma in any number of infinite universes to those who dwell in their own heavens and to whom worship, propitiation, and veneration could be directed. Some of these celestial Buddhas included Vairocana (in the pure land of Akanistha) or Amitābha (in the pure land of Sukhavati). Mahayana places equal emphasis on compassion and wisdom.[11] Mahayana teachings expand the Theravada nonself (*anatta*) doctrine in the form of emptiness (*shunyata*), which is the noninherent existence of all phenomena, as well as the positing of Buddha nature, which is the intrinsic potential of all beings to become a Buddha (*tathagatagarbha*). It also teaches the doctrine of the three bodies (*trikaya*) of the Buddhas, which consist of manifestation (*nirmanakaya*); the archetypal, subtle, cosmic form (*sambhogakaya*); and the ultimate, unconditioned, empty nature (*dharmakaya*).[12]

The final significant contribution to the Buddhadharma occurs in the form of Tantra, a tradition found in Buddhism and Hinduism. Commonly known as Vajrayana (the Diamond Path), Tantric Buddhism emerged around AD 750 and relied on the tantras, teachings written by the Buddha or other Buddhist deities that were hidden and revealed to (select) humans at appropriate times and places. Tantric Buddhism includes a number of what may be termed magical and supernatural practices including the recitation of mantras (magical formulae to evoke a deity, protect from demonic forces, and nurture spiritual advancement), mudras (ritual hand gestures), mandalas (visions of totality of the mind and the universe depicted in magic circles), and the introduction of a vast number of new deities including spirits, demons, protectors, and other spiritual beings whom one could invoke, propitiate through liturgy, and visualize union. Five Buddhas (or *Tathagatas*) were especially considered central to Buddhist tantric cosmology: Vairocana, Ashksobhya, Rantnasambhava, Amitābha, and Amoghasiddhi. Vajrayana can be found primarily in Tibet, Bhutan, Mongolia, Nepal, China, and Japan. Unique among the Buddhist traditions is the pivotal role of the guru, or realized teacher who mediates the attainment of enlightenment.[13]

Over the long history of Buddhism there have been, and still exist, many schools, sects, and traditions that emerged, flourished, disappeared, and emphasized different aspects of the historical Buddha's teachings; interpreted or reinterpreted what he taught; and addressed aspects of the teachings that were overlooked or neglected by other interpretations and vary in their interpretation of texts, soteriological practices, and traditions. Nevertheless, the basic teachings found within the Pali Canon, especially the Four Noble Truths, are found within every tradition and will be described briefly in this chapter.[14]

Conceptualizing Illness and Healing: Buddhist Perspectives

As the description of the Buddha's life and the traditions that developed since his passing clearly demonstrate, suffering and illness (or more precisely mental illness) is closely tied to the functioning of our mind. Suffering is the result of perceptual and cognitive distortions that yield a number of harmful emotional states and the associated actions. Without insight into the cause of our suffering and the role that we play in our mental health and wellness, then we are doomed to repeat the conditions that can only lead to suffering for ourselves and others. The insight that authentic health can be attained only by a disciplined reorientation of our mental life (rather than focusing solely on the outside world as a solution to our mental suffering) can begin the process of healing the wounds we acquire through life and foster our responsibility for our own health and well-being. It is not surprising that the Buddha's final advice to his followers was to work diligently on realizing the nature of the mind (empty and impermanent).

The Development of Buddhism and Healing in the Modern World

The core teachings of the Buddha can be considered his instruction advice on attaining true health, healing the emotional suffering and dissatisfaction that each of us is sure to experience and for which no solution can ever be found "out there." Indeed, the teachings of the Buddha present a radical psychology that situates the deepest states of bliss and happiness and wholeness "in here," in the workings of our mind.

The Four Noble Truths

The **Four Noble Truths** (or insights or realizations) summarize the first major teaching of the Buddha following his enlightenment and, if properly understood, can be considered to contain his entire psychology, psychotherapy, and soteriology. In some presentations of the Four Noble Truths, an explicit medical model is adopted with the Four Noble Truths corresponding to the diagnosis, etiology, prognosis, and cure of suffering, respectively. As such, the model of the Four Noble Truths represents an analysis of the human condition and its causes (the first two truths), its profound healing through the prescriptions summarized in the fourth Noble Truth culminating in enlightenment, or, more accurately, authentic health, the third Noble Truth.[15]

Noble Truth 1: There is Suffering

The Ubiquity of Suffering

The essential teaching of the first Noble Truth is that suffering or sorrow is an inescapable fact of life. This does not mean that everything is just suffering or that there is only suffering, a common misunderstanding of the first Noble Truth and Buddhism in general. Within the broad compass of the term commonly translated as suffering, *dukkha*, is a focus on what today we might consider primarily to be psychological or emotional suffering: anguish, stress, agony, disappointment, unfulfilled, etc.[16] These aspects of suffering are unavoidable as long as one clings to specific perceptual and cognitive distortions (or illusions). This is the human condition. Our body can be the source of endless and excruciating suffering (hence, the dedication of vast amounts of financial, intellectual, and human resources toward the amelioration of suffering in our society). Suffering can also accompany all of our remaining senses, including mental suffering. In other words, we have the potential to suffer at any moment in a myriad of ways. Pain may be inescapable (e.g., disease, accident, violence), but suffering—the way we interpret, react, work with the pain—is within our power. It is this type of suffering that is the primary focus of the Buddha's teaching.[17]

The Illusion of Permanence

All phenomena, mental and physical, are finite from the most majestic mountain ranges to the subtlety of a flame, from thoughts and perceptions to the universe itself. The intrinsic quality of all phenomena is change, transformation, movement, process, and flow. Impermanence is often concealed by apparent continuity—many things seem to be the same day after day—or change very slowly (e.g., a table). The constant arising and subsiding of every moment of cognition whether it is a thought, emotion, sensation, perception, or action, can be easily perceived. Aging, from the moment we are born to our final dissolution, is the most emotionally powerful example of impermanence.[18]

The Delusion of Essence

While suffering and impermanence may become obvious to any intuitive observer, the Buddha's core insight, which underpins both suffering and impermanence, is a cognitive one and much more subtle. The Buddha came to understand that suffering and impermanence were based on the utter conditionality (or causal interdependence) of all phenomena. All appearance is conditioned and composite, created or caused by the coming together of specific elements and components and that disappears when those components dissolve. There is only appearance and no ultimate reality behind what we perceive, including the human being. The truth of nonself suggests that there is not essence, substance, or inherent existence to any phenomenal experience.[19] While objects appear as if they really do exist, they would cease to if the conditions that brought them into appearance change. To present this doctrine in a more positive way, the existence of phenomena is conditional, dependent, contextual, including the self. In a sense, the Buddha advocated a contextual realism. Everything exists in the sense that they are real and have real effects in the world, but they lack essence or substance. There is no thing in itself "behind" the appearance. Our subjective reality is the outcome of an interconnected interaction between the external world, as detected by our senses, and the interpretive processes of our mind.[20]

Noble Truth 2: The Cause of Suffering Is Craving

The Buddha told us that the condition or cause for mental and emotional suffering lies in the activity of the mind. He adopted the term *craving* and compared it to thirst (*tanha*) to describe it. However, craving is not the same as simple desire (*kama*). But what exactly is craving, and why is it the basis of suffering? Craving is bidirectional as it includes both a compulsive desire *for* something as well as a compulsive aversion against something. It can be understood as a very strong, intensive, obsessive, or compulsive projection of our needs upon the world. When in the state of lustful craving, desirable properties are viewed as inherent in the object of our craving. The craved object is considered a real source of happiness, pleasure, or well-being. When in the state of aversive craving, undesirable properties are viewed as inherent in the object of our craving and the avoidance of the object is considered a real source of happiness, pleasure, and well-being. The Buddha described three types of craving:

- *Sense experience* (*kama tanha*; e.g., pleasure, hedonism) refers to the compulsive desire for pleasurable sensory experience (or the removal of unpleasant ones). Craving for sensation expresses the belief that happiness is inherent in pleasure and the objects that give pleasure. As a result, we fixate, seek, and cling to objects that we are convinced will give us pleasure or eliminate pain. Any of the senses may be the focus of our sensory craving.
- *Being or existence* (*bhava tanha*) refers to the strong belief, desire, or obsession to become greater than we are, to become "somebody," to achieve, overcome, attain, accomplish, etc. This craving is often motivated by a desire to satisfy others and cultural expectations. It is important to distinguish normative efforts to achieve success in life versus craving. This distinction lies in the attribution or projection onto the goal or target of our efforts an excessive or exaggerated function or significance (without consideration of the costs that must be borne to achieve this goal or target) and that we fervently believe is needed to achieve happiness.
- *Nonbeing or nonexistence* (*vibhava tanha*) refers to the strong desire, obsession, or compulsion to escape from experience, existence, being, to become "nothing," to reduce stimulation, to die (e.g., absorb, merge, unite, be one, sleep, avoid, numb out, escape, "veg," dissociate, be reckless, be suicidal, do drugs). *Vibhava tanha* encompasses all the activities that diminish or attenuate consciousness. As with other cravings, there is a normal or healthy form of *vibhava*. This occurs when we wish to sleep, rest, reduce stimulation, relax, or withdraw from the world

> temporarily. When we crave nonbeing, our goal is to eliminate sensation, perception, cognition, and any other form of subjective experience even if doing so may harm ourselves or others.[21]

The second Noble Truth situates genuine healing within our mind. Healing the suffering we endure can be achieved only through a recognition that health and wellness arises from our own subjectivity. Only by correcting the delusional beliefs that the Buddha identified as underlying suffering can the authentic health be attained.[22]

Noble Truth 3: Cessation of Suffering

The first two Noble Truths or insights describe the human condition under the sway of ignorance (or lack of awareness). If the Buddha had stopped at describing the first two insights, then he could be accused of presenting a very pessimistic view of human nature. The last two Noble Truths or insights describe the human condition under the sway of wisdom (or awareness). The third Noble Truth or insight induces hope without which there would be no escape from the inevitability of suffering. Within the medical or psychological model of the Four Noble Truths, the third Noble Truth or insight is the positive prognosis for the elimination of mental suffering and illness. There is a way of realizing genuine health and happiness. The third Noble Truth is often expressed as nirvana or enlightenment. When one has understood nirvana, one is able to remain free of the perceptual, cognitive, and affective distortions that create continuous suffering, ill-health, and misery. We are able to encounter our world with wisdom and discernment. Nirvana is genuine health.[23]

Noble Truth 4: The Path to the Cessation of Suffering

Having discussed the human condition and the potential for liberation, the Buddha described a method (i.e., the cure or treatment) for realizing nirvana that places the responsibility for true health squarely upon ourselves. The Buddha delineated the **Eightfold Path**, a systematic approach to transforming the personality, beginning with perception and culminating with our place in the world. The Eightfold Path is neither prescriptive nor moralistic, but it is ethical and intersubjective. How we relate to others is central to the fourth Noble Truth and is critical to lasting health.[24]

Skillful View

Skillful view retrains our perceptions. It encompasses the realization of the suffering, impermanence, and nonself that characterize all phenomena; the law of cause and effect; and the Four Noble Truths. The full realization of the wisdom of skillful view acknowledges that the roots of our suffering are to be found in the most basic way that we encounter the world. The realization of the insights of skillful view on its own might culminate in a depressive realism, or nihilism, unless these insights are allowed to mature within the insights of the remaining aspects of the Eightfold Path.[25]

Skillful Thought

Skillful thought focuses on the relationship we develop with the world around us but in particular with others.[26] This path strongly emphasizes intention, which reflects the goal of our action and the quality of the mind that engages in that action. The Buddha described three types of skillful thought or intention to cultivate: (1) our relationship toward sensation or perception should avoid craving; (2) an attitude of goodwill (*metta*), benevolence, and kindness toward ourselves as well as to those whom we know and like (e.g., family), those to whom we may be indifferent (i.e., strangers), and those to whom we dislike (e.g., "enemies"); and (3) an attitude of nonharming and compassion toward others and wishing to relieve their suffering (*karuna*). We are encouraged to be empathically mindful of our behavior, speech, attitudes toward others that might cause them harm. *Metta* advocates a genuine desire for others to be happy and successful. Both *metta* and *karuna* require that we realize our mutual interconnectedness. Without authentic relationships with others, durable health is not possible.[27]

Skillful Speech

Unskillful speech (e.g., lying; gossip; divisive, deceitful, denigrating, humiliating, critical, abusive, insulting, sarcastic, demeaning language) is a contributor to almost all interpersonal conflict. Language can generate destructive emotions within oneself and in others. Speech reflects and shapes our views of others and ourselves.[28] Authentic happiness must guard against destructive speech patterns. Such speech directed at oneself can produce feelings of anger, rage, anxiety, or depression and may culminate in acts of self-destruction (e.g., addiction, suicide, self-mutilation). When such speech is directed toward others, we can generate similar emotions in others and intensify emotions that may lead to enactments (e.g., violence).[29]

Skillful Action

The Buddha encourages us to avoid the following activities if we are to attain the kind of genuine health that requires harmonious, benevolent, compassionate relationship with others.[30] Skillful action is directly related to skillful thought and skillful speech:

- Killing is the intentional harming of other beings and is prohibited. Unintentional harm may still occur (e.g., we may hurt or kill someone inadvertently) but is less harmful to our well-being than the type the Buddha is describing.

- Lying refers to intentional deception that violates trust and can harm others.
- Stealing includes activities beyond the act of taking something that does not belong to oneself but also includes other forms of stealing such as fraud, plagiarism, or other efforts to deceive, manipulate, or extort others in order to obtain what they possess.
- Sexual misconduct refers to sex with sentient beings who cannot consent, who are emotionally attached to others, or who may be hurt or deceived.
- Intoxication disinhibits mental processes that can readily lead to other harmful activities; it is to be avoided.[31]

Skillful Livelihood

Most of our waking lives are eventually spent in a form of work. The Buddha cautions that the need to earn a living should not include the harming of others. This can be difficult to discern at times and will always need a judgment on the part of the individual, especially when the harms may not be directly obvious. While some forms of livelihood (e.g., working in a gun factory or abattoir, running computer scams, dealing drugs) are clearly unskillful, in other cases it may be difficult to discern (e.g., certain types of scientific research, sex trade, farming).[32]

Skillful Effort

Skillful effort is concerned with mental training and the effort required to master harmful emotional states. Harmful mental states are those that disturb calm, insight, equanimity, and tranquility. They interfere with the development of authentic self-understanding and impact our relationships with others. Since action is closely tied to feeling, we are advised to skillfully address negative emotions by preventing their occurrence and by terminating them when they should arise. The Buddha identified five specific classes of harmful emotions that may impede emotional health: (1) craving attachment, (2) ill will, (3) depression, (4) anxiety, and (5) confusion.[33]

Skillful Mindfulness

In order to undermine the tendency to identify with interpretive narratives (*vicara*), the Buddha encouraged the cultivation of present-moment awareness.[34] This interpretive process elaborates, embellishes, and otherwise distorts perceptual events (*vitarka*) and fosters an inner commentary that can strongly influence our emotional states. Once *vicara* is active, it is difficult to remain aware of the original perceptions that form the bases of our interpretations. If the narrative is dysfunctional, intense emotional suffering can result (e.g., depression, anger, anxiety). Through the interruption of such narratives by grounding attention by recollecting present-moment awareness, such emotional states can be attenuated.[35]

Skillful Concentration

Concentration encourages in maintaining one-pointedness attention on an object. It unifies the mind. Through sustained concentration on a meditative object (such as the breath), deep states of relaxation and absorption can be attained (e.g., *samadhi*). Skillful concentration nurtures unbroken attentiveness and induces tranquility and is a natural antidote to emotional suffering.[36]

The Nature of the Self

In describing nonself, it is important to clarify that the Buddha did not say that the **self**, or our sense of who we are, does not exist. The Buddhist teaching is that our self (our sense of unique subjective reality) is, like all other phenomena, also compounded, composite, and conditional, devoid of any unique ontological status or essence. The self is a process, not an essence or substance. The notion of nonself is central to Buddhist psychology. The Buddhist teaching of self is described in the teaching of the five psychophysical elements (*skandhas*) that comprise the self.[37]

- Form (*rūpa*) includes our physical body and all of its functions, including the five sense organs and their objects. The form aspect our self is in constant transformation from the moment we are conceived in the womb until our death.
- Feeling (*vedanā*) is composed of three hedonic qualities that the Buddha said accompanies every moment of subjectivity: (1) pleasure, (2) aversion, and (3) neutrality. Since there are six senses, there are 18 feeling states.
- Perception–cognition (*samjñā*) refers to discernment, analysis, recognition, judgment, and thinking arising from contact with objects. This aspect of our self is intimately connected with memory and can be affected by expectations, our current emotional state, habits or karma, experience, and conditioning.
- Conditioning (*samskara*) is our embodied conditioning. It includes what is normally called the personality (e.g., mental activities, volition, action, will, reflexes, dispositions, habits).
- Consciousness (*vijñāna*) consists of six types, five sense consciousnesses and mental consciousness. This *skandha* allows us to be aware and conscious. Without consciousness, we would have no awareness of anything else although one could imagine having a physical self without consciousness (e.g., asleep, coma, deep intoxication).

Conclusion

The Buddha's description of the human condition summarized in the Four Noble Truths can be summarized in the following way: The pervasive dissatisfaction, lack of fulfillment, and mental suffering and illness that is part of life (first Noble Truth) is caused by the strong tendency to look for happiness, satisfaction, and reality in the phenomenal world that, by definition, cannot provide such dissatisfaction (second Noble Truth). The Buddha demonstrated that phenomenal experience, due to its transience and conditionality, can never provide us with genuine health and happiness but only conditional states of mind. As a result, we repeatedly encounter mental suffering. However, through discipline and discernment (fourth Noble Truth), one can develop a new *experiential* understanding of oneself, our social relationships, and the "world" based on uncontrived acceptance and equanimity rather than obsessive clinging and fear (third Noble Truth). The discipline described in the Eightfold Path outlines a reconditioning of our life through a healthier attitude toward others, effective regulation of emotions, cognition and behavior, and insight into the perceptual patterns of our minds, all to be applied with effort, mindfulness, and one-pointed concentration. The outcome of this process is a durable, intuitive, direct, authentic understanding into the nature of our own subjectivity that it is open, unbound, aware, flexible, and skillfully responsive. This describes the traditional Buddhist notion of health and happiness.

DISCUSSION QUESTIONS

1. What challenges might arise in the comprehension of the core Buddhist notion of nonself (or emptiness) outside of the Buddhist context? How might nonself be misunderstood? Are there potential dangers in this concept (e.g., nihilism, lack of meaning)?
2. Although considered a religion, the nontheistic emphasis of Buddhism places the emphasis of self-development squarely on the individual. Might there be limitations to the value the Buddhist perspective in cultures that are strongly founded on theistic religions? Does the focus on self-determination ignore historical, social, and cultural oppression?
3. As Buddhism grows outside of its original Asian cultural context, what are potential challenges to its preservation in very different multicultural environments? Does the growth of Buddhism in the West and its emphasis on science challenge the notion of the nature of Buddhism?
4. Buddhism makes bold claims about the ability to end suffering through disciplining of the mind. Does the psychological emphasis of Buddhism ignore or minimize other variables that influence suffering (e.g., systemic racism, homophobia)? Does the psychological perspective reflect an incomplete analysis of the nature of emotional suffering?

REFERENCES

1. Mishra, P. (2004). *An end to suffering: The Buddha in the world*. New York, NY: Picador; Olendzki, A. (2003). Buddhist psychology. In S. R. Segall (Ed.), *Encountering Buddhism*. Albany, NY: SUNY Press.
2. Gowans, C. W. (2003). *Philosophy of the Buddha*. London, England: Routledge; Laumakis, S. J. (2008). *An introduction to Buddhist philosophy*. Cambridge, England: Cambridge University Press; Olendzki, Buddhist psychology.
3. Laumakis, *An introduction to Buddhist philosophy*; Mishra, *An end to suffering*.
4. McGovern, W. M. (1997). *An introduction to Mahayana Buddhism*. New Delhi, India: Munshiram Manoharlal; Mishra, *An end to suffering*.
5. Schumann, H. W. (1989). *The historical Buddha*. London, England: Arkana; Smith, J. D. (2006). *The essence of Buddhism*. London, England: Arcturus; Williams, P. (2000). *Buddhist thought: A complete introduction to the Indian tradition*. London, England: Routledge.
6. Ibid.
7. McGovern, *An introduction to Mahayana Buddhism*; Mishra, *An end to suffering*.
8. Lopez, D. S. (2002). *The story of Buddhism: A concise guide to its history and teachings*. New York, NY: HarperOne; Smith, *The essence of Buddhism*; Williams, *Buddhist thought*.
9. McGovern, *An introduction to Mahayana Buddhism*.
10. Hanh, T. N. (1998). *The heart of the Buddha's teaching*. New York, NY: Broadway Books; Lopez, *The story of Buddhism*; Seager, R. H. (2012). *Buddhism in America*. New York, NY: Columbia University Press.
11. McGovern, *An introduction to Mahayana Buddhism*.
12. Laumakis, *An introduction to Buddhist philosophy*; Lopez, *The story of Buddhism*; Seager, *Buddhism in America*.
13. Laumakis, *An introduction to Buddhist philosophy*; Lopez, *The story of Buddhism*; Seager, *Buddhism in America*; Smith, *The essence of Buddhism*.
14. Laumakis, *An introduction to Buddhist philosophy*.
15. Laumakis, *An introduction to Buddhist philosophy*; Mishra, *An end to suffering*.
16. Mishra, *An end to suffering*.
17. Lopez, *The story of Buddhism*; McGovern, *An introduction to Mahayana Buddhism*; Seager, *Buddhism in America*.
18. Laumakis, *An introduction to Buddhist philosophy*; Mishra, *An end to suffering*; Williams, *Buddhist thought*.
19. Gowans, *Philosophy of the Buddha*; Mishra, *An end to suffering*.
20. Gowans, *Philosophy of the Buddha*; McGovern, *An introduction to Mahayana Buddhism*; Mishra, *An end to suffering*; Williams, *Buddhist thought*.
21. Mishra, *An end to suffering*; Olendzki, Buddhist psychology; Smith, *The essence of Buddhism*.
22. Gowans, *Philosophy of the Buddha*; Lopez, *The story of Buddhism*, Olendzki, Buddhist psychology; Smith, *The essence of Buddhism*.
23. McGovern, *An introduction to Mahayana Buddhism*; Olendzki, Buddhist psychology.
24. Gowans, *Philosophy of the Buddha*; Hanh, *The heart of the Buddha's teaching*; Lopez, *The story of Buddhism*; Williams, *Buddhist thought*.
25. Ibid.
26. Mishra, *An end to suffering*.
27. Gowans, *Philosophy of the Buddha*; Hanh, *The heart of the Buddha's teaching*; Lopez, *The story of Buddhism*; Williams, *Buddhist thought*.
28. Mishra, *An end to suffering*.

29. Gowans, *Philosophy of the Buddha*; Hanh, *The heart of the Buddha's teaching*; Lopez, *The story of Buddhism*; Williams, *Buddhist thought.*
30. Mishra, *An end to suffering.*
31. Gowans, *Philosophy of the Buddha*; Hanh, *The heart of the Buddha's teaching*; Lopez, *The story of Buddhism*; Williams, *Buddhist thought.*
32. Ibid.
33. Gowans, *Philosophy of the Buddha*; Hanh, *The heart of the Buddha's teaching*; Lopez, *The story of Buddhism.*
34. Mishra, *An end to suffering*; Smith, *The essence of Buddhism.*
35. Gowans, *Philosophy of the Buddha*; Hanh, *The heart of the Buddha's teaching*; Lopez, *The story of Buddhism*; Williams, *Buddhist thought.*
36. Ibid.
37. Gowans, *Philosophy of the Buddha*; Mishra, *An end to suffering*; Olendzki, Buddhist psychology.

SUGGESTED READINGS

Gowans, C. W. (2003). *Philosophy of the Buddha.* London, England: Routledge.

This is an excellent overview of the Buddha's core teachings and the underlying philosophical assumptions. An especially noteworthy feature of this book is an in-depth and articulate description of the notion of nonself, an aspect of the Buddha's teaching that can be challenging to fully comprehend

Laumakis, S. J. (2008). *An introduction to Buddhist philosophy.* Cambridge, England: Cambridge University Press.

This book surveys the breadth of Buddhist traditions and teachings with chapters on later developments of the Dharma. A useful aspect of this book is the description of the cultural conditions that led to the emergence of Buddhism.

Lopez, D. S. (2002). *The story of Buddhism: A concise guide to its history and teachings.* New York, NY: HarperOne.

In addition to an overview of the core teachings of Buddhism, this book also explores the structure of the Buddhist universe and the emergence of the Mahayana. In addition, a detailed exposition of the monastic life and the practices of the laity is excellent.

Schumann, H. W. (1989). *The historical Buddha.* London, England: Arkana.

The teachings of the Buddha are closely associated with the life of the Buddha. This excellent text surveys in detail the Buddha's life and his teachings and the social, religious, and political conditions that led to the development of Buddhism in the centuries following his death and the establishment of the ordained *sangha.*

4 Qigong and Healing (Based on Taoist Philosophy)

Amy L. Ai

Introduction

Qigong (QG) is a branch of traditional Chinese medicine (TCM), alongside its other major aspects (i.e., herbs, acupuncture, and tuina massage).[1] The term *qigong* is the phonetic juxtaposition of two Chinese characters: (1) *qi* (氣), meaning "flow of air," in a literal sense, or "vital force or energy," in a symbolic sense, and (2) *gong* (功), meaning "perseverant practice." In general, QG can be classified into two systems: (1) internal QG, a self-care practice to harmonize healthy *qi* flow and balance, and (2) external QG, the transformation and manipulation of healing force by a master to balance the *qi* pattern of recipients. The concept of vital energy is the very essence of TCM, as manifested in its two Chinese characters, *zhong yi*. While *yi* (醫) refers to "medicine," *zhong* (中) means "middle," or more precisely, a "golden mean" of internal equilibrium. TCM is an Eastern health and longevity practice aiming at achieving the inner balance of vital energy, rather than an oriental version of medical treatment for disease, as is Western medicine.[2] Accordingly, QG is an inner mind–body–spirit healing exercise, using various breathing exercises and meditative movement to achieve the goal of longevity.

To fully comprehend the essence of QG, it is imperative to address the core idea, the ever-changing patterns of *qi*, or energy, in the universe and in human life, contained in its guiding philosophy, Taoism. Taoism offers a dialectical worldview that undergirds theory and practice of TCM and QG. This philosophy is highlighted as the fundamental ground of the healing practice in this chapter, because it represents the original ideology of QG rooted in the ancient China. Tao (道), refers to the way, or the universal order, to be followed in life and in nature.[3] The world's reputed *Tao Te Ching* (道德經; *The Classic of the Universal Order* or *The Way of Virtue*) states the following: "When the consistency of the Dao is known, the mind is receptive to its states of change.[4] It also states this: "Man's laws should follow natural laws, just as nature gives rise to physical laws, whilst following from universal law, which follows the Dao."[5] Thus, Tao is the ultimate, indefinable principle that underlies all energetic movements and all processes in the universe. As Laozi (老子; 4th–5th century BC; also Lao-Tzu), an eminent Taoist philosopher in the Zhou dynasty (1028–221 BC), stated, "The Dao is abstract. . . . Without form or image, without existence, the form of the formless . . ."[6] In keeping with its image as an invisible yet perceivable "flow of air," the word *qi* serves as a vivid metaphor to illustrate constant energy movements in an interaction between the universe and human life.

What is the uniqueness of QG? While many forms of Eastern healing arts (e.g., Buddhist meditation, yoga) have shared a meditative component, Taoist QG is uniquely centered on the patterns of "change" in all vital force, based on a philosophical view that takes energy as the primary in everything and their relationship with the universe. Accordingly, the TCM and QG framework does not simply offer the guidance for healing practice but rather provides a more important grounding philosophy for one's life, health, and longevity. This chapter will address the following questions: (1) How did the ancient idea of Taoist QG emerge in China and later move to the world? (2) How did the Taoist worldview determine the theory and practice of QG? (3) How can TCM and QG enrich contemporary practice of health and healing in the West?

From an Ancient Idea of Healing in China to Its Modern World Practices

The Origin of QG

In *Tao Te Ching*, Laozi described the key characteristics of QG, such as concentration, emptiness of desire, quiescence, flexibility, and infant-like breath. His disciple Zhuangzi (莊子, 369–286 BC; also Chuang-Tzu or Zhuang Zhou), also a legendary Taoist philosopher, delineated the spiritual and intellectual function of this healing practice as the art of longevity, spirituality, and intuitive wisdom, all derived from contemplation and intuition in state of tranquil mind.[7] At their own time, early Confucianist and Legalist schools also emphasized tranquility and peace through sitting in meditation, viewed as the fasting of mind. In TCM and QG theory, *qi* is thus characterized with respect: (a) the rationale that activities of vital force are fundamental to the well-being of both human and the surrounding environment, (b) a framework involving a web of multilevel energy patterns as the central concern regarding holistic health, and (c) the description of pathways (meridian systems) through which circulations of *qi* occur and are to be balanced.[8]

However, essential components of QG practice emerged long before its systematic description by Taoists and other ancient scholars in China, where its dynamic or gymnastic component can be traced back to early ceremonial dances during the Zhou dynasty. A pottery jar over about 5,000 to 6,000 years ago there demonstrated an image of a dancing human figure in the posture of breathing exercise. *Qi*-based meditative practice originated in neolithic shamans' religious observances and New Year's dancing ritual. In their acting on, shamans mimic animal actions to drive out demons, a process recorded on rock art panels during the New Stone Age. Accordingly, many forms of QG were named after animals (***wu-chin-his***). Unlike various world's folk medicine or shamanism, however, TCM and QG neither involve supernatural and magic healing, nor attribute diseases to witchcraft, demons, or ghosts. Rather, they describe ailments and dysfunctions in a systematic approach to numerous perniciously physical and emotional disturbances.

The original quieting and tranquil component of QG was presented in other terms, such as **Dao Yin** (導引), meaning "leading and guiding the vital energy," following Tao. The Taoist Canon (AD 1145) is compiled of 1,120 volumes, including a volume donated to the classic edition of Dao Yin, which contains all the principles involved in QG. *Huangdi Neijing* (黄帝内经, *The Emperor's Inner Canon*), the Chinese medical text, summarized the fundamental doctrinal source for the basic theory and practice of TCM and QG for over 2 to 3 millennia.[9] The Neijing classics demonstrate the human being in both cosmic and geographical terms. It stated that the ultimate aim of Dao Yin is to become ancient, sage-like individuals who had been tranquilly content in nothingness, given their possession of true vital force (Zheng Qi) preserved within humans to prevent entry of any illness elements. Wang Ziqiao (ca. 220 BC), a royal Taoist sage from Qin state, performed the crane dance to achieve immortality. In *Huainanzi* (淮南子; *The Masters/Philosophers of Huainan*), a Taoist classic, Liu An, also a grand prince in the early Han dynasty (206 BC–AD 220), presented QG postures (e.g., bathing duck, leaping monkey, and turning tiger) with core theories in TCM (e.g., *yin* and *yang*, the five elements—metal, wood, water, fire, and earth). During this dynasty, medical applications of QG were promoted by the two most eminent TCM sages, Hua Tuo (c. AD 140–208), with his Dao Yin medical exercise, *Wu Qin Xi* (五禽戲, *Five Animal Dances*), and Zhang Zhongjing (AD 150–219), who first used the term *dantian* (丹田, "elixir field") in describing the circulation of *qi*.

Globalization and Modernization

QG entered Japan with TCM during the Shui and Tang dynasties (AD 582–907). In 1779, Taoist QG texts were first introduced to Europe by the Jesuit Pierre-Martial Cibot's translation of the documents into French.

The idea of vital energy in Taoist exercise may later have led to a major influence on the development of modern medical gymnastic by Per Henrik Ling (1776–1839). From the early 1950 to the 1960s, QG flourished and has been integrated into modern treatment as a means of rehabilitation and health promotion in China.[10] Newly established QG rehabilitation institutes evidenced therapeutic effects of internal QG practice on hypertension and neurasthenia. After the Cultural Revolution (1966–1976), China witnessed the second renaissance of QG in terms of medical QG, with more ambitious attempts to heal physical illness carrying Western diagnoses and health promotion. This was demonstrated by a senior QG master, Guo Lin, an artist cancer survivor. Guo Lin was brought up by her grandfather, a Taoist priest, who taught her ancient QG healing techniques. From the 1970s to 1980s, with thousands of followers, including cancer patients, she demonstrated Hua Tuo's *Wu Qin Xi*, which was believed to be long extinct in China, at the Center Station of Television in Beijing.

In 1980, scientific investigation of QG was endorsed by Qian Xuesen, the MIT-trained "father of Chinese space technology." Such celebrity advocacy led to millions of people joining QG healing practices in China. The vast and rapid revival of QG practices and studies reached the American continent at that time.[11]

Eastern Versus Western Worldview: Where Is Energy-Based Healing Embraced?

Different Views Regarding the Building Block of the World

Why did energy healing art emerge in ancient China but not in ancient Greece? Why did theory and practice of TCM and QG focus on energy rather than the structure of the body as it does in Western medicine? The answer to these puzzles lies in foundationally different philosophical worldviews undergirding two sides. The divergence involves both ontology (nature of being, existence, or reality) and epistemology (the way of knowing), dating back to the early Western versus Eastern civilization when Taoist and Greek philosophies formalized their outlooks of the world. Ontologically, the Taoist energy-based view presents remarkably different outlook from the operative philosophy of classical science in the West. The Western ontology originated especially in Aristotelian empirical materialism, which largely provided the rationale underlying the scientific foundation for Western medicine. This perspective views the world in systematic structures of which the basic unit of natural substances lies in the atom, a notion imagined and conceived by Democritus, a pre-Socratic philosopher (ca. 460–370 BC). An offspring of this outlook, allopathic medicine, thus focuses primarily on the material structure of the body (e.g., systems, organs, tissues, cells, chromosomes, genes, and molecules), enabling standardized diagnosis and specialized treatment.

In the East, the Taoist ontology views the world and humans in an interactive energy system, a multilevel *qi* system with ever-changing patterns. According to Laozi, in his *Tao Te Ching*, "All living things are formed by being, and shaped by their environment, growing if nourished well by virtue; the being from nonbeing."[12] Stated differently, an invisible energetic force, viewed as the origin of the world, existed before all material substances emerged and is the constant reality of the world. One the other hand, all visible materialistic aspects of the world are merely transitory phenomena in a cosmic sense. Based on this worldview, Tao, or the natural law, governs the dynamic relationship between formless energetic aspect, termed *nonbeing*, and the formed substantive aspects of all things, termed *being*. Nonbeing is also described in terms of nothingness, which Democritus called the void, whereas being refers to things. This Eastern worldview considers the former as the primary reality, the seemingly "nonexistence," meaning the formless and timeless dynamic vital force. In contrast, the latter is seen as the secondary reality, the visible "existence," referring to material structures involving everything with a certain space–time form in the universe. If this view seems to be perplexing, the closest and comprehensible analogy may be found in the contemporary challenge of dark energy phenomenon in modern cosmology. As Laozi stated, "All things are born of being; being is born of non-being."[13] While one could not scientifically define nonbeing, the term in name of *qi* can be considered as a legitimized intervention point for human health.

Eastern Genesis and Ways of Knowing

Why doesn't the creation of the world have a creator in the Chinese worldview? The Taoist view about the essence of the world actually reflects the original Chinese genesis that was summarized as this: The one created the two, the two created the three, and the three created everything. This phrase must be understood in energy-based terms: The one refers to Tao (the universal principle governing all forces of the word); the two refers to *yin* and *yang* (the polarized forces within all phenomena in the universe); and the three refers to heaven (the universe), earth (the surrounding environment in nature and society), and human being (the totality of mind–body–spirit). In this unique Eastern perspective, the world is created without a creator but with Tao. The image of Chinese creation is the counterpart to that in the ancient Hebrew Genesis, which claims God as the creator of humans with the universe and the guide of their life and death. Because ancient Chinese view both the universe and human life based on energy creation, the maintenance of the world's order and human health are inevitably subjective to the orderly movement of *qi*. The very idea, *qi*, in Taoist worldview thus paves the way to an energy-centered framework of TCM and its healing art, QG.

This perspective is also illustrated in the oldest Chinese classics, *The I Ching* (易經, *Classic of Changes* or *Book of Changes*), around the third millennium BC. The law of nature is not perceived as a fixed order but as a continuous flow, as symbolized by *qi*, in the constant movement of both nonbeing and being aspects. The law of the universe, not of human logic, is what Taoism intends us to comprehend philosophically, to appreciate aesthetically, or to worship spiritually. The concept of *qi* refers not only to the essence of all material objects but also to their dynamic interactions in terms of the rhythmic alternation of two forces, *yin* (陰) and *yang* (陽), similar to positive and negative electric charges. *The Tao of Physics*, by Capra, not only well presents this fundamental West–East worldview difference but also depicts the similarity between the idea in Taoism and that in modern quantum physics.[14] In modern terms, both perspectives posit that (a) all forms of substance are nothing but materialization of energy and (b) the dynamic patterns of energy are primary, whereas substantive aspects are secondary.

Central to Taoist dialectical perspective are three different interrelated principles: (1) change, (2) contradiction, and (3) holism. Specifically, the first principle asserts that reality is in constant flux. The second principle claims that reality is full of paradoxes. The third principle declares that all things are interdependent and interactive. In this view, Taoist epistemology values dialectic thinking for wisdom over linear rational thinking and deductive reasoning central to formal logics. In this view, Taoist Laozi and Zhuangzi offered insights into human existence in the universe, such as this in *Tao Te Ching*: "When living by the Dao, awareness of self is not required, for in this way of life, the self exists, and is also non-existent, being conceived of, not as existentiality, nor as non-existent."[15] From this Taoist perspective, the order of the world, including that of humans, follows a path of three rules: (1) uncertainty, (2) mutuality, and (3) a circling pattern that links the individual part to the whole. The last principle (holism) is the essence of Taoist dialectical thinking and the consequence of the first two. Thereby, truth is often presented in a fluid sense in relation to its context or to opposite but related aspects rather than as something isolated and absolute. Based on these principles, TCM and QG address health promotion and disease prevention through balancing approaches, involving energy-oriented diagnosis, interactive patterns, and personalized healing.

Understanding Coded Eastern Principles as the Key Application for the West

Symbols and Codes for Eastern Healing Principles

Following the Taoist worldview, a master healer must understand the moving patterns of *qi* not only within the body but at hierarchical levels in order to provide effective healing. The symbol of *taiji* (太極圖) aptly exhibits the principles of change, contradiction, and holism observed in this Eastern dialectic outlook that connects humans' *qi*, the essence of life, with that in the nature. The S-curve dividing line of this symbol implies change, meaning the constant cyclical movement of opposing pairs between its two halves. The black-and-white parts, symbolized by *yin* and *yang*, imply contradiction, meaning the dynamically conflicting but mutually controlling opposite forces in everything. The totality of the symbol implies holisms, meaning that the universe, including humans, depends on reciprocal influences and transforms between opposite but interdependent energetic forces in the ever-changing world. As such, parts become meaningful only in relevance to the whole context. From this relativist and artistic perspective, everything about health and, especially, disease prevention should correspond to the movement of *qi* and, accordingly, the healing process of energy practices.

The interactive and cyclical patterns of *qi* are systematically elaborated within the TCM and QG theory as noted in the previous chapters, in which all things in the universe are energetically interrelated and affect other matters. Detailing all the complexities is beyond the scope of this chapter, but principles of TCM and QG can be understood through the basic information-processing or coding system and be applicable to modern healing. Unlike science and Western medicine, based on experiments and mathematic approvals, Taoist TCM are embraced in experiential intuition and wisdom, as summarized with its basic coding system tracing back to *The I Ching*. The book is entirely devoted to the ordering patterns of change with respect to the dynamic system of the universe and has tremendous influence on TCM and QG.

Energy System Among Functional Organs

The coding system for TCM and GQ did not evolve to classical Newtonian science or modern medicine because it was not based on the defining system of a materialistic world. Rather, this energy-based perspective may help comprehend the principle holism, regarding *qi* movement among basic organ functions. This Taoist position is exemplified in TCM, in which all phenomena are viewed within a complex hierarchical web of *qi*, rather than as a system of isolatable structures. Humans are seen to be inseparable from their surrounding environment, because one's vital energy (*qi*) is constantly dancing with forces existing in the universe. Health and longevity can be maintained only in the harmonic interactions of individuals' internal and external energetic *qi* patterns. The pair concept, *yin* and *yang*, in TCM, is used to organize and, thereby, to predict *qi*-centered health patterns, alongside the five-element theory, as emerged in the Han dynasty around the 2nd or 1st century BC. Unlike four elements in ancient Greek, taken as basic components of the world's structure, ancient Chinese took the five elements (metal, wood, water, fire, and earth) to symbolize the holistic principle in *qi* movement of the universe, including those along its channel daily within the human body—that is, the meridian system linking all organ pairs.

In TCM and QG theory, this parsimonious framework displays circling interconnections among five paired organ systems, symbolized by the five elements. To illustrate, they are metal–lung or large intestine, wood–liver or gall bladder, water–kidney or small intestine, fire–heart or pericardium, and earth–spleen or stomach. In name of "organs," the system describes how *qi* constantly moves between their represented systems, involving generating (i.e., mother–son relationship, curve lines forming a circle) and consuming (e.g., controlling relationship, direct lines forming the pentagon). The system involves its flowing and ebbing of *qi* in paired organ systems and corresponding meridians, while each system has its peak *qi* time around a circadian system covering a 24-hour cycle (**Zi-Wu-Liu-Zhu**, 子午流注). Yet, this circling pattern can be apprehended only in terms of functioning, partly related to modern knowledge on various hormonal and neuroendocrinological functional circles in terms of daily time. For example, Stomach Qi (its mental components including thinking function) is abundant between 9:00 a.m. and 11:00 a.m., corresponding to the peak function of the adrenal line. To enhance its *qi*, healers may practice at certain times daily at the peak functioning time of an "organ," to enhance its weakened *qi*, or at the turning point between systems (*qi* transition between key meridians), to maintain the energetic equilibrium or holistic health in the body.

Energy Interaction Between Mind and Body

The coding system links physical health with changing moods of emotions as well as behaviors, sexuality, spirituality, contextual factors such as lifestyle and food, and components in one's environment. TCM and QG theories employ five organs to pair cognition or emotions with their hosted organs, including liver–anger, heart–joy, spleen–contemplation or concentration, lung–grief, and kidney–fear or sadness. The functional relationship within each mind–body system pair can also be symbolized by *yin–yang* with *yin* referring to nonlocalized emotions and *yang* to the localized organ's functioning system. As such, TCM and QG do not follow the Cartesian dualism of mind and matter (*res cogitans/res extensa*) separation but the Taoist holism of *yin–yang* force interaction, including mind–body interaction.

The mind–body–spirit phenomena are viewed in a complex hierarchical web of energy, rather than as the collected function of isolatable physical structures. Accordingly, the approach of QG is psychosomatic, which performs mental activities to balance both emotions and the *qi* flow, spontaneously affecting physical health. The TCM and QG theory thus enables perplexing energy movement in humans to be comprehensible, physical well-being to be inseparable from emotional well-being, and illness conditions to be preventable through self-healing practice and other interventional approaches. Health is maintained only when mind–body–spirit as a whole harmonically balance each other rather than being mere absence of pathology.

Energy Interaction Between Humans and the Universe

In keeping with Taoist ontology, TCM and QG theory views each person as an energetic cosmos in miniature that is energetically interacting with and corresponding to change in the holistic environmental system (i.e., nature, society, and cosmos). One's energy movement manifests the same pattern as does that of the universe, also registered by the same coding system on daily, monthly, seasonally, and yearly bases. In terms of time and space, this Easter healing system is literally the systematic elaboration on changing patterns of *qi* with respect to the interconnectedness of the body–mind–spirit totality with the multilevel nature's contexts. Paired organs, tissues, meridians, pulse, tongue status, sounds, tastes, colors, seasons, directions, planets, temperament, herbs, food, and external pathogens are orderly linked together by the coding system along with their interconnected relationships. This practical principle is in a sharp contrast to Western exercise that tends to target the sides of muscles with forced movements.

In one Taoist diagram of "the regeneration of the primary vitalities" in internal alchemy, major organ parts and energy centers (e.g., *dantian*) are demonstrated with the changing image of the moon alongside key meridians (e.g., *renmai* and *dumai*), across the 24 fortnightly circles based on the Chinese lunar calendar. These moon images illustrate circadian energy patterns of *qi* movement in the body, literally synchronized with that of the cosmic patterns. Following Taoist epistemological principles, QG is essentially a self-care approach to longevity and to spiritual cultivation, with an emphasis on breathing technique for holistic health. As stated in the *Tao Te Ching*, by breathing as a sleeping babe, one can maintain harmony and achieve enlightenment.[16]

Conclusion

QG as an ancient Eastern healing art is based on an energy-centered worldview. Following the basic laws of uncertainty, mutuality, and a circling pattern, three Taoist principles—changes, contradictions, and holism—provide guidance in the entire *qi*-based framework of the TCM and QG theory and practice. According to the principle holism, illness conditions are often individually assessed and addressed using multiple principles concerning one's (or the patient's) whole energy system rather than a standardized diagnosis and assessment for structural abnormality. Because of the principle contradiction, health and well-being are not viewed as the state opposing to disease or the absence of psychopathology but rather as an uncertain process of constantly balancing normal and abnormal *qi* patterns. Given the principle of change, healthy and illness conditions can be transformed into each other, depending on interaction between the ailment stage and an individual's health practice. In this dynamic perspective, health and well-being are maintained only when overall internal and external *qi* movements are harmonized. Based on the Taoist *qi*-centered worldview, everything is initially created and exists in the form of energy that is the driving force of materialized aspects, including human health. The holistic position in TCM and QG theory need to be understood in dialectic and interconnected patterns within which the biophysical, neuroendocrine, psychobehavioral, environmental, and cosmological levels operate as one coherent system. Taking an open-mined perspective, the principles demonstrated in its coding system may illuminate the modern healing practice of psychotherapy in which psychopathology is largely not structural based even in the renewed *DSM–5*.[17]

DISCUSSION QUESTIONS

1. What are the fundamental principles of Taoism? Briefly state how the history and philosophy of Taoism contributed to the ways in which we understand Asian healing practices.
2. Qigong (QG) is an inner mind–body–spirit healing exercise based on the inner balance of vital energy. Discuss this concept, and also explain how this idea differs from the mind–body idea of the Cartesian dualism.
3. Discuss how you would go about applying the principles of QG to contemporary counseling and psychotherapy practice. Offer a SWOT (strengths, weaknesses, opportunities, threats) analysis of integrating QG into psychological practice.
4. Traditional Chinese medicine (TCM) and QG theory view each person as an energetic cosmos in miniature that is energetically interacting with and corresponding to change in the holistic environmental system (i.e., nature, society, and cosmos). Discuss.

REFERENCES

1. Ai, A. (2010). Qi gong. In M. S. Micozzi (Ed.), *Fundamentals of complementary and alternative medicine* (4th ed.). St. Louis, MO: Saunders.
2. Yuan, C. H. (2015). "Chinese medicine" is not the abbreviation of the medicine of China: *I Ching* expert. Lui Dajun's definition of "Chinese medicine." *Chinese News*, *28*(23), 199 (in Chinese).
3. Yuan, "Chinese medicine."
4. Tzu, Lao. (6th century BC). *Tao Te Jing* (S. Rosenthal, Trans.; Chapter 16). Retrieved from http://web.clas.ufl.edu/users/gthursby/taoism
5. Tzu, *Tao Te Jing* (Chapter 25).
6. Tzu, *Tao Te Jing* (Chapter 14).
7. Capra, F. (2000). *The Tao of physics: An exploration of the parallels between modern physics and Eastern mysticism* (4th ed.). Boston, MA: Shambhala Publications.

8. Ai, Qi gong.
9. Ibid.
10. Ibid.
11. Ibid.
12. Tzu, *Tao Te Jing* (Chapter 51).
13. Tzu, *Tao Te Jing* (Chapter 40).
14. Capra, *The Tao of physics.*
15. Tzu, *Tao Te Jing* (Chapter 7).
16. Tzu, *Tao Te Jing* (Chapter 10).
17. American Psychiatric Association. (2013). *Diagnostic and statistical manual of mental disorders* (5th ed.). Washington, DC: Author.

SUGGESTED READINGS

Bloom, A. (1968). *The republic of Plato: Translated with notes and an interpretive essay.* New York, NY: Basic Books.

The Republic, a Socratic dialogue written by Plato around 380 BC, concerning the definition of justice, the order and character of the just city-state and the just man. For this reason, ancient readers used the name *On Justice* as an alternative title.

Capra, F. (2000). *The Tao of physics (4th ed.).* Boston, MA: Shambhala Publications.

This book presents the similarity between philosophies underlying theoretical physics and Eastern mysticism.

Hammer L. (2003). *Dragon rises, red bird flies: Psychology & Chinese medicine* (Rev. ed.). Seattle, WA: Eastland Press.

This book provides a psychological insight into the mind–body–energy interaction concepts in TCM. They are the fundamental energy constructs of Chinese medicine.

The I Ching (also known as the *Classic of Changes* or *Book of Changes* in English) is an ancient divination text and the oldest of the Chinese classics—an influential text read throughout the world, providing inspiration to the worlds of religion, psychoanalysis, business, literature, and art. The hexagrams in this text have often acquired cosmological significance and paralleled with many other traditional names for the processes of change such as *yin* and *yang* and *Wu Xing.*

Tzu, L. (6th century BC). *Tao Te Jing* (S. Rosenthal, Trans.). Retrieved from http://enlight.lib.ntu.edu.tw/FULLTEXT/JR-AN/an142304.pdf

This is a Chinese classic text. Its name comes from the opening words of its two sections: 道 "dào" and "way."

5 *Ki* (氣) and Healing

Tadashi Ogawa and Mami Ishii

The Eastern concept of *ki* (or *qi*), which is often translated into English as "vital force" or "life energy," has received attention in the Western world for some time now. In Asian countries, *ki* is understood as a fundamental dimension of the relation between human beings and the world. Because all cultures evolve their own traditions, mythology, habitude, history, and language, this concept is also spelled differently as *ki, qi,* and *ch'i* in different cultures. It is called *qi* in China and *ki* in Japan. They both have a special character "氣" and the pronunciation is almost the same. We will use the word *ki* when referring to all types of such energy in this chapter.

This word *ki* appears in the oldest book of Japanese history and mythology, *Kojiki*, as well as in many Chinese classics, such as the *Medical Classic of the Yellow Emperor*. In modern Japanese society, many everyday words contain *ki*, such as *kibun* for mood and *funiki* for atmosphere. They are used in various ways to describe the types, states, conditions, and maneuvers of *ki*. As it is a word reflecting one's energy state, *ki* is also an essential concept necessary to understand one's health. In fact, the state of good health is called *genki* (original *ki*), and illness or diseased health is called *byoki* (sick *ki*). One's awareness of being in the present moment or consciousness is called *shoki* (right ki), and the mental or emotional status or mood is called *kibun* (*ki* divided). Emotional energy can be described as a type of *ki* (e.g., *doki* for anger, *yoki* for cheerfulness).[1]

Based on this concept of universal energy, *ki*, Asian countries have developed and practiced such healing methods for a few thousand years. Even though *ki* functions as an essential source of human living, behaviors, and cognitive patterns, it is also an ambiguous concept. Due to its invisible nature and the paradigm difference between the East and West, it can be challenging for many to understand what exactly *ki* actually is.

In this chapter, we will explore the challenge by defining and conceptualizing *ki* in terms of its history, healing, and development in Asia (mainly China and Japan) and the West.

Defining the Various Manifestations of *Ki*

Ki is the foundation of the universe's infinite manifestation of the world and the life of everything—minerals, plants, and animals, including human beings. The body and mind create a vortex of *ki* in its various manifestations by interacting with each other to form an organism. It is a versatile concept, which can mean and turn into multiple directions. *Ki* is the infinite collection of infinitely small particles so that *ki* can be a part but also a whole of something. At the foundation of all is *ki*; everything is the manifestation of *ki* in varying degrees of materiality.[2]

Ki has dimensionality and exists in two forms. The first form is the energy materialized into some form of being or expression of objects and living creatures such as human flesh, the soul, and feelings (*kimochi*). The other form of *ki* is formless, such as *kimochi* for feelings and *tenki* for weather. The first type of *ki* is a vital spiritual power, which is embodied in the living flesh of humans and other beings. For human beings, it is the core of their being, behaviors, thoughts, and emotions and has effects at each level of mind–body–spirit to exchange energy, material, and/or information. Traditional Chinese medicine (TCM) calls the vessels of this energy in the human body as meridians and uses them in the practice of acupuncture.[3]

Ki is a connective power that exists between heaven and the earth. This *ki* is neither subjective nor objective but is the deepest aspect of the relation of human and environmental world. *Ki* is something natural around human beings, like vapor and steam, or mist and fog. Another word like ***futei*** (literally meaning "wind–body") specifically denotes the mood surrounding a person. The letter used for *ki*, written as "氣" reflects a type of steam moving outward in eight directions. When there is a certain type of steam around a person, it is called *funiki*, meaning "atmosphere." This connective energy is also considered as a spiritual power and is sometimes called Reiki (meaning "spiritual energy"). As spirit has no concrete shape, it is often seen or considered as gaseous.[4]

Another way of looking at *ki* is its degree of materialization. At the basis of all is *ki*. Everything is the manifestation of *ki* in varying degrees of materiality, ranging from the completely material, such as body fluid, to the totally immaterial, such as mind.[5] *Ki* is phantasmagoric, existing and filling the space in everything such as the sky, mountains, flowers, and air. It originally had no form, but it can give form to something by filling the object or space.

Timely observation can categorize *ki* according to its various functions.[6] In the theory and practice of TCM, there are many types of *ki* affecting our bodies and minds, ranging from the subtle and rarefied to the very dense and coarse. All the various types of *ki*, however, are ultimately one *ki*, merely manifesting in different forms. For example, the *yin–yang* theory explains the bipolarity of *ki* while the five elements classify *ki* based on five different organs and its subsequent pairs (e.g., liver *ki* & gallbladder *ki*). The refined energy produced by the internal organs are also named according to their function (e.g., gathering *ki*). Among all of them, a mind with mental and emotional energies has the most nonmaterial type of *ki*.[7]

Moreover, individual *ki* can also be the indicator of its bigger manifestation. The world situation is disturbed when *ki* is not in order. In today's world, people usually use this word *ki* in reference to our own bodies, yet wisdoms of ancestors in Asia formerly spoke of the personal body as reflecting the world and saw them as one.

Folk Nosology and Healing in *Ki*

The original thinkers in ancient China were concerned with concept of "vital force" or "life energy" and eventually referred to it by the philosophical technical term: *ki*. The influential Chinese Taoist philosopher Zhuangzi (or Chuang-Tzu or Zhuang Zhou) mentioned that *ki* means both to live life and its movement itself. This definition, however, would not give us a concrete sense of *ki*.

Mencius was probably the first person to realize the deep and relevant philosophical meaning of *ki* in the relationship between human beings and the world. He said that *ki* fills in the body and is commanded by the will. As a philosopher of voluntarism, he expressed the importance of the integration of willpower, in order to control *ki*. Mencius used a word *hao jan chih chi* (*kozen no ki* in Japanese) to describe the strong moving force of human mental and spiritual power. This *ki* means literally "the moving powerful wind" or "breathing of the great and large openness."

Ki could be nourished in two ways into something so great, so vast, and so strong. The first way was the "rightness" as an accumulation of right deeds. The second way was the formless space that unfolds between heaven and the earth. This was supposed to be the way of truth, opening up to the world. Mencius believed that these two ways of *ki* between the individual and the universe were connected by one's willpower.[8]

The influence of Mencius's Confucianism concept also had an ethical–political dimension and affected the medical thinking and practice in East Asia. This strong notion of *ki* was well understood because *ki* signified the mental and spiritual state of the living flesh that lived in the world. It was important to recognize and remember for people that *ki* means originally the human living flesh, which is, through breathing, combined with the outer world.

Along with Confucianism, Taoism was another ancient Chinese style of living, religion, and philosophy. According to Taoism, *ki* is the material that creates Tao, a path, as well as everything existing in the universe. Through exercise and movement, material transforms into objects with energy.

When there are two different beings, energy is created naturally (i.e., men and women, strength and weakness). After *yin* and *yang* energy are completely mixed into a balanced way, a third neutral *ki* is created and eventually turned into the harmonious four-dimensional existence of heaven and the earth.[9]

The idea of *ki* migrated to Japan in the 7th century, where it mingled and fused with Buddhist philosophy to describe the energy that drives cycles of life and death in both the human and supernatural worlds. The concept of *ki* shifted with the advent of the samurai and martial arts (MA) in the late 14th century. The Mito School in Japan integrated the concept of *ki* from ancient China and explained *ki* as the mental and spiritual strength that fills the space between heaven and the earth. *Ki* was also perceived as an ethical concept, important in maintaining relationships amongst people.[10]

Worldwide, even though each culture has its own term to explain *ki*, the content and meaning of the *ki* is quite similarly universal and foundational. For example, this energy is called *prana* in the Ayurvedic medicine; *pneuma* in ancient Greece; *mana* in Pacific culture; *lüng* in Tibetan Buddhism; *ruah* in Hebrew culture; and vital energy, mood, or atmosphere in Western philosophy.

Conceptualizing Health, Illness, and Healing in *Ki*

In East Asia, the philosophical and phenomenological concept of *ki* was applied and developed further into many different areas of life including medicine, lifestyle, and MA as a core principle. In order to understand the role of *ki* in health and wellness, it is important to see the simultaneous universality and particularity of *ki*. Since *ki* is the foundation of life, where the energy of human beings connects with the universal energy between heaven and the earth, there is death when the communication or breathing stops. Therefore *ki* is present and continuously in motion as long as a person is alive.[11]

The maintenance of the *ki* balance is the key to one's health and wellness so that it is evaluated through the careful observation and assessment of the person's constitution and other possible contributing factors such as diet and lifestyle, presence of trauma, and living climate at the different levels of the human architecture (i.e., mind–body–spirit, *yin–yang*, five elements, and internal organs). In practice, it also requires people to be able to distinguish between the different types of *ki* (e.g., essence, original *ki*, and stomach *ki*).[12] The *yin–yang* qualities of *ki* as opposites was also mentioned in the "Great Meditation" by Kaibara to create movements or stillness resulting in a state of balance. He believed that the essence of health is the flow of *ki*, as saying "*ki* wo *hashirasu*" ("let the *ki* run") because both reducing and obstructing *ki* could be the cause of any disturbance of life force.[13]

Ki is also transformative to promote the holistic health and wellness of human being. Human physiology is essentially based on the transformation of *ki*, which can assume different forms depending on its states of aggregation or dispersal, and it is the motive force of all physiological processes. There is health when *ki* is shifting and flourishing to keep its balance, while there is disease when *ki* is weak or when it is moving into the wrong direction or stagnating to cause imbalance. *Ki* is an energy that manifests simultaneously on multiple levels.[14] Thus, the proper process and direction of movement of *ki* are the basis of human physiology including movement of bodily fluids and body parts, excretion of wastes, digestion and absorption of nutrients, moisture of skin, and resistance against exterior pathogenic factors.

While Western medicine uses the explanation of neurobiochemistry for psychiatric disorders, Asian traditional medicine still uses the concept of *ki*. In terms of mental health and illness in Asia, the explanatory model was historically a possession by other spirits, such as ghosts and demons.[15] It has been common for Chinese patients to visit a Buddhist temple, a fortune-teller, or *feng shui* master to engage the spiritual healing services. TCM doctors use a set of complicated methods to diagnose *ki* disturbance or stagnation rather than simply relying on the enacted symptoms and disease characteristics.[16] There are several conditions that are similar to depression in the West, and they are usually caused by stagnation of *ki*. Anxiety is a modern term that does not have an exact equivalent in Chinese medicine but can be described as rebellious *ki*, when *ki* moves toward the opposite direction. The state of mania or psychosis is also related to the state of mind, either obstructed, unsettled, or weakened depending on the insightfulness, energy, sleep, and emotions.[17]

The causes of *ki* disharmony can be internal or external. Internal causes of disease are usually emotional factors that can upset the movement and transformation of *ki* and affect the exterior of the body first. Emotional stress is considered to be the main cause of psychological problems, and the other factors are usually only contributory. They often originate from different times in one's life: the period in the womb, childhood, and adulthood.[18] The seven emotions identified in TCM are (1) anger, (2) joy, (3) sadness, (4) worry, (5) pensiveness, (6) fear, and (7) shock. The first effect of emotional stress on the body is to affect the proper circulation and direction of *ki*, leading to stagnation of *ki*. For example, anger makes *ki* rise while joy slows *ki* down.

The pathology of *ki* transformation can be explained by the direction of movement of the various types of *ki*.[19] The specific *ki* directions associated with internal organs in TCM have the unique reciprocal relationships that are different from what Western medicine defines about organ systems. Each *ki* moves into a certain direction to perform unique functions so that any disruption of *ki* transformation needs to be viewed as the dysfunction of the internal organs, causing the manifestation of various symptoms and illnesses such as anxiety and depression.[20] The movement of *ki* is essentially determined by how we use or not use our energy through different activities and the state of emotion being experienced. Prolonged and extra expenditure of a great deal of *ki* reduces *ki* into the deficiency state, and also, the long-term sedentary work obstructs *ki*. Failure in moving toward the right direction also causes the stagnation of *ki* flow.[21]

In terms of healing practices, rather than simply treating the symptoms being presented, identifying the cause of illness is essential in the healing practices of TCM.

The power of knowing is actually emphasized and valued in its practice so that people can avoid, minimize, and prevent recurrence of the illness after or along with the healing. Therefore, the relationships between healers and patients are more directive and didactic in nature, rather than the insight-oriented, client-centered approaches of Western medicine.[22] As to produce health, diet, movement (exercising body), and **meditation** (quieting mind) have been practiced to unite the mind and body.

In terms of the effect of *ki* healing, it also acts on each and every level of the body, mind, and spirit, the holy trinity of human being. At the physical level, *ki* may work to alleviate or eliminate symptoms such as pain and inflammation. At the psychological level, the mood of a person can be elevated, or negative emotions, such as anxiety and frustration, can be sedated and removed. Also, a sense of exhilaration and even catharsis can be achieved, as if playing sports or listening to music through the *ki* healing. At the spiritual level, healing is promoted through the resonance between the person's spirit and universal nature or priest or spiritual practitioners who strike the souls of others.[23]

The Development of *Ki* and Healing in the Modern World

Despite the foundational differences in the practice of healing and medicine, the concept of *ki* has in recent years been more accepted and incorporated into the West. The way *ki* is translated and practiced depends on the particular viewpoint taken. Most modern physicists would probably agree that *ki* is presumed as a type of energy since *ki* expresses the continuum of matter and energy.[24] The integration of Eastern traditional healing components is usually safe and therapeutic through delivery of culturally competent care that acknowledges the client's social and relational world.[25] Major traditional treatment modalities utilizing the concept of *ki* include Qigong (QG), MA, acupuncture, acupressure, herbal medicine, nutritional therapy (dietetics), spiritual healing, and the use of religions such as Buddhism.

QG is a relatively new umbrella term, developed to call a variety of energy-based healing practices based on the theory of *ki*. In general, QG is a way to practice directing the flow of *ki* energy either internally or externally through the body in a more balanced and healthful manner, rather than a treatment for a certain condition. With the physical and spiritual discipline, QG has an emphasis on specialized breathing exercises that have been developed to help move energy through the body and to clear the mind.[26] The internal QG focuses on the internal processes through meditation, visualization, and breathing, while the external QG focuses on interpersonal healing practices. Visualization exercises and ritualistic movement in QG practice may encourage a change of unconscious by using the transcending phenomenon of some sort.[27] QG and other healthy regimens are prescribed to balance and promote circulation of *ki* for the practitioner's physical, mental, emotional, and sexual health.[28]

The basic principles of QG—meditation, awareness, movement, and breathing—underlie several complementary energy exercises that are practiced in the Western health care settings.[29] Researchers have shown the positive therapeutic effects of QG in the mental health area, including relieving stress; positive influence on anxiety, mood, and several physiological variables such as blood cortisol levels; and strengthening personal control of mind energy.[30]At the same time, some studies also mentioned that QG induces temporary psychosis, characterized by the appearance of auditory hallucinations and delusions. This condition typically resolves itself after cessation of QG.[31]

Practicing QG or from QG-derived exercises is not only beneficial in attaining better health but also provides the opportunity of finding our own authentic selves, in the answer to the fundamental question of who we are. This valued perspective of personal spiritual development in Asian traditional cultures is similar to the concept in transpersonal psychology.[32] It integrates the spiritual and transcendent aspects of the human experiences as the sense of self-identity is considered to extend beyond personal to bigger aspects of human experiences such as psyche and universal consciousness.[33] The manifestation of *ki* is not only life but also one's soul.[34] Through various life experiences, a person learns and cultivates skills to manipulate *ki* to shine his or her soul. In the East, people strongly believe that this soul is something that remains after the death of the body and reincarnates to continue its journey to grow continuously.

Both QG and psychotherapy have an ability to bring a specific awareness and realization to individuals who are facing some challenges.[35] Such certain phenomena of attraction brought by *ki* are called *kizuki*, literally meaning "attaching *ki*" or "awareness." By increasing awareness of one's own *ki* state through a practice of meditation or other form of restoring and promoting the flow of *ki,* a person may realize the relationship among their thoughts, actions, and things happening externally. This may be equated to the existence of the unconscious that Freud mentioned in his psychoanalytic view of psyche.[36]

In Japan, this collective term for the use of *ki* to restore health is *reijutsu,* including laying on hands as well as direct hand touch and religious or spiritual ritualistic healings.[37] Because of the component of spiritual healing, hypnotherapy, and visualization, *reijutsu* was considered as a kind of psychotherapy before the Second World War. *Reijutsu* literally means "the art of spirit (human psyche or mind)" or "the art of a mental healing." *Ki* can also mean "spirit," so *reijutsu* can also be understood as the art of *ki*. A viewpoint of *reijutsu* is that the diseases can be healed by the power of human mind (will), which gives the directional movement to *ki*. The spirit (*ki*) in spoken words is called *kotodama* and is often utilized by the *reijutsu* healers. One relatively recognized example of this energy healing in the West is Reiki, and it has been widely used in different medical settings.[38]

MA (or martial arts) are physical techniques to manipulate *ki*, using the essence of the theoretical and spiritual teachings from esoteric Buddhism, Taoism, and Confucianism. Tai Chi (TC) is a type of MA derived from QG. Another MA form, *aikido*, meaning "the way of Spiritual Harmony," has been practiced to induce a state of harmony (*ai*) and spirit (*ki*) that also can be described as flow, higher states of consciousness, and peak experiences.[39]As MA also can be described as moving meditation, it requires stilling the mind, even if the body is in action. Therefore, in the psychological literature, MA has been seen as a useful approach to both physical and mental health.[40] As a useful supplement to verbal psychotherapy, MA can foster and expose feelings, enhance self-esteem through the provision of physical activity and group experience, and teach relaxation, concentration, assertiveness, and honesty in communication. Moreover, the practice of MA can also provide an experiential grounding in spirituality, which can be beneficial for both therapists and clients in practice.[41]

Acupuncture and acupressure are based on the assumption that *ki* flows along the meridians in the body, and their flow can be restored by stimulating peculiar points on the body. They are intended to affect and balance the energetic system of the body in order to treat the human body, mind, emotions, energetic field, and spirit.[42] The medical acupuncture model is practiced through the adaptation of traditional methods based on modern medical knowledge. Evidence from research so far published has mixed results and suggestions. The most commonly used acupuncture protocol in mental health is probably the National Acupuncture Detoxification Association (NADA) protocol, developed for drug and substance abuse and dependence.[43] Some other studies indicate some promise, especially when combining acupuncture with conventional prescribed medications for cases of schizophrenia, anxiety, depression, cognitive disorders, and post-traumatic stress disorder (PTSD).[44] In addition, very few serious side effects have been reported, so acupuncture could be considered a relatively safe intervention.[45]

Besides the therapeutic use, the East Asian cultures emphasized the self-cultivation of *ki* for maintenance, prevention, and optimization as self-responsibility. In terms of cycle, it is suggested practicing a lifestyle following the natural *ki* flow, such as bipolar *yin–yang* phenomenon (i.e., waking up at the same time with the sunrise and staying awake during the day so that *ki* flows throughout the day).[46] These habits are intended to be incorporated into various aspects of lifestyle or even prescribed in order to consume in positive *ki* and release negative *ki* in a simple manner by resonating and being in harmony with nature. Many modern practices of *ki* moderation include utilization or modification of sound (music), environment, sleep, diet, and sexual behavior.[47] In addition to these points, we cannot forget to consider the effects of singing songs. To sing a song means the inspiration and the expiration of our spirit, namely the wind. It is an essential practice of the phenomenology of wind.

Dietetics is important as specific food items carry certain *ki* so that both cooking and consuming them requires special attention to utilize *ki* from them. *Ishoku Dogen* is an idea originating in Asian medicine, and it means that the source of diet and medicine is the same. The medicinal effects exist even in the most basic daily diet so that it is wise to choose food items according to the *ki* type that they possess.[48] Understanding the relationship of *ki* between self and the environment is believed to assist the wellness of a person and is a core value of Asian tradition.[49] Taking in and harmonizing the essence of natural environments is known as ***feng shui***, which is literally translated as "wind–water."

Moreover, there is a saying in Japanese—***yamai wa ki kara***—that means an illness is coming from *ki*. This can be explained by the modern science of psychoneuroimmunology that the mood (*kibun*) and emotion (*kimochi*) of a person strongly influence the self-healing power to be either stagnated or flourished. Therefore, it is often the core of lifestyle suggestions to enjoy life moments and to fulfill desires and dreams in order for a healthy and happy life through the spiritual unity and harmony with Mother Nature.[50]

Lastly, the therapeutic utilization of energy, such as *ki* seen in TCM, is considered as a practice of vibrational medicine today. It is an integrative method of theories and practices of modern medicine and ancient teachings.[51] Vibrational medicine recognizes and employs the use of different forms of energy including homeopathy, flower essences, color and light, magnetobiology, radionics and distant healing, and other hands-on healing practices. Other types of energetic modalities that have a psychological impact may include music therapy, art therapy, and aromatherapy.[52] Because *ki* is the energy, we may be able to say that those are all related to the therapeutic use of *ki*.

Conclusion

The ancient philosophical and healing concept of *ki* is still valid and practical today to assist people to overcome certain types of suffering but also to support fulfillment of life. As *ki* is the foundation of everything, including basic human physiology and actions such as breathing, moving, eating, and singing, a therapist can also incorporate the concept into the practice of psychotherapy. Learning the concept of *ki* may provide a more comprehensive understanding of the individual condition as a whole and his or her relationship to the environment for both therapists and clients themselves. Moreover, incorporating this concept of *ki* into therapy provides individuals the transcending opportunity to look deeper into their own existence and into all dimensions of being, beyond just the "mind" or "emotion." When this energy is freed to flow naturally, healing occurs as needed at the optimal pace, intensity, and timing so that individuals can be in harmony within as well as with the universe.

DISCUSSION QUESTIONS

1. *Ki* is the central concept in Asian traditional culture and healing practices. What is the historical significance of *ki* in one's health and wellness regardless of the state of being?
2. What is a role of *ki* in one's challenged mental health state, such as anxiety, depression, and psychosis? What are the clinical methods you would use to approach mental health based on your understanding of *ki*?
3. How would you apply the concept of *ki* in counseling and psychotherapy? How could the current practice of psychotherapy be modified to change the state of *ki* and ultimately the mental health of clients?
4. *Ki* is more than just a mind–body connection. Discuss how the concept of *ki* and healing contribute to the discourse of counseling and psychotherapy in theory, practice, and research.

REFERENCES

1. Ogawa, T. (1996, November). Philosophy of *ki* and atmosphere: An essay of the phenomenology of wind. *Aurora*, 281–290; Ogawa, T. (1998). Qi and phenomenology of wind. *Continental Philosophy Review*, *31*, 321–335.
2. Ogawa, Philosophy of *ki*; Ogawa, Qi and phenomenology; Maciocia, G. (2005). *The foundations of Chinese medicine: A comprehensive text for acupuncturists and herbalists* (2nd ed.). Philadelphia, PA: Churchill Livingstone Elsevier.
3. Maciocia, *The foundations of Chinese medicine.*
4. Ogawa, Qi and phenomenology.
5. Maciocia, *The foundations of Chinese medicine.*
6. Tobioka, K. (1998). *Reading the essence of ki.* Tokyo, Japan: Kawade Shinsha Shobo Publishers.
7. Maciocia, *The foundations of Chinese medicine.*
8. Ogawa, Philosophy of *ki*; Ogawa, Qi and phenomenology.
9. Maciocia, *The foundations of Chinese medicine*; Tobioka, *Reading the essence.*
10. Ogawa, Philosophy of *ki*; Ogawa, Qi and phenomenology.
11. Tobioka, *Reading the essence.*
12. Maciocia, *The foundations of Chinese medicine.*
13. Ogawa, Philosophy of *ki*; Ekken, K. (2009). *Yojokun: Life lessons from a samurai* (S. W. William, Trans.). New York, NY: Kodansha USA.
14. Maciocia, *The foundations of Chinese medicine*; Tobioka, *Reading the essence.*
15. Kua, E. H., Chew, P. H., & Ko, S. M. (1993), Spirit possession and healing among Chinese psychiatric patients. *Acta Psychiatrica Scandinavica*, *88*(6), 447–450.

16. Maciocia, *The foundations of Chinese medicine.*
17. Maciocia, G. (2008). *The practice of Chinese medicine: The treatment of diseases with acupuncture and Chinese herbs* (2nd ed.). Philadelphia, PA: Churchill Livingstone Elsevier.
18. Ibid.
19. Tobioka, *Reading the essence.*
20. Maciocia, *The foundations of Chinese medicine.*
21. Maciocia, *The foundations of Chinese medicine*; Tobioka, *Reading the essence.*
22. So, J. K. (2005). Traditional and cultural healing among the Chinese. In R. Moodley & W. West (Eds.), *Integrating traditional healing practices into counseling and psychotherapy* (pp. 100–111). Thousand Oaks, CA: Sage.
23. Tobioka, *Reading the essence.*
24. Gerber, R. (2001). *A practical guide to vibrational medicine: Energy healing and spiritual transformation.* New York, NY: HarperCollins.
25. Yayama, T. (1995). *Humanology of ki* (14th ed). Tokyo, Japan.
26. Gerber, *A practical guide.*
27. Yayama, *Humanology of ki.*
28. Maciocia, *The foundations of Chinese medicine*; Yayama, *Humanology of ki.*
29. NMJ Contributors. (2010). An evidence-based review of *Qi gong* by the natural standard research collaboration. *Natural Medicine Journal, 2*(5).
30. NMJ Contributors, An evidence-based review; Lee, M. S., Kang, C. W., Lim, H. J., & Lee, M. S. (2004). Effects of *Qi*-training on anxiety and plasma concentrations of cortisol, ACTH, and aldosterone: A randomized placebo-controlled pilot study. *Stress and Health, 20*, 243–248.
31. NMJ Contributors, An evidence-based review.
32. Walsh, R., & Vaughan, F. (2003). On transpersonal definitions. *Journal of Transpersonal Psychology, 25*(2), 125–182.
33. Ibid.
34. Yayama, *Humanology of ki*; Nakagawa, M. (2009). *Ki: The energy of light to fill the body, mind, and soul.* Tokyo, Japan: Bio Magazine.
35. Yayama, *Humanology of ki.*
36. Ibid.
37. Imura, H. (2014). *Golden era of Reijutsu-ka.* Kanagawa, Japan: Being Net Press.
38. Vitale, A. (2007). An integrative review of *Reiki* touch therapy research. *Holistic Nursing Practice, 21*(4), 167–179.
39. Faggianelli, P., & Lukoff, D. (2007). Aikido and psychotherapy: A study of psychotherapists who are Aikido practitioners. *The Journal of Transpersonal Psychology, 38*(2), 159–178.
40. Ibid.
41. Ibid.
42. Maciocia, *The foundations of Chinese medicine*; Gerber, *A practical guide.*
43. Carter, K. O., Olshan-Perlmutter, M., James Norton, H., & Smith, M. O. (2011). NADA acupuncture prospective trial in patients with substance use disorders and seven health symptoms. *Medical Acupuncture, 23*(3), 131–135.
44. Carter et al., NADA acupuncture; Shen X., Xia J., & Adams C. E. (2014). Acupuncture for schizophrenia. *Cochrane Database of Systematic Reviews*, 10, CD005475. doi:10.1002/14651858.CD005475.pub2
45. Carter et al., NADA acupuncture; Edwin, L. F. G. (1986). The psychotherapeutic utilization of acupuncture (counseling, Eastern philosophy, mental health, medicine) (Doctoral dissertation). Available from ProQuest Dissertations and Theses database. (Paper AAI861203)
46. Tobioka, *Reading the essence.*
47. Maciocia, *The foundations of Chinese medicine*; Tobioka, *Reading the essence.*

48. Ibid.
49. Tobioka, *Reading the essence.*
50. Maciocia, *The foundations of Chinese medicine*; Tobioka, *Reading the essence.*
51. Gerber, *A practical guide.*
52. Tobioka, *Reading the essence.*

SUGGESTED READINGS

Böhme, G. (1993). Atmosphere as the fundamental concept of a new aesthetics. *Thesis Eleven, 36*(1), 113–126.

Böhme explores a concept of *ki* as atmosphere in the area of aesthetics and arts. The book describes the environmental perspective of *ki* and its influence on the perception of people. Therefore, *ki* can be described in many subjective ways that are personal or collective.

Ekken, K. (2009). *Yojokun: Life lessons from a samurai* (S. W. William, Trans.). New York, NY: Kodansha USA.

Kaibara combines his knowledge of holistic health, the principles of *ki*, and *jin* (human-heartedness), Buddhism, Confucianism, and the art of living in this book. The book addresses various concerns from mental and physical health to spiritual matters and how one can achieve healthy and rewarding life, which is based on nourishing one's own *ki*. He implies that the breath is the act that unites human beings and *ki* between heaven and the earth.

Ogawa, T. (1996, November). Philosophy of *ki* and atmosphere: An essay of the phenomenology of wind. *Aurora,* 281–290.

It is the first article written to describe the phenomenology of cultural universalism that combines the Gospel of John and *Kozen-no-Ki* by Mencius, the relational triad of heaven, the earth, *ki*, and *pneuma*, which leads to the development of *ki* of atmosphere. Ogawa discusses and compares the versatility of *ki* characteristics from multiple philosophical and historical perspectives.

Ogawa, T. (1998). *Qi* and phenomenology of wind. *Continental Philosophy Review, 31*(3), 321–335.

This paper was written to clarify the state of things and appeared in the context of the wide atmosphere in terms of the relationship between the mind and the atmosphere. *Ki (qi)* is discussed from the philosophical and environmental perspective to describe its intimate relationship between life of humans and the surrounding nature and breath as what connects between them.

PART B

Integrating Asian Healing Traditions Into Clinical Practices

6 Infusing Asian Healing Traditions Into Counseling Psychology

Ben C. H. Kuo and Beatriz Rodriguez-Rubio

Despite the growing attention and openness toward indigenous, cultural forms of healing and the prevalent use of traditional methods of healing worldwide, exposure to and analysis of the intersection between traditional therapies and the practices of counseling psychology remain very limited. At the present time, there have been only a handful of published articles specifically addressing the interconnection and infusion between **indigenous healing**, which include Asian traditions and counseling psychology.[1] In fact, a recent survey of the contents of multicultural course syllabi in counseling psychology and counselor education graduate programs in the United States showed that the topic of traditional healing practice across cultures was largely overlooked in the current multicultural training curriculum.[2] The authors of the study found that among the 54 course syllabi identified and reviewed in the study only 4 (i.e., 7%) indicated "indigenous forms of healing" as part of the course content.

Clearly, at the present time, there remains a significant disconnect among the prevalence of age-old traditional indigenous healing practices among the general population; the growing therapeutic interest in infusing Asian forms of healing into psychological treatment interventions; and the extent to which these issues are presently being addressed in the practice, the research, and the training of counseling, counseling psychology, and other mental health professions. Yet the impetus in search of traditional healing methods alternative to modern medicine and the movement toward indigenization of psychology, counseling, and psychotherapy internationally are expected to grow.[3] These developments have begun to challenge the ways in which psychology and psychological treatments have been applied to work with culturally and nationally diverse groups and individuals.[4] Consequently, counseling and mental health practitioners and scholars have advocated concerted and renewed efforts to better understand traditional cultural healing practices and to discern the implications these therapies hold for the practices of counseling, counseling psychology, and mental health services.[5]

As a case in point, Asian traditional forms of healing in particular have existed for thousands of years as means to treat ailments, diseases, and problems.[6] However, only recently have the assumptions, the philosophies, the concepts, and the applications of these traditional methods begun to make their way into the practice and the discourse of mainstream counseling psychology, clinical psychology, and psychiatry disciplines.[7] Recent literature distinctly attests to this developing trend, as evidenced by the rising interest in East–West therapy integration, including a growing body of published works on the research and the application of **mindfulness**, meditation, yoga, Qigong (QG), Buddhist principles, etc., for psychological and mental health interventions.[8]

Cast within the perspectives described previously, the present chapter explores the issue of infusion and integration of Asian traditional healing into counseling, counseling psychology, and mental health interventions. The specific goals of this chapter are to review and survey the past and the present scholarly and professional discourses on Asian and other cultural healing traditions within the fields of counseling and counseling psychology and to explore ways in which more systematic efforts of integrating traditional wisdom and practices into these fields might be achieved into the future.

To these ends, this chapter examines the prevailing discourse on traditional healing by exploring two key issues. We first ask this question: How are traditional or indigenous forms of healing in general and Asian traditional healing more specifically currently being viewed, portrayed, and considered within counseling, counseling psychology, and mental health professions? To address this question, we review and highlight critical discussions being forwarded by proponents of **traditional and conventional therapy integration** in association with the multicultural counseling movement. Next, we raise and attempt to address this second question: What future directions and approaches might the fields of counseling and counseling psychology undertake to further the pursuit of a greater infusion and integration of Asian traditional healing into counseling and psychotherapy practices, research, and training? We attend to this question by offering a summary and synthesis based on the existing literature as well as our own observations and experiences as active researchers, instructors, and practitioners of multicultural counseling training and therapy. Finally, we conclude the chapter by providing a concrete, illustrative case example of Asian traditional therapy integration. It is based on an actual short-term group therapy for patients with obsessive–compulsive disorder (OCD) conducted by the second author of the chapter within a graduate-level clinical therapy practicum. The case study illustrates the incorporation of acceptance and commitment therapy (ACT), meditation, and Buddhist principles into group treatment of patients with OCD.

Counseling Psychology in Relation to Traditional Healing Practices

A scan of the literature shows that the ongoing discourse on the intersection of Asian and other cultural forms of indigenous practices and professional psychology has been noticeably sporadic and haphazard. The initial attention on indigenous forms of healing within counseling psychology specifically began with the early works of a few multicultural counseling scholars.[9] This increasing attention was strongly tied to the fledgling cross-cultural counseling or multicultural counseling movement at the time.[10] Three key developments have contributed and fueled the prevailing discourse and debate about the role of traditional therapies and indigenous healing practices in counseling psychology: (1) the multicultural counseling competency movement, (2) the internationalization of counseling psychology movement, and (3) the indigenization of counseling or psychotherapy movement.[11] In the following sections, we provide a review of the influences each of these movements have on the increasing call for therapy integration between traditional healing methods and conventional counseling and psychotherapy practices. Given that the extant counseling and multicultural counseling literature typically speaks to traditional healing practices and therapy integration inclusively, beyond ethnic, cultural, or regional specifications, the ensuing discussion will refer to "traditional" or "indigenous" therapies in generic terms.

Contemporary Ways in Which Traditional Healing Is Considered in Counseling Psychology

The multicultural counseling movement, which began in the United States following the civil rights movement, represents one of the earliest and the most influential forces that pressed counselors and psychologists to give attention to traditional forms of healing.[12] For example, pioneering multicultural counseling scholars have beckoned the counseling field to research and examine in-depth nonconventional, culturally and spiritually based forms of helping when supporting clients from diverse racial and ethnic backgrounds.[13] As early as the 1990s, the prominent African American counseling scholar Vontress studied, analyzed, and published research on traditional healing methods in Africa based on his field trips to four African countries.[14] As a strong advocate of traditional healing methods and therapies, Vontress heeded that the infusion of indigenous healing into counseling is imperative for counseling to be truly relevant to the increasingly diverse immigrant populations in North America in the 21st century.[15]

Around the same time, we began to see the inclusion of traditional healing being formally included in the definition of **multicultural counseling**

competencies. In 1992, Sue, Arredondo, and McDavis published the landmark, seminal document of "Multicultural Counseling Competencies and Standards: A Call to the Profession" in the *Journal of Counseling and Development*.[16] Of particular relevance to our current discussion, this document stipulated that (a) "Culturally skilled counselors respect indigenous helping practices and respect minority community intrinsic help-giving networks" and (b) "Culturally skilled counselors are not averse to seeking consultation with traditional healers or religious or spiritual leaders and practitioners in the treatment of culturally different clients when appropriate" (pp. 482–483).[17] While the use of words such as *respect* and *not averse to* was quite cautious and discreet, the article nevertheless represents a significant step forward at a time when strong suspicions about indigenous and traditional therapy by Western-trained counselors and psychologists were often the norm. As such, these calls alerted and set the field in motion in striving for a more holistic helping approach that would give consideration to the mind–body–spirit connection of health and well-being.[18]

Despite these early efforts, the progress toward integrating indigenous and spiritual healing approaches into the practice of mainstream counseling, counseling psychology, and other mental health professions has been subtle. In fact, more recent discourse around traditional healing and counseling practices reflects the concern over the inadequacy of the current multicultural counseling movement and the movement's lack of cultural and clinical relevance in meeting the changing needs of immigrants and minority populations.[19] For instance, in recent expositions by Moodley and his colleagues, these scholars expressed a grave concern about the limited scope and focus of the present-day multicultural counseling movement in the United States and Canada. Indeed, criticisms have been levied against the narrow attention the contemporary multicultural counseling movement placed on race, culture, ethnicity, and psychopathology as well as the multicultural practitioners' and scholars' tendency to reduce cultural competencies to a composite of "therapeutic techniques."[20] The consequences of this delimited focus are being observed in the perpetual underutilization of the mainstream mental health services by immigrants and racial and ethnic minorities, including Asians in the United States and Canada.[21]

Moodley, Sutherland, and Oulanova observed that the concepts and the practices of traditional healing continue to be highly prevalent among immigrants and ethnic minorities due to several factors: immigration, multiculturalism, inadequacy of Western allopathic medical treatments, improved availability of traditional healers in urban areas, and increased popularity of dual interventions help-seeking patterns (accessing Western health and traditional healing methods concurrently).[22] These sociodemographic trends are expected to continue. Thus, they stress the need for a paradigm shift on the part of psychological service and mental health providers to adopt new ways of conceiving and delivering culturally responsive counseling and psychotherapy interventions.[23] Moodley and West said the following:

> We believe that a creative move(ment), a small paradigm shift—the inclusion and integration of traditional healing methods into mainstream counseling and psychotherapy—will not only make a difference to (an ailing) multicultural counseling movement but will also add a new lease of life to psychotherapy and counseling generally. (p. 149)[24]

According to these assertions, a systematic adaptation and purposeful accommodation of cultural healing traditions and practices by the fields of counseling and counseling psychology should constitute the next critical frontier in the advancement of the multicultural counseling movement.

The Internationalizaton of Counseling Psychology and the Indigenization of Counseling

The discourse concerning **traditional healing practices** within counseling and counseling psychology was further enhanced by two additional intellectual transformations: (1) *the internationalization of counseling psychology movement* and (2) *the indigenization of counseling movement*.[25] Both of these developments arose out of the main multicultural counseling movement. Leung et al. characterized the internationalization movement of the counseling profession in terms of the following three objectives and features: (1) adaptation and nurturance of a global perspective in all counseling activities, (2) facilitation of cross-cultural and national collaboration among counseling professionals globally, and (3) indigenization of counseling profession within a given region by incorporating culturally specific elements into the practice of counseling.[26] Henceforth, the indigenization of the counseling movement, the third transformation, really grew out of this larger, global vision of internationalizing counseling psychology. That is, understanding and examining psychological and healing phenomena from the specific perspective of a given social and cultural milieu embody one of the principal goals of the internationalization of counseling psychology initiative.[27] These emerging models of thinking compel the disciplines of counseling, counseling psychology, and clinical psychology to look "outwardly" with openness (between cultures) while at the same time to look "inwardly" with depth and discretion (within culture).

Taking East Asian cultures as a case in point, these emerging conceptual shifts and the associated literature are observable in the growing trend of indigenous counseling in several East Asian countries, such as Chinese-speaking regions including Hong Kong, Taiwan, and China.[28] As such, in recent years, there have been increasing interests and published research and book volumes authored by counseling and mental health researchers and practitioners who are native to East Asian countries (e.g., Japan, Korea, China, and Taiwan). These writings have offered unique insights and explanations into indigenous forms of healing methods being practiced in various Asian countries and elsewhere around the world, from local, cultural insiders' perspectives.[29] Proponents of internationalization and indigenization of counseling psychology have long argued for the need to integrate Asian traditions into the implementation of counseling and psychotherapy. For example, in the case of counseling with Chinese people, Leung and Chen made this contention poignantly clear.[30] These authors stressed that it is essential for counseling psychologists to consider Chinese indigenous practices and their effects on the health and well-being of Chinese individuals and communities. Using QG as an example, Leung and Chen noted the following:

> These culture-specific practices are reflections of prevalent beliefs, values, and preferences that are deeply rooted in traditional Chinese and Asian culture. The effects of indigenous cultural practices and the integration of these practices into the counseling treatment process (e.g., through the use of an interdisciplinary treatment team) should receive a stronger dose of attention from counseling psychology researchers and practitioners in Chinese communities. (p. 954)[31]

Similarly, other scholars have regarded combining and assimilating Asian cultural values, **worldviews** (e.g., Taoism, Confucianism, Buddhism), and traditional helping methods (e.g., acupuncture, herbal medicine) into psychological interventions to be essential in providing effective treatment with Asian immigrants and Asian nationals.[32] For instance, in a recent in-depth case study, Kuo, Hsu, and Lai revealed that an effective crisis counseling for a native Taiwanese family requires skillful but measured adaptation and interweaving of indigenous values and beliefs into the counseling process by culturally competent counselors.[33] Such a culturally adapted counseling approach involves an active and tactful assimilation of traditional Taiwanese beliefs and indigenous assumptions about social status; hierarchy; reverence for authority; filial piety; saving face (*mainzi*); shame and stigma; social relationships (*kuansei*); and harmony, superstition, ritual, etc., into the therapist role as well as the helping process.

Furthermore, active infusion efforts of Asian philosophies and practices with Western clinical interventions are most visible in the growing body of research on culturally modified cognitive behavioral therapy (CBT) and treatment. In fact, this corpus of literature has seen a proliferation of empirical research on this form of culturally based therapy integration for a wide variety of populations and purposes, including culturally modified CBT for Asian Americans and mindfulness meditation treatment with substance abuse patients, to name a few.[34] In Liu and Leung's recent review, they noted the striking compatibility between Zen Buddhism and the cognitive approach to therapy and the efficacy of integrating both in treating clients of Chinese backgrounds.[35] According to these authors, the current infusion of Buddhism into conventional therapeutic approaches is evident in the emerging fields of ACT, which uses mindfulness and a commitment to values as agents of change, and dialectical behavior therapy (DBT).[36]

Recommendations for Integration and Future Directions

In this following section, we now turn to our second question for this chapter: What future directions and approaches might the fields of counseling and counseling psychology undertake to further the pursuit of a greater infusion and integration of Asian traditional healing into counseling and psychotherapy practices, research, and training? We endeavor to offer some recommendations in terms of ways in which counselors, psychologists, researchers, and educators might consider and participate to promote and advance the integration of Asian healing traditions into three key professional domains: (1) counseling and clinical practice, (2) research, and (3) training.

The practical implications of considering cultural and spiritual healing methods when working with racially and ethnically diverse populations have been explicitly outlined by the American Psychological Association (APA). The APA *Guidelines on Multicultural Education, Training, Research, Practice and Organizational Change for Psychologists* urges psychologists to broaden their clinical perspectives by including non-Western healing and helping approaches into their treatments and interventions.[37] The guidelines recommend psychologists "learn about helping practices used in non-Western cultures within as well as outside the North American and Northern European context" and to recognize that "culture-specific therapy (individual, family, and group) may require nontraditional interventions and (that psychologists) should strive to apply this knowledge in practice" (pp. 391–392).[38]

Along similar lines, Yeh, Hunter, Madan-Bahel, Chiang, and Arora have offered a series of practical strategies and skills for promoting therapy integration.[39] First of all, Yeh et al. proposed that counselors should challenge themselves to be open-minded about traditional forms of healing, to examine their own assumptions and beliefs about traditional therapeutic and healing practices, to inquire about their clients' views about traditional curative methods in order to assess the usefulness and relevance of these practices to their clients' healing, and, finally, to actively learn and seek out more information about traditional forms and methods of healing familiar to their clients.[40] Secondly, to take a step further, Yeh et al. recommended that counselors develop connections with indigenous healers in the local community; share and discuss with indigenous healers about the commonalities and differences between traditional therapy and Western counseling; involve indigenous healers in the counseling process; and nurture a positive therapeutic alliance and working relationship among the client, the healer, and the counselor.[41] Thirdly, Yeh et al. suggested that counselors explore and nurture their own "spirituality and connection to others, the cosmos, and nature," in order to develop a therapy framework that is congruent with their own personal beliefs (p. 415).[42]

On the basis of their clinical work with Native Americans, Native Canadians, and Hmongs in Southeast Asia, Jilek and Draguns noted that it would be profitable for counselors to extract, mimic, and foster some of the curative "ingredients" of traditional cultural healing in counseling racially and culturally diverse clients.[43] For instance, similar to the holistic healing framework assumed by traditional healers, counselors are challenged to expand their therapeutic and conceptual perspectives by giving consideration to the psychological, the medical, and the spiritual well-being of their clients and the mutual connections and implications among these critical dimensions. Similarly, to the extent that traditional and spiritual healers regularly offer concrete advice to clients, counselors who are working with clients who endorse traditional healing methods, such as less acculturated Asian immigrant clients, for example, would do well in providing tangible suggestions and timely advice to their clients whenever appropriate.

Research

In terms of research, at the present, empirical research pertaining to the infusion between Asian traditional healing practices and conventional therapy has been dominated mainly by works in Asian cultural adaptation of psychotherapy and treatment interventions, such as the incorporation of Asian philosophical traditions and practices based on Buddhist principles and practices.[44] This development is evident in the rise of clinical research on mindfulness-based cognitive therapy (MBCT), ACT, and DBT for diverse clinical concerns and populations as described elsewhere and in other chapters of this book. It is anticipated that the advancement of this kind of research will continue to evolve and expand in the future. However, as we conducted a literature review in preparation for this chapter, we found that the majority of the currently available, published psychological literature on this subject is heavily represented by descriptive writings on depicting different forms of Asian healing methods. Consequently, empirical and quantitative scholarly investigations of Asian and other traditional healing methods are still significantly lacking.

Potential directions for advancing research in this area, however, have been identified. In terms of content areas for research, scholars have recommended empirical inquiry into (a) studying healers who administer and deliver traditional forms of healing, (b) studying clients who have experienced the traditional cultural healing, (c) investigating and explicating thc nature and the inner working mechanisms of traditional therapies, and (d) examining the effects of indigenous therapy or integrated therapy as compared to conventional counseling or psychotherapy.[45] With respect to research methodology, these same scholars have advocated for the use of both qualitative and quantitative approaches to address these potential areas of research and to examine indigenous healing and its implications for mental health services.

Moreover, we recommend future research in this area to take cues from the latest emerging concepts of the indigenous counseling psychology movement. As a case in point, in a recent paper, Hwang articulated a framework to pursue indigenous counseling psychology with Chinese communities—a culturally specific counseling that is grounded in and infused with traditional Chinese values and worldviews of Confucianism, Taoism, and Buddhism.[46] To "indigenize" counseling and counseling research within the Chinese context, Hwang heeded counseling and psychology researchers and scholars (a) to use sensitive empathy in studying or understanding the cases in question, (b) to construct indigenous theories and to conceptualize these cases from local cultures, (c) to develop psychological measures to assess unique local phenomena, and (d) to devise new forms of counseling and psychotherapy methods and techniques by referring to all the available cultural heritages associated with a case.[47] We contend that the same recommendations can be applied to help guide future empirical scholarly works and to bridge the existing gap between Asian traditional healing practices and the practices of mainstream counseling and counseling psychology.

Training and Teaching

With respect to training and teaching, the subject of traditional healing practices remains to be a profoundly neglected area within the current psychology graduate curriculum in North America. Many mental health professionals and training programs remain suspicious and skeptical about the topic. Therefore, conscious efforts are required on the part of graduate programs and course instructors to bridge this gap, to highlight the current knowledge base on traditional healing, and to dispel any misinformation and misunderstanding about traditional therapies. A specific way to do this would be to encourage students and therapist–trainees to explore Asian curative traditions, such as meditation, mindfulness, yoga, acupuncture, QG, herbal remedy, etc., and to reflect on and discuss how these traditions can be integrated within their therapeutic frameworks. Graduate students should be exposed to and familiarize themselves with the latest counseling and clinical literature on nontraditional therapies, as well as prevailing scholarly discourse and debates concerning therapy integration. This can be accomplished through required reading assignments, conducting literature reviews, and optionally encouraging students and therapist–trainees to explore and experience some widely available traditional healing practices firsthand by themselves (e.g., yoga, acupuncture, meditation).

Further, students should be given numerous opportunities to examine their subjective experiences, views, beliefs, and positions about indigenous and spiritual forms of healing. Relatedly, students should be supported to openly explore and define their own stance on the broader issues of spirituality, religion, metaphysical matters, and the connection among mind–body–spirit in class or during clinical supervision. For training purposes, it is important for counseling and clinical students to be cognizant of their own perceptions and biases on different and not yet scientifically supported healing methods and how their perceptions and positions might influence their counseling work with clients who believe in them.[48] The first author of this chapter who has taught several graduate-level multicultural courses in his clinical psychology program for over a decade requires his students to engage in the aforementioned reflection and critical thinking exercises with the intent to help students internalize their learning. Through such a critical, self-reflective learning, students are more able to communicate their own biases and attitudes about nonconventional healing methods and then to articulate a plan or framework to help them address these issues with their clients in the future.

Additionally, to promote East–West therapy integration, hands-on, experiential learning opportunities should be included as part of the curriculum. Yeh et al. recommended training programs to consider (a) inviting local traditional or indigenous healers and helpers (e.g., Asian herbalist, acupuncturist, Buddhist monk, meditation practitioner) as guest speakers to present and speak with graduate students, (b) having these traditional healers and helpers explain and demonstrate their methods of practice in class, and (c) having students conduct interviews with traditional healers and helpers in the local community.[49] Lastly, it would benefit counseling and clinical graduate training programs and faculties to establish some collaboration and partnership with local indigenous healers and practitioners, spiritual and religious clergies, ethnic or cultural community leaders, etc. These initiatives will serve to model for student trainees the value of community-based collaboration and to deliver culturally responsive counseling and mental health services to multicultural clients.

Conclusion

In this chapter, we reviewed and examined in some detail the historical contexts and the contemporary positions and methods of infusing Asian and non-Asian traditional healing approaches into the practices and the training within the fields of counseling and counseling psychology. Specifically, we highlighted the growing interest in the integration of traditional and spiritual curative methods and counseling or mental health practices. This development can be attributed to the inadequacy of Western medical and mental health interventions in meeting the needs of immigrants and diverse populations; the rise of the multicultural counseling movement; the advent of increasing professional and ethical mandates for the provision of culturally competent and responsive psychologist services to diverse clients; and the calls for counselors and psychologists to be more flexible, inclusive, and holistic in their practices and training. It is anticipated that clinical research on integrating Buddhist principles into conventional therapy, such as ACT and DBT, will continue to evolve and expand way into the future. However, given the nascent nature of the current discourses and empirical research on East–West therapy integration, intentional and systematic efforts are imperative on the part of counseling practitioners, educators, and the profession to sustain the current interest and momentum on this subject. To this end, we argue and offer a number of concrete ideas and strategies for advancing therapy infusion in the areas of counseling and clinical practice, research, and training and teaching. We hope these recommendations and this chapter can serve as catalysts for further discourse, pursuit, and implementation of interweaving and infusing Asian traditional healing with conventional counseling and psychotherapy practice and training.

Case Study

Mia is a 55 year old White woman and is a practicing Catholic. She is unemployed due to her obsessive–compulsive disorder (OCD) and anxiety struggles. She had access to funding for her disability. Mia struggled with OCD for about two decades, and she had been in therapy for many years. Despite having received individual therapy for years, Mia continued to struggle with OCD symptoms. However, Mia's years of psychotherapy did give her deep insights into her OCD, and she had a good sense of humor about her struggle. Mia entered therapy with the second author, who is knowledgeable about Buddhist philosophy and a regular practitioner of yoga. The therapy group (four men and three women) participated in a weekly group for people with OCD.

Mia's compulsions centered on cleanliness; in addition, she had elaborated rituals, which she carried out every time before she left her house. Mia asserted that her rituals were very important to her. On one occasion, a fire occurred at her apartment, and she refused to evacuate until her rituals were completed. Mia was also extremely socially isolated due to her OCD symptoms. The group therapy Mia attended was based on an acceptance and commitment therapy (ACT) framework integrated with principles of self-compassion. ACT has many parallels with Buddhist philosophy, including the following: the view that suffering is a part of life, placing an emphasis on acceptance (of inner experience) and nonattachment (defusion from thoughts), and promoting the concept of "right action" and "valued living." On the other hand, the concept of self-compassion is borrowed directly from Buddhist teachings. It is being characterized as an alternative to self-esteem, and it helps shed light on the understanding of healthy psychological functioning. Self-compassion involves being open to experiencing one's pain without avoidance in a nonjudgmental, understanding, and accepting way. One's experiences are also understood as part of the larger human experience as opposed to in

(*Continued*)

(Continued)

isolation. Self-compassion was emphasized throughout the session of this group therapy. In addition, a brief, guided meditation was conducted every session. During Session 1, the group leaders or therapists focused on creating a safe space for the group members. The emphasis on the importance of community building was inspired by the Buddhist Sangha. Mia and the other participants were given the opportunity to share their experiences, and subsequently, they became aware of how their OCD symptoms were part of the larger human experience. They became aware that others shared their suffering. Having the opportunity to share was meaningful for Mia and the participants, as most of them had kept their symptoms a secret throughout their lives. During Sessions 2 and 3, the therapy focus was placed on defusing and accepting thoughts and letting go of one's illusion of control. Mia found this concept challenging but useful as she stated that she was not used to "letting go." In Session 4, Mia and the other group members concentrated on accepting their inner experiences without suppression and on mindful eating. In Session 5, Mia was introduced to the concepts of being nonjudgmental and valued living. Then, in the following two sessions, Mia was challenged to identify her personal values and then to strategize more meaningful ways of living her life. At the concluding session, Mia and the other group members were supported to integrate their new learning in the group, to implement it in their lives, and to practice self-compassion and patience with themselves when life adversity arose.

Mia was a consistent member of this therapy group who attended nearly all the sessions. Mia reported that attending this ACT group helped remove her from her rigid and repetitive rituals, such that the group intervention was a form of "built-in" exposure therapy for her. Through this ACT–self-compassion integrated approach, Mia reported feeling better able to tolerate anxiety, viewing struggles in a more compassionate and understanding way, and feeling more open to learning from others in the group. Mia spoke about wanting to take her life in more "valued" directions, meaning to take more risks such as leaving her house more often and expanding her circle of friends. In retrospect, the effectiveness of this ACT-based intervention for Mia and the others could be attributable to the therapy's emphasis on taking action to engage in change rather than waiting until Mia felt "cured" before she engaged in change, and the learning of accepting her undesirable feelings. This is consistent with the Buddhist principles of right action, right effort, and right mindfulness. Clearly, the integration of Asian healing traditions and philosophies and modern psychological concepts and therapies, as illustrated in Mia's experience, holds a great deal of promise for infusing Asian healing traditions into counseling and clinical psychology.

DISCUSSION QUESTIONS

1. Have you had any experiences with nonconventional therapies or medical treatments either personally or through someone you know (e.g., family, friends, colleagues)? What is your personal belief about Asian traditional healing practices specifically and traditional forms of healing more generally? Explain the basis of your belief on this issue.
2. In what ways do you think counseling and psychotherapy can benefit from the infusion and the integration of Asian traditional healing assumptions and practices?

What do you think are the challenges, or barriers, to moving toward such a therapy integration?

3. If one of your clients were to ask you for your opinion about her thinking of seeking help from an indigenous spiritual healer (e.g., a local Hindu priest) for the same problem she has been working with you through counseling, what would you say to her? What would be the important information and message that you would want to convey to the client before involving the indigenous healer?
4. The present chapter describes several ideas and strategies for counselors and psychologists to work toward a better infusion and integration between Asian healing practices and the practices of counseling and clinical psychology. Identify what strategy or strategies you can incorporate into your own practices as a counselor or psychologist toward such an integration, and explain why.

REFERENCES

1. Moodley, R. (1999). Challenges and transformations: Counseling in a multicultural context. *International Journal for the Advancement of Counseling*, *21*, 139–152; Yeh, C. J., Hunter, C. D., Madan-Bahel, A., Chiang, L., & Arora, A. K. (2004). Indigenous and interdependent perspectives of healing: Implications for counseling and research. *Journal of Counseling and Development*, *82*, 410–419.
2. Pieterse, A. L., Evans, S. A., Risner-Butner, A., Collins, N. M., & Mason, L. B. (2009). Multicultural competency and social justice training in counseling psychology and counselor education: A review and analysis of a sample of multicultural course syllabi. *The Counseling Psychologist*, *37*, 93–115. doi:10.1177/0011000008319986
3. Moodley, R., Sutherland, P., & Oulanova, O. (2008). Traditional healing, the body and mind in psychotherapy. *Counseling Psychology Quarterly*, *21*, 153–165. doi:10.1080/09515070802066870; Hwang, K.-K. (2009). The development of indigenous counseling in contemporary Confucian communities. *The Counseling Psychologist*, *37*, 930–943.
4. Vontress, C. E. (2001). Cross-cultural counseling in the 21st century. *International Journal for the Advancement of Counselling*, *23*, 83–97.
5. Yeh et al., Indigenous and interdependent perspectives.
6. Liu, W.-S., & Leung, P. W.-L. (2010). Psychotherapy with the Chinese: An update of the work in the last decade. In M. H. Bond. (Ed.), *Oxford handbook of Chinese psychology*. Hong Kong: Oxford University Press.
7. Moodley, R., & West, W. (Eds.). (2005). *Integrating traditional healing practices in counseling and psychotherapy*. Thousand Oaks, CA: Sage.
8. Zgierska, A., Rabago, D., Chawla, N., Kushner, K., Koehler, R., & Marlatt, A. (2009). Mindfulness meditation for substance use disorders: A systematic review. *Substance Abuse*, *30*, 266–294. doi:10.1080/08897070903250019
9. Lee, C. C., Oh, M. Y., & Mountcastle, A. R. (1992). Indigenous models of helping in nonwestern countries: Implications for multicultural counseling. *Journal of Multicultural Counseling and Development*, *20*, 3–10; Vontress, C. E. (1991). Traditional healing in Africa: Implications for cross-cultural counseling. *Journal of Counseling and Development*, *70*, 242–249.
10. Sue, D. W., & Sue, D. (2013). *Counseling the culturally diverse: Theory and practice* (6th ed.). Hoboken, NJ: John Wiley.

11. Liu & Leung, Psychotherapy with the Chinese; Gerstein, L. H., Heppner, P. P., Ægisdóttir, S., Leung, S. A., & Norsworthy, K. L. (2009). *International handbook of cross-cultural counseling: Cultural assumptions and practices worldview.* Thousand Oaks, CA: Sage; Hwang, The development of indigenous counseling.
12. Yeh et al., Indigenous and interdependent perspectives.
13. Lee et al., Indigenous models of helping.
14. Vontress, C. E. (1999). Interview with a traditional African healer. *Journal of Mental Health Counselling, 21*, 326–339.
15. Vontress, Cross-cultural counseling.
16. Sue, D. W., Arredondo, P., & McDavis, R. J. (1992). Multicultural counseling competencies and standards: A call to the profession. *Journal of Counseling and Development, 70*, 477–486. doi:10.1002/j.2161-1912.1992.tb00563.x
17. Ibid.
18. Lee et al., Indigenous models of helping.
19. Vontress, Cross-cultural counseling.
20. Moodley, Challenges and transformations; Moodley & West, *Integrating traditional healing practices.*
21. Kuo, B. C. H., Kwantes, C. T., Towson, S., & Nanson, K. M. (2006). Social beliefs as determinants of attitudes toward seeking professional psychological help among ethnically diverse university students. *Canadian Journal of Counseling, 40*, 224–241.
22. Moodley et al., Traditional healing.
23. Vontress, Cross-cultural counseling.
24. Moodley & West, *Integrating traditional healing practices.*
25. Moodley et al., Traditional healing; Leung, S. A., & Chen, P.-H. (2009). Counseling psychology in Chinese communities in Asia: Indigenous, multicultural, and cross-cultural consideration. *The Counseling Psychologist, 37*, 944–966.
26. Leung, S. A., Clawson, T., Norsworthy, K. L., Tena, A., Szilagyi, A., & Rogers, J. (2009). Internationalization of the counseling profession: An indigenous perspective. In L. H. Gerstein, P. P. P. Heppner, S. Ægisdóttir, S. A. Leung, & K. L. Norsworthy (Eds.), *International handbook of cross-cultural counseling: Cultural assumptions and practices worldview* (pp. 111–123). Thousand Oaks, CA: Sage.
27. Ibid.
28. Hwang, The development of indigenous counseling; Leung & Chen, Counseling psychology in Chinese communities.
29. Moodley & West, *Integrating traditional healing practices*; Gerstein et al., *International handbook.*
30. Leung & Chen, Counseling psychology in Chinese communities.
31. Ibid.
32. Hwang, The development of indigenous counseling; Kuo, B. C. H., Hsu, W.-S., & Lai, N.-H. (2011). Indigenous crisis counselling in Taiwan: An exploratory qualitative case study of an expert therapist. *International Journal for the Advancement of Counselling, 33*, 1–21. doi:10.1007/s10447–010–9108-y
33. Kuo et al., Indigenous crisis counseling.
34. Leung & Chen, Counseling psychology in Chinese communities; Liu & Leung, Psychotherapy with the Chinese; Zgierska et al., Mindfulness meditation.
35. Liu & Leung, Psychotherapy with the Chinese.
36. Ibid.

37. American Psychological Association. (2003). *Guidelines on multicultural education, training, research, practice and organizational change for psychologists.* Retrieved from http://www.apa.org/pi/oema/resources/policy/multicultural-guideline.pdf
38. Ibid.
39. Yeh et al., Indigenous and interdependent perspectives.
40. Ibid.
41. Ibid.
42. Ibid.
43. Jilek, W. G., & Draguns, J. G. (2008). Interventions by traditional healers: Their impact and relevance within their cultures and beyond. In U. P. Gielen, J. G. Draguns, & J. M. Fish (Eds.), *Principles of multicultural counseling and therapy* (pp. 353–370). New York, NY: Routledge.
44. Liu & Leung, Psychotherapy with the Chinese.
45. Yeh et al., Indigenous and interdependent perspectives.
46. Hwang, The development of indigenous counseling.
47. Ibid.
48. Yeh et al., Indigenous and interdependent perspectives.
49. Ibid.

SUGGESTED READINGS

Gerstein, L. H., Heppner, P. P, Ægisdóttir, S., Leung, S. A, & Norsworthy, K. L. (2009). *International handbook of cross-cultural counseling: Cultural assumptions and practices worldview.* Thousand Oaks, CA: Sage.

This compendium presents the latest developments and debates around the internationalization of counseling movement. The book describes the profession of counseling and how it is being practiced internationally in countries across all continents of the world. The chapters explore topics including the history of counseling; the relationship among culture, religion, and counseling; diverse clients and presenting problems; indigenous frameworks of counseling; cross-national research collaboration; challenges; and future directions for the internationalization of counseling movement.

Moodley, R., & West, W. (Eds.). (2005). *Integrating traditional healing practices in counseling and psychotherapy.* Thousand Oaks, CA: Sage.

This edited volume introduces readers to the diversity of beliefs and perceptions about mental health problems and curative methods to address them. The book describes in some detail about the various traditional, indigenous, and spiritual beliefs and practices around the world, including shamanic healing, aboriginal healing, South Asian healing, African healing, Chinese healing, etc.

Sue, D. W., & Sue, D. (2016). *Counseling the culturally diverse:* Theory and practice (7th ed.). Hoboken, NJ: John Wiley.

This is the most widely used textbook and reference on multicultural counseling and multicultural counseling competencies. It provides a comprehensive review of the field and surveys critical issues related to dimensions of multicultural counseling, sociopolitical nature of mental health practice, practice of multicultural counseling, and counseling with diverse multicultural populations.

7 Integrating Asian Healing Traditions Into Psychotherapy

Boon-Ooi Lee

Introduction

The main argument for integrating Asian traditional healing into psychotherapy is the differences in worldview between non-Asian therapists and Asian clients. Worldviews are beliefs, assumptions, and values that describe reality, human nature, the meanings of life, and one's relationships with the world.[1] Since the main source of therapists' worldviews is derived from their theoretical orientations that have been mainly developed in the Euro-American sociocultural contexts, it is important to question how relevant psychotherapy is to Asian clients. A shared worldview between clients and therapists is associated with positive therapeutic outcomes through the effects of alliance and expectations.[2]

However, although non-Asian therapists and Asian clients may hold different views of the self, communication patterns, emotional expressiveness, and family structure, psychotherapy is not completely irrelevant to Asian clients.[3] It is not useful to view Western and Eastern cultures as two opposite entities given that all cultures are dynamic and constantly interact with each other. Contemporary Asian communities have become more multicultural due to globalization. In China, for example, under the influence of the Western mental health concepts, the younger and urbanized Chinese have become more open to Western psychotherapies.[4] However, rather than accepting all Western approaches, Chinese clients are more receptive to the problem-solving approach in cognitive behavioral therapy (CBT) rather than to the self-exploration in insight-oriented therapies.[5] Nonetheless, the Socratic dialogue may put the Chinese off, as they may feel ashamed for not being able to answer the "why" and "what" questions. Similarly, although the humanistic approach in person-centered therapy is consistent with the Korean worldview, its emphasis on an egalitarian counseling relationship is in conflict with the Confucian beliefs of social hierarchy.[6] Thus, the question does not lie in the compatibility in worldviews per se but in which aspects of the therapists' worldviews are compatible with Asian clients. Since Asian traditional healing is embedded in Asian worldviews, can therapists learn from traditional healing to culturally sensitize Western psychotherapy?

However, when a contemporary Asian community becomes more culturally diverse, local people may even reject their own traditional healing practices. For example, Asians believing in Christianity are less likely to consult shamans. Hence, any effort in integrating traditional healing into psychotherapy must consider the multicultural factors. Although there are some incompatibilities between the worldviews of psychotherapy and Asian clients, we do not have to discard psychotherapy altogether. Although some concepts of Western psychotherapy are relevant to Asian clients, we should not apply them uncritically. A better approach is to understand the similarities and differences between the psychotherapeutic and Asian worldviews and to identify a middle path for a creative integration between psychotherapy and traditional healing.

This chapter seeks to explore the contexts, challenges, and opportunities of integrating traditional healing into psychotherapy. It begins with a brief discussion on Asian healing traditions—particularly those from East Asian cultures—followed by the integration of traditional healing into Western mental health care, the challenges for such integration, and methods for integration.

Asian Healing Traditions in Health and Mental Health

Since the 1980s, there has been a movement in China to develop a branch of traditional Chinese medicine psychotherapy (TCMP).[7] This is an attempt of repackaging traditional Chinese medicine (TCM) into a form of psychotherapy. The TCMP practitioners attribute psychological problems to the imbalance of the seven modes of emotion (joy, anger, shock, anxiety, thinking, fear, and sorrow), personality factors (classified according to the five elements; *yin* and *yang*), organic functional factors (e.g., the interactions between the seven modes of emotion and their respective metaphorical organs, the imbalance of *qi*), and environmental factors (e.g., wind, air). The treatment methods include talk therapy (e.g., psychoeducation, rational thinking), emotional rebalance and control, work and rest, change of personality types through moral education and herbal treatments, Qigong (QG), *taiji*, herbs, and acupuncture. Previous studies have mostly focused on herbal treatments and acupuncture rather than on other aspects of TCMP. One meta-analysis showed that certain TCM herbs were better than placebos and as effective as antidepressants in reducing depressive symptoms.[8] However, due to the small number of studies with sufficient methodological quality, it is premature to conclude the benefits of TCM herbs for treating depression.

The therapeutic potentials of TCM for mental health issues appear to be inconclusive and may largely be due to placebo effects. However, the strong placebo effects may reflect the roles that nonspecific therapeutic factors play in these indigenous practices—for example, the therapeutic relationship, client expectations, faith, hope, and shared worldviews.[9] Psychotherapists can learn from traditional healing to activate these therapeutic mechanisms to enhance their treatment effectiveness.

In Asian cultures, especially those under the influence of Confucianism and Buddhism, well-being is not simply a matter of mind and body but also about social relationships. In traditional Chinese culture, there is no institutionalization of health care (e.g., hospital); the family is the center of health care. Although psychiatric-like symptoms were documented in ancient medical texts, TCM has never treated emotional suffering in isolation from a larger context comprising metaphorical organs, social relationships, and nature. Emotional suffering is associated with character deficiency and is an integral part of life. From a Buddhist perspective, emotional suffering is an inescapable part of existence that has to be accepted. As such, emotional suffering is not classified into diverse mental disorders, but it is represented in everyday life language—for example, resentment, greed, fear, pride, hatred, jealousy, attachment, or "heart problems." Heart problems arise when people are too independent and are not being integrated into social groups.[10] Since emotional suffering is not construed as sickness but a relational issue, it is managed though personal cultivation and the maintenance of harmonious relationships. Thus, when working with Asian clients, the focus of psychotherapy should move from psychological disorders to social disorders based on Confucian, Taoist, and Buddhist philosophies. Several Asian indigenous psychotherapies have been developed for this purpose, such as Onmeum counseling in South Korea, **Chinese Taoist cognitive psychotherapy (CTCP)** in China, and Morita and Naikan therapies in Japan.[11] In CTCP, clients are taught Taoist doctrines (e.g., "Benefiting without hurting others," "Being in harmony with others and being humble") as part of psychoeducation. In Morita therapy, clients follow a natural life path and immerse in current life experiences rather than focus on thoughts and emotions. Naikan therapy focuses on character development and penance as well as expressing one's guilt and reshaping one's interpersonal relationships. These Asian indigenous psychotherapies can be potentially integrated into psychotherapy. To date, only one study has evaluated the efficacy of CTCP, which found that CTCP with or without benzodiazepines was a more effective, although slower, method for treating generalized anxiety disorder (GAD) than the use of benzodiazepines.[12] Neither Morita therapy nor Naikan therapy has been evaluated with Asian clients.

Integrating Spiritual Beliefs Into Psychotherapy

Although there has been a significant advancement in infusing spiritual concepts into various theoretical models of psychotherapy, most of these spiritual concepts are derived from Christianity. Religious beliefs in Asian communities comprise not only Christianity but also Buddhism, Hinduism, Judaism, Islam, and shamanism. Previous studies have found that CBT combined with Islamic beliefs was more effective than CBT alone for Muslim clients.[13] In one case study, a Malaysian client sought help from a Western-trained psychotherapist for her grief after her mother's suicide.[14] With her therapist's support, she consulted a Buddhist nun who reassured her that her mother would not return as a revengeful spirit. The therapist creatively applied the empty-chair technique to invite her "mother" to join the session. Through dialogue and confession, the client found a sense of closure by seeking her mother's forgiveness. This case illustrates how a Western technique can be used to enact a cultural script in line with the client's spiritual beliefs. The spiritual healing process also resonates with the Asian relational healing discussed earlier. The client symbolically reconciled with her mother so that she could move on in life. In fact, human relationships can be symbolically transformed through religious means, which are otherwise not possible in actual life situations.

Methods and Strategies for Integration

In psychotherapy, several models have been developed for integrating different theories, such as technical eclecticism, theoretical integration, common factors, and **multitheoretical psychotherapy** (MTP).[15] Regardless of which model is used, it is essential to know the rationale for integration. An unsystematic or an atheoretical integration does not help in advancing our knowledge in the integration. Likewise, the integration between traditional healing and psychotherapy should be based on a sound theoretical rationale. However, not all integration models are suitable. Eclecticism, which combines different theories to explain human behaviors, has been criticized for lack of consistency. The theoretical integration, which is aimed at synthesizing theories to eventually develop a new perspective, may not be useful for fusing psychotherapeutic and traditional healing theories because of their contrasting worldviews (e.g., the concept of organismic self in person-centered therapy vs. *yin* and *yang* in TCM). By contrast, common factors and MTP provide a more systematic and pragmatic framework for integrating psychotherapy and traditional healing without the need for reconciling their conflicting worldviews.

A Common Factors Approach

As mentioned earlier, the main rationale for integrating traditional healing practices into psychotherapy is to foster a shared worldview for the therapist and client to work together. This rationale is consistent with the tenet of common factors, which proposes that a shared worldview provides client and therapist with a common framework to work together.[16] To foster a shared worldview, a therapist has to be culturally competent, to adopt a perspective that each theory in psychotherapy does not represent an objective reality, and to recognize that psychotherapy is more concerned about meaning rather than truth.

Being culturally competent means that, first, therapists become more aware of their worldviews so as to prevent their assumptions from interfering with their therapy work.[17] Second, they learn to accept their clients' worldviews in a nonjudgmental manner. Acceptance does not mean an agreement with or the need for adopting the client's worldview but rather being respectful of the client's worldview. For example, a therapist whose religious belief is Christianity may support her Taoist client for attending Taoist rituals for atonement. These two cultural competencies are built on the premise that people construct and live in different realities rather than in a single objective world. Similarly, each theory of psychotherapy does not mirror an objective reality but it is a collection of rich cultural language invented in its historical and cultural context. Therapists are encouraged to perceive all healing systems, including biomedicine, psychotherapy, and traditional healing practices, as different forms of symbolic healing constructed in different mythic worlds.[18] A myth, or rationale, provides explanations for the client's issues and prescribes interventions for addressing them. The form of a mythic world varies across healing systems. It may take a scientific form in contemporary psychotherapy or a supernatural form in ritual healing. The question does not lie in whether a particular myth is truer than the other but in whether it is socioculturally meaningful to both practitioner and client. Therefore, psychotherapy is more concerned with meaning rather than truth. This meaning-centered tradition is linked to the interpretive and social constructivist philosophy, which adopts a critical challenge to the subject–object dualism, positivism, and a singular truth advocated in the scientific mode of inquiry.

By following a meaning-centered tradition, the therapists are able to move between various mythic worlds by temporarily suspending their own worldviews. They will not attempt to replace the concepts (e.g., spirit possession) in one myth (e.g., a supernatural realm in shamanistic healing) with the concepts (e.g., dissociative identity disorder) from another myth (e.g., a scientific realm in psychotherapy). If they do so, they are imposing Western values on the indigenous culture. The therapist must be able to explain and label the client's predicaments with a cultural category that makes sense to the client—for example, imbalance of energy. The therapist then attaches the client's experience to certain healing symbols (e.g., acupunctural points) derived from the mythic world (TCM) and then manipulates these symbols to transform the client's experience. If a therapist believes that only biomedicine or psychotherapy is scientifically valid and dismisses traditional healing as quackish or superstitious, she is less likely to see the value of integrating traditional healing into her practice. When a therapist becomes more aware of her own worldview, has knowledge about her client's worldview, and does not hold a view of absolute truth, she will be able to use appropriate intervention strategies, including traditional healing, consistent with her clients' worldviews.

A shared worldview is also related to the therapist's ability in tailoring the therapeutic relationship to clients' needs and expectations. Research on the interactional patterns between traditional healers and their clients suggests how a therapeutic relationship should be culturally defined. Asian clients are more comfortable with therapists who actively play the role of an expert or a problem solver than with those who subscribe to nondirective approaches.[19] This role expectation reflects the hierarchical social order in Asian culture in which professionals are accorded a higher social status. In a form of Chinese ritual healing, the spirit medium behaves as an authoritative figure, telling his devotees what to do and how they should behave—even to the extent of scolding and disciplining them.[20] Therefore, a psychotherapist should not be hesitant to be authoritative or directive with her Asian clients so long as she treats them with respect.

Because of its individualistic approach, the therapeutic relationship in psychotherapy tends to focus on the therapist and her client. By contrast, many forms of traditional healing are conducted at a communal level. For example, the Chinese ritual healing, as mentioned, is not performed in a private room but in the presence of family members and other devotees.[21] Privacy or confidentiality is not observed; everyone can watch and listen to the consultation. This form of communal healing, which reflects the collectivistic worldview emphasized in Asian culture, has implications for the issue of boundary and confidentiality in psychotherapy. When an Asian client attends a psychotherapy session, her family members may want to know what has been covered in the session. Since personal problems are usually managed at the group level in the traditional Asian family, privacy and confidentiality should be defined at a group level rather than at an individual level. With this broader sense of confidentiality and boundary, relevant social supports can be mobilized to alleviate individual predicaments.

A Multitheoretical Integration

Similar to the common factors approach, MTP offers a pragmatic framework for integrating Asian traditional healing and psychotherapy without the need for reconciling their contrasting worldviews. A systematic approach is employed to formulate an integrative treatment plan. The therapist identifies markers in the client's presenting concerns, which suggest the possible focal dimensions for intervention. These focal dimensions include thoughts, feelings, actions, biology, interpersonal patterns, social systems, and cultural contexts. Relevant interventions are then applied to address the corresponding focal dimensions. For example, cognitive therapy is applied to manage cognitive distortions whereas interpersonal psychotherapy is applied to manage interpersonal conflicts.

However, MTP does not include spirituality and the relationship with nature in its focal dimensions, even though Western psychotherapy has long recognized their important roles in mental health. These two focal dimensions are relevant to Asian traditional healing. The correspondence between microcosm (human) and macrocosm (physical environment, nature, spiritual forces, and cosmos) is an important principle in Asian health beliefs.[22] Thus, these two focal dimensions should be added to MTP for the purpose of integrating relevant traditional healing practices.

To illustrate how Asian traditional healing can be integrated into MTP, Chinese healing practices are used as an example here. Various Chinese healing practices can be employed to target several focal dimensions. TCM, *taiji*, QG, or meditation may be used to address issues related to thoughts, feelings, actions, behaviors, and physical functions. Since *taiji*, QG, and meditation involve bodily actions and sensory experiences, they may produce corresponding mental states. This is because bodily states can influence cognitive states.[23] Inducing a still body in meditation may trigger a stilling and calm effect on the mind, whereas the slow bodily movements in *taiji* and QG may help slow down the cognitive and emotional processes such as rumination and anxiety. Taoist and Confucian doctrines can be taught to regulate negative thoughts and interpersonal relationships, using CTCP or Naikan therapy. For clients who wish to achieve a sense of transcendental freedom, detachment, and spiritual enlightenment, they may resort to Buddhist and Taoist philosophies, in a way similar to the Western existential therapy. In view of the connectivity between humans and the physical environment or nature, clients can be taught the Taoist doctrines on the relationship between humans and nature or referred to a *feng shui* master.

Research and Future Directions

Although the common factors and MTP may be appropriate integrated approaches, research is needed to empirically substantiate their effectiveness. In fact, research on the integration between Asian traditional healing and psychotherapy is generally limited. Most of the studies, particularly those on traditional medicine, have focused on the relevance of traditional healing concepts to mental health rather than on integration. Although researchers have cited case examples to illustrate the usefulness of integration, they have not offered a systematic framework for integration as mentioned before. There are several research challenges for the integration of Asian healing traditions into psychotherapy.

First, given the diverse theoretical orientations in psychotherapy, which are the models that can be integrated with Asian traditional healing, for what types of problems, and under which circumstances? Conceptual analyses and case studies have suggested that Asian clients prefer CBT to nondirective approaches. However, this observation has not been substantiated by clinical trials with large samples. Research should be conducted to evaluate CBT in comparison with other theoretical orientations in Asian clients. Only through this line of study will we know which theoretical models can be meaningfully integrated with traditional healing.

Second, is there any evidence to support the efficacy of traditional healing practices? Do such practices provide additional benefits over and above the benefits that psychotherapy has already offered? Thus far, research information is limited. Research evidence derived from clinical trials is required to convince the professional organizations, mental health practitioners, and even clients of the benefits for integrating traditional healing into psychotherapy. However, there are some challenges for evaluating traditional healing because of the difficulty in operationalizing and measuring its concepts (e.g., the humors, *qi*, and the loss of soul). Another challenge is whether it is appropriate to evaluate the effectiveness of traditional healing (e.g., acupuncture) for a target problem framed in Western diagnostic categories (e.g., major depressive disorder) given the epistemological differences between the two systems. Would it be more appropriate to frame a target problem in an indigenous category, for example, *yu* (depressive-like symptoms) according to TCM? The improvement of *yu* can then be assessed by palpating the pulse or the abdomen.

Third, what is the evidence of the efficacy of the integration between Asian traditional healing and psychotherapy? Although qualitative research helps elicit the subjective experiences of the clients and practitioners, its findings may not be generalizable.[24] No clinical trials have been conducted on the outcomes of the collaboration or on the systematic integration of Asian traditional healing and psychotherapy.

Since mental health professionals may not understand their clients' belief systems and are usually not trained in traditional healing practices, a better solution is to collaborate with traditional healers, resembling the multidisciplinary approach that has already taken place in mental health care. Through collaboration, traditional healers and mental health professionals can learn from each other. However, some traditional healers may not be familiar with the roles of mental health professionals whose work is relatively new to non-Western cultures. They are more familiar with the roles of biomedical physicians and are prepared to make referral to the latter. To achieve a constructive collaboration, informal meetings or conferences may be useful platforms for traditional healers and mental health professionals to understand each other's roles and work. Mental health professionals can also be exposed to traditional healing by attending courses such as multicultural counseling or medical anthropology.

In general, future research, using both qualitative and quantitative methods, should focus on three levels of inquiry. First, more research should examine specific psychotherapy approaches that are effective with Asians clients in Asian countries. The theoretical approach of CBT and non-Asian clients have been overrepresented in psychotherapy research. Even research findings from Asian clients in Western countries may not be generalizable to Asian clients in other regions due to sociopolitical and geographical differences. Although the **common factors model** proposes that the effectiveness of the many psychotherapeutic approaches is due to their similarities rather than specific factors, whether this observation can be generalized to Asian clients remains unknown. Second, research would need to examine the effectiveness of traditional healing for mental health issues. Previous research in this area is inconclusive due to methodological shortcomings. Indeed, information derived from these two levels of research can then pave way for studies on the effectiveness of integration. Currently, the most well-researched psychotherapy based on Asian spiritual traditions is mindfulness-based therapy. Traditional mindfulness practices have been secularly incorporated into various Western models of psychotherapy. However, since these mindfulness approaches have been culturally adapted for Western clients, they may not be necessarily suitable for Asian clients given their focus on independent self-construal, direct communication, and emotional expressiveness.[25]

Conclusion

The main argument for integrating Asian traditional healing into psychotherapy is to bridge the gap between the perceived differences in worldview between Western trained therapists and Asian clients. Through this integration, psychotherapy may become more culturally relevant for Asian clients seeking this form of healing, which in turn may increase the utilization of mental health services and therapeutic effectiveness not only for Asian clients but for clients from other communities as well.

Case Study

Mei Ling (pseudonym), aged 46, is a Chinese Singaporean. She has worked as an administrator for 20 years. She is single and lives with her aging parents. All her siblings have moved out after getting married. One year ago before coming to see me (the author), her mood deteriorated after having conflicts with her supervisor, Mr. Ang. She believed he wanted to consolidate his power to eventually become a departmental head. Since he had never had a

(*Continued*)

(*Continued*)

good working relationship with her, he wanted to force her to resign. He had given her a lot of work and isolated her in the department. All of these office politics, she claimed, had led to her depression. She consulted a psychiatrist who diagnosed her with major depressive disorder. Besides prescribing an antidepressant, he referred her to a social worker for counseling. She did not find the medication or the counseling helpful. She could not tolerate the side effects of the medication. She was very uncomfortable with the confrontational method the social worker had recommended. The social worker advised her to speak up and assert herself confidently in front of Mr. Ang. She stopped the medication and counseling, hoping that I could teach her other methods to manage her interpersonal problems and depression. One of the challenges for working with Mei Ling was her difficulty in expressing her thoughts and feelings. She did not respond well to cognitive therapy or the gestalt two-chair technique. Although recognizing the importance of thinking positively, she slipped into rumination whenever facing Mr. Ang. Rather than coming up with her own solution, she wanted me to tell her what to do. For her, the rationale for talking to an empty chair by imagining Mr. Ang sitting there was completely absurd.

Although she did well for her high school examination, Mei Ling chose to continue her study at a vocational school rather than a college so that she could start work early to support her family. After graduating, she joined her present company as a clerk and worked toward her current position as an assistant administrator. She is not socially active and prefers to be on her own, reading and watching TV. She has a small circle of friends who she occasionally meets. She describes herself as a simple person without any life ambition. Since adolescence, Mei Ling had experienced some mild anxiety with depressive symptoms, such as negative outlook in life, low energy, and insomnia. These symptoms are not associated with any specific causes. In general, they did not significantly affect her life. Her financial condition is stable, allowing her to hire a maid to take care of the house chores and her parents. Since she does not find psychotherapy helpful and given her Buddhist and Taoist beliefs, I encouraged her to learn meditation to regulate her moods and thoughts. Although meditation helped to mitigate her depressive symptoms to some extent, she slipped into depression and anger whenever she went to work. I asked her if she wanted to try a Taoist ritual at a temple. The purpose of this ritual is to ward off bad luck, including villains. During the ritual, offerings are made to the tiger god, which include a piece of tofu, a duck egg, some yellow noodle, a piece of fat meat, paper money, tea leaves, and *gui-ren-zhi* (a form of incense paper for summoning a benefactor). Performance of this ritual is different at other temples where the participants use an object to beat a paper figure that represents a villain to stop the villain from causing harm. The temple that I recommended does not encourage this behavior. It adopts a more compassionate approach. Rather than "beating the villain", participants pray to transform the villain into a benefactor. Mei Ling hoped the ritual would transform Mr. Ang's character. Interestingly, after the ritual, her relationship with Mr. Ang improved. She believed the ritual was effective. I also referred her to a traditional Chinese physician for regulating her anxiety, depression, and insomnia. Her symptoms reduced after she received herbal treatments and acupuncture. After about six months, her scores on the Beck Depression Inventory indicated mild depressive symptoms.

Although past research has suggested that Asians are generally receptive to cognitive therapy, it does not work with Mei Ling. The analytical process involved in Socratic dialogue is not meaningful to her. In fact, she became more depressed after going through a series of cognitive exercises. By contrast, the Taoist ritual probably works because it has symbolically transformed her emotional experiences within a culturally legitimate myth consistent with her Taoist and Buddhist worldviews. Her emotional experience was attached to the transactional symbols (ritual) derived from the myth. These symbols, in turn, transformed her emotional and cognitive experience. By converting the villain (Mr. Ang) into a benefactor, the burning of *gui-ren-zhi* symbolically changed her attitude toward him. A positive attitude may, in turn, lead to a more positive interaction with him. Given her difficulty in expressing her thoughts and feelings, the ritual allowed her to regulate inner experiences through nonverbal actions. This passive yet effective ritual helped her to avoid confrontation in an actual social situation. In Chinese culture, a face-saving and nonconfrontational strategy is often used to preserve social harmony, which is more culturally sensitive than the self-assertiveness training recommended by her previous therapist. The herbal medicine and acupuncture offered her another way to regulate mind and body without requiring her to express negative emotions and thoughts. Her traditional Chinese medicine (TCM) physician told her how the herbs and acupuncture had balanced her *qi* and *yin* and *yang*. Most importantly, these remedies did not lead to intolerable side effects. Interestingly, meditation did not help her much even though it does not require her to express her inner thoughts. Perhaps, it requires a certain degree of effort that a client has to put in to see the effect. By comparison, self-effort is not required much in the Taoist ritual and TCM treatments that another person administers, namely, the priest and the physician. Taken together, this case illustrates how nonverbal and culturally sensitive therapies are useful for Asian clients who do not respond well to Western talk therapies.

DISCUSSION QUESTIONS

1. Have you sought help from an Asian traditional healer before? If yes, what prompted you to do so? What were your experiences? If you have never consulted a traditional healer, would you consider visiting one in the future, and why?
2. Has someone you know ever sought help from an Asian traditional healer? What was his or her experience? How does his or her experience affect your views of traditional healing practices?
3. As a mental health professional, what thoughts do you have about the roles of Asian traditional healing practices in psychotherapy and mental health care?
4. Have you attempted to integrate Asian traditional healing concepts and processes into your own therapy work? What was the rationale for doing so? What were your and your clients' experiences? If you have never made such integration, would you consider doing so? If yes, what would be your rationales and integration approach?

REFERENCES

1. Koltko-Rivera, M. E. (2004). The psychology of worldviews. *Review of General Psychology*, *8*, 3–58.
2. Wampold, B. E. (2015). How important are the common factors in psychotherapy? An update. *World Psychiatry*, *14*, 270–277.
3. Sue, D. W., & Sue, D. (2016). *Counseling the culturally diverse: Theory and practice* (7th ed.). Hoboken, NJ: John Wiley.
4. Kolstad, A., & Gjesvik, N. (2014). Collectivism, individualism, and pragmatism in China: Implications for perceptions of mental health. *Transcultural Psychiatry*, *51*, 264–285.
5. Chen, S. W. H., & Davenport, D. S. (2005). Cognitive-behavioral therapy with Chinese American clients: Cautions and modifications. *Psychotherapy: Theory, Research, Practice, Training*, *42*, 101–110.
6. Lee, S. M., & Yang, E. (2013). Counseling in South Korea. In T. H. Hohenshil, N. E. Amundson, & S. G. Niles (Eds.), *Counseling around the world: An international handbook* (pp. 137–144). Alexandria, VA: American Counseling Association.
7. Lee, B. O. (2002). Psychotherapy in Chinese medicine: A theoretical review. In A. G. Tan & M. Goh (Eds.), *Psychology in Singapore: Issue of an emerging discipline* (pp. 124–146). Singapore: McGraw-Hill.
8. Yeung, W. F., Chung, K. F., Ng, K. Y., Yu, Y. M., Ziea, T. C., & Ng, B. F. L. (2014). A systematic review on the efficacy, safety and types of Chinese herbal medicine for depression. *Journal of Psychiatric Research*, *57*, 165–175.
9. Wampold, How important are the common factors in psychotherapy?
10. Kolstad & Gjesvik, Collectivism, individualism, and pragmatism.
11. Lee & Yang, Counseling in South Korea; Zhang, Y., Young, D., Lee, S., Li, L., Zhang, H., Xiao, Z., . . . Chang, D. F. (2002). Chinese Taoist cognitive psychotherapy in the treatment of generalized anxiety disorder in contemporary China. *Transcultural Psychiatry*, *39*, 115–129.
12. Zhang et al., Chinese Taoist cognitive psychotherapy.
13. Amer, M. M., & Jalal, B. (2012). Individual psychotherapy/counseling: Psychodynamic, cognitive-behavioral, and humanistic-experiential models. In S. Ahmed & M. M. Amer (Eds.), *Counseling Muslims: Handbook of mental health issues and interventions* (pp. 87–118). New York, NY: Routledge.
14. Ting, R. S. K., & Ng, A. L. O. (2012). Use of religious resources in psychotherapy from a tradition-sensitive approach: Cases from Chinese in Malaysia. *Pastoral Psychology*, *61*, 941–957.
15. Jones-Smith, E. (2012). *Theories of counseling and psychotherapy: An integrative approach*. Thousand Oaks, CA: Sage.
16. Wampold, How important are the common factors in psychotherapy?
17. Sue & Sue, *Counseling the culturally diverse*.
18. Dow, J. (1986). Universal aspects of symbolic healing: A theoretical synthesis. *American Anthropologist*, *88*, 56–69.
19. Sue & Sue, *Counseling the culturally diverse*.
20. Lee, B. O., Kirmayer, L. J., & Groleau, D. (2010). Therapeutic processes and perceived helpfulness of *dang-ki* (Chinese shamanism) from the symbolic healing perspective. *Culture, Medicine & Psychiatry*, *34*, 56–105.
21. Ibid.
22. Lee, Psychotherapy in Chinese medicine.
23. Barsalou, L. W., Barbey, A. K., Simmons, W. K., & Santos, A. (2005). Embodiment in religious knowledge. *Journal of Cognition & Culture*, *5*, 14–57.

24. Ting & Ng, Use of religious resources.
25. Hall, G. C. N., Hong, J. J., Zane, N. W. S., & Meyer, O. L. (2011). Culturally competent treatments for Asian Americans: The relevance of mindfulness and acceptance-based psychotherapies. *Clinical Psychology: Science and Practice, 18*, 215–231.

SUGGESTED READINGS

Frank, J. D., & Frank, J. B. (1991). *Persuasion and healing: A comparative study of psychotherapy*. Baltimore, MD: Johns Hopkins University Press.

This book offers a theoretical framework for understanding the common therapeutic features that many healing practices share and how they may evoke placebo effects. These healing practices include biomedicine, psychotherapy, and traditional healing practices.

Gielen, U. P., Fish, J. M., & Draguns, J. G. (Eds.). (2004). *Handbook of culture, therapy, and healing*. Mahwah, NJ: Lawrence Erlbaum.

This book brings together the work of scholars from psychology, anthropology, psychiatry, and related disciplines. They focus on how the interaction of cultural, psychosocial, and biological factors influences psychotherapy and traditional healing practices. The authors provide an overview of healing traditions, psychotherapies, and religious and spiritual practices in Asia, the Americas, and Africa.

Kleinman, A. (1980). *Patients and healers in the context of culture*. Los Angeles: University of California Press.

This book presents a theoretical framework for studying the relationship among culture, medicine, and psychiatry in a pluralistic health system. Although the field materials were mainly drawn from Chinese culture, the theoretical concepts that Kleinman discusses are applicable for analyses in other cultures as well. These concepts include clinical reality, cultural construction of illness experience, explanatory models, and relationships among professional, patient, and family.

Moodley, R., & West, W. (2005). *Integrating traditional healing practices into counseling and psychotherapy*. Thousand Oaks, CA: Sage.

This book provides a critical analysis on the relevance of traditional healing practices to mental and physical health. It argues persuasively that to develop culturally sensitive psychotherapy and counseling, mental health professionals should understand and learn from the worldviews, experiences, and ideas of indigenous healing traditions. The materials and theories presented are multidisciplinary, coming from psychology, anthropology, and social work. The traditional healing practices covered include those in North America, Africa, and Asia.

Acknowledgments:

Preparation of this article was supported by a grant from the National Institute of Education, Nanyang Technological University (SUG 9/14 LBO).

8 Integrating Asian Healing Traditions Into Biomedicine

Tenzin Lhundup and James H. Lake

Asian healing traditions and biomedicine are the most widely practiced systems of medicine globally. Asian medicine is becoming an accepted alternative approach to diagnosis and treatment in many Western countries, while acceptance of biomedicine is growing in Asia. The confluence of Western medicine and Asian healing traditions in both Western countries and Asia presents many challenges and opportunities with regard to the safe and appropriate uses of disparate approaches to diagnose and treat both medical and psychiatric disorders. Increasing numbers of Western and Asian patients receive both biomedical therapies and Asian medical treatments concurrently; however, few efforts have been made to establish clinical guidelines for rationally *integrating* therapeutic approaches from these disparate systems of medicine. Asian healing traditions offer many potential benefits to biomedicine, including a graduated series of therapies, improved management of adverse effects caused by potent pharmaceuticals, great coherence in healing and clinician–patient interactions, a more holistic framework, and an improved prescriptive methodology. By the same token, biomedicine offers many potential benefits to Asian systems of medicine including improved accuracy in diagnosis and symptom management, improved recognition of adverse effects, potent therapies addressing severe or acute symptoms, better tracking of outcomes; and continuous emergency and inpatient care. This chapter develops arguments for integrating Asian medicine and Western biomedicine in the context of their respective strengths and limitations.

Biomedicine in Mental Health Care

Disparate systems of medicine are based on different conceptual models of illness. Biomedicine is the dominant medical model in Western culture. The

Western perspective *constructs* disorders from symptom patterns attributed to underlying physical or psychological causes. Diagnosis entails the confirmation of a particular symptom pattern by a qualified medical professional. Biomedicine borrows concepts from physics, chemistry, and biology; equates health and sickness with normal and abnormal biological functioning, respectively; and assumes that symptoms reflect dysregulation in biological processes in the human body. **Biomedical psychiatry** holds that mental illness can be explained as the dysregulation of neurochemical processes in the brain. Many non-Western systems of medicine reject this assumption. In contrast, Asian systems of medicine rest on fundamentally different assumptions about the nature of the human body; the role of consciousness in healing; and the influences of biological, psychological, or postulated "energetic" factors in health and illness. This difference has resulted in important problems for biomedical researchers attempting to *objectively* evaluate approaches used in Asian healing traditions.

Biomedicine evaluates its theories and methods in light of emerging findings in physics and the life sciences that call into question some of the core tenets of contemporary science. Recent scientific advances are yielding novel theories that may eventually explain mechanisms underlying nonbiomedical treatments, including "energy" medicine. The conceptual foundations of science will continue to evolve resulting in increasing acceptance of Asian healing traditions by Western-trained researchers and physicians.

How Biomedicine Is Practiced Today: Advantages and Limitations

In spite of its impressive advances, broad sociocultural and economic issues limit the ability of biomedicine to provide adequate health care. These include the limited availability and high cost of pharmaceuticals in many world regions and restrictions placed on treatments by insurance companies. Widespread dissatisfaction over the quality of biomedical care has arisen out of concerns over cost, safety, and effectiveness as well as complaints about managed care that often result in short and impersonal contact with patients.[1] Growing dissatisfaction with biomedicine as currently practiced together with the increasing cost of obtaining care have led to increased uses of complementary and alternative medicine (CAM) approaches to treat medical and mental health problems.[2] This emerging paradigm of integrative medicine employs evidence-based therapies from all systems of medicine while emphasizing *person-centered* care and engaging each patient in the process of changing his or her lifestyle to achieve improved health.

Millions of people inflicted with severe mental illnesses rely on psychotropic medications in order to function; however, there are increasing concerns over the safety and efficacy of psychotropic medications. When unpublished findings are taken into account, the efficacy of many widely used antidepressants is not greater than placebos.[3] Several medications for depression, anxiety disorders, and bipolar disorder have serious safety problems. In fact, safety risks associated with antidepressants may outweigh their beneficial effects.[4] These issues are made worse by the high cost of newer antidepressant and antipsychotic medications not covered by insurance.

In biomedical psychiatry, there is an entrenched belief that mental illness is caused by dysregulation of neurotransmitters. Until recent decades, unquestioned acceptance of the neurotransmitter theory as the central dogma of biomedical psychiatry has resulted in a paucity of research on promising CAM treatments. In this medical landscape, change is beginning to take place in medical education, research, and in popular attitudes toward CAM. Core competencies in integrative medicine are now being taught in the majority of U.S. medical schools and residency training programs.[5] Approximately half of U.S. physicians endorse acupuncture, chiropractic, and homeopathy as valid medical principles and frequently refer patients to CAM practitioners.[6] Increasing numbers of physicians are becoming certified in one or more areas of CAM, including acupuncture, herbal medicine, and homeopathy.[7] In parallel with these changes, the National Center for Complementary and Integrative Health of the National Institutes of Health is addressing the imbalance between the entrenched paradigm and CAM by funding research on promising CAM therapies.

Changes in the public perception and use of biomedicine are related to shifting values, economic factors, renewed emphasis on healthy lifestyles, and research findings supporting treatments outside of biomedicine, including acupuncture.[8] The increasing use of CAM in developed countries reflects an increasingly consumer-driven health care environment in the context of increasing medical diversity. Persons diagnosed with any psychiatric disorder are significantly more likely to use CAM compared to the general population.[9] One third of persons who experience generalized anxiety, mood swings, or psychotic symptoms use CAM.[10] Two thirds of severely depressed or anxious persons use both biomedical and CAM therapies concurrently, and 9 out of 10 see a mental health professional but only one third of those who use CAM disclose this information to their physician.[11]

Relationship and Collaboration With Western Mental Health Care

In North America, Europe, Australia, and other developed world regions, most persons who seek treatment from an Asian medical practitioner have previously been diagnosed by a conventionally trained medical practitioner.

Many are already taking prescription medications for one or more "disorders." Persons being treated by a practitioner of Asian medicine seldom disclose this information to their Western-trained medical provider. By the same token, the majority of individuals who are taking a biomedical treatment do not disclose this information to a practitioner of Asian medicine treating them concurrently. Persons treated by practitioners trained in different healing traditions elect *not to disclose* their treatments to their various providers for many reasons including a desire to avoid being seen as naive or ignorant. Nondisclosure of information pertaining to treatment has many risks, including being misdiagnosed, taking a treatment that may worsen health or interfere with appropriate treatments, and having adverse effects or toxic interactions.

After decades of widespread use of Chinese medicine in Western countries, there is still little information on which herbals and prescription medications may be combined safely. Practitioners trained in biomedicine or traditional Chinese medicine (TCM) acknowledge the risks associated with combining certain Chinese herbals and prescription medications—for example, *ma huang* (which contains ephedrine) and antidepressants or blood pressure medications, both of which can have serious potentially fatal consequences. Even less is known about the risks of combining prescription medications with herbal treatments used in Ayurveda, Tibetan medicine, and Japanese traditional medicine (Kampo). Emerging research findings on the pharmacological actions of Asian herbal formulas will guide clinicians when treating psychiatric disorders. A review of pharmacologic studies of TCM herbal formulas used to treat mental illness found that Western psychopharmacology and TCM herbal formulas used to treat mental illness rest on mechanisms of action involving the same neurotransmitters including serotonin, norepinephrine, GABA, and others. Such findings are providing a strong empirical basis for further integration of Asian medicine and biomedical psychiatry by identifying select herbal formulas that are safe and effective treatments of particular psychiatric disorders when used alone or in combination with psychotropic medications.[12]

It is important that practitioners of biomedicine and Asian systems of medicine carefully review the research literature on efficacy and safety when considering using integrative approaches that consider recommending combinations of treatments from two disparate systems of medicine. In view of the limited information about the safe, synergistic combinations, I encourage clinicians to err on the side of caution and to avoid combinations that could potentially result in serious adverse effects. Finally, when recommending a treatment strategy that is not supported by good research evidence in the published medical literature, it is important to obtain informed consent from the patient and to carefully document this in the patient record. The following concise review of the strengths and limitations of Asian medicine and biomedicine is offered as a general framework for clinicians advising their patients about mental health care.

Comparing Biomedicine and Asian Systems of Healing

Every system of medicine has strengths and limitations with respect to diagnostic and treatment approaches used when approaching a particular symptom or disorder. All treatments used in Asian medicine and conventional biomedicine have beneficial effects and potential adverse effects. When comparing the relative benefits and shortcomings of different treatments important considerations include the research evidence for a particular treatment with respect to a unique patient's current symptoms, the patient's history of treatment response, cost issues, and personal preferences. In world regions where Asian medicine and biomedicine are used, patients choose treatments based on perceptions of comparative effectiveness, convenience, cost, and adverse effects.[13] Biomedicine rests on advanced diagnostic technologies that guide both research and clinical decision making, including, for example, functional magnetic resonance imaging (fMRI) and other functional brain imaging technologies as well as the genetic analysis of disease. Advanced technological approaches do not currently play a role in Asian systems of medicine. As a general rule, biomedical therapies have more potent and more rapid effects than Asian herbal medicines, acupuncture, and other treatment modalities.

When approaching individuals with severe mental illness, it is prudent to treat the patient with potent prescription medications or, when there is a question of suicide risk, to urgently refer them to the nearest emergency room. After a patient afflicted with a severe mental illness has responded to prescription medications, it may be appropriate to try an Asian medical treatment including herbal formulas, acupuncture, or others, when there is evidence of both efficacy and safety for the treatment being considered. There is a growing body of research on herbal formulas used in TCM and Ayurveda to successfully treat neuropsychiatric disorders including depressed mood, schizophrenia, and neurodegenerative disorders.[14] Unlike Asian systems of medicine, around-the-clock biomedical services are available to individuals seeking urgent care in Western hospitals and emergency rooms. This is especially important for individuals with severe mental illnesses who may require rapid stabilization and hospitalization for their safety. An important attribute of all Asian systems of medicine is the provision of disparate therapies that result in a series of responses ranging from subtle effects with few or no adverse effects, to more potent therapies resulting in marked physiological or energetic changes that may have more frequent or more serious adverse effects. The same general principle is at the heart of conventional Western biomedicine, which has the parallel goal of achieving an adequate therapeutic response via the safest available interventions addressing a postulated disease-causing agent. This principle is embodied in a fundamental principle of biomedicine, *primum non nocere* ("first, do no harm"), which warns physicians against using interventions for which the potential risk may outweigh likely benefits. Research advances in biomedicine and neuroscience have yielded a steady flow of powerful drugs that have revolutionized mental health care providing newfound hope to millions of individuals afflicted with severe mental illness. By the same token, many widely used psychotropic medications are associated with serious adverse effects. In some cases, the risks associated with psychotropic agents may outweigh their potential benefits. Examples include both older antipsychotics such as haloperidol and chlorpromazine and recently introduced so-called atypical antipsychotics like risperidone, quetiapine, clozapine, olanzapine, and ziprasidone. The chronic use of antipsychotics may result in a debilitating permanent movement disorder, life-threatening cardiac arrhythmia, or toxic **metabolic syndrome** that increases the risk for obesity and diabetes. Treatment used in both traditions restores *balance* when skillfully administered by a trained clinician but may also cause pathological imbalances and adverse effects when applied erroneously or by a poorly trained clinician.

The belief that good health is a reflection of harmony is embedded in many world healing traditions and is an easy concept for non-Asians to grasp. Unlike biomedicine, Asian systems of medicine treat the *whole* person, not a particular symptom, organ, or illness condition based on the concept that the body is an integrated whole and that the core causes of illness can be eliminated only when the entire organism is restored to a healthy state of harmony with nature. In contrast to biomedicine, which uses highly technical language to convey information to patients, Asian systems of medicine rely on simple metaphors referring to "energy" that are easy to understand and help patients visualize a disease process or the health-promoting benefits of treatment. In Asian systems of medicine, illness is a manifestation of loss of energetic harmony between oneself and the world. According to this metaphor, curing illness entails making changes in lifestyle or taking treatments that restore life to its natural state of *harmony* with the universe. "Wind" is an important metaphor used to describe the energetic principle of ***rlung*** in Tibetan medical theory related to balance or harmony.[15] According to the *Rgyud bzhi* ("Four Tantras"), depending on the particular causes involved, disorders of wind can manifest as a wide range of neuromuscular and psychosomatic disorders including the "life-wind illnesses," which are syndromes that resemble depressed mood, panic disorder, and generalized anxiety.[16]

All Asian healing traditions are patient-centered, and when practiced according to traditional principles, each patient receives treatments that address the unique imbalances that manifest as physical or mental symptoms. The highly individualized, or "person-centered," approaches used to assess and treat symptoms in Asian healing traditions are performed to ensure a close match between the underlying causes of symptoms and the effects of treatments at various levels of body and mind. When a skillful physician or Asian medical clinician arrives at an appropriate treatment choice, there is a close match between a specific treatment and the causes' underlying symptoms. The match between the energetic pattern of symptoms and treatments ideally results in few or no adverse effects.

A comparative analysis of the three major Asian systems of medicine with respect to mental health care is beyond the scope of this chapter. The reader is referred to several excellent reviews.[17] When skillfully administered, external therapies such as acupuncture, energetic massage, and somatic therapies practiced in Chinese medicine, Ayurveda, and **Sowa-Rigpa** (traditional Tibetan medicine) are seldom associated with adverse effects. In contrast to such "external" therapies, herbal formulas may carry a significant risk of adverse effects; however, the majority of herbal formulas used in Asian healing traditions are compounded from unrefined herbal materials or other natural products and have limited physiological potency and are thus associated with relatively little risk of adverse effects. Further, Asian herbal formulas are typically prescribed on an individual basis, reflecting each patient's unique constitutional pattern. All of these factors result in few or no adverse effects when Asian herbal formulas are prescribed by skilled medical practitioners. Asian systems of medicine rest on a pattern-based prescriptive methodology in which a particular *disease* is a reflection of the energetic *pattern* of the body as a whole. A practical consequence of this concept is that *good* treatments are associated with few or no adverse effects. Applying the general concept to diagnosis in biomedicine may lead to *more accurate identification of the underlying patterns of disease*, resulting in more individualized treatments with fewer adverse effects. Applied to the pharmacologic management of psychiatric symptoms, this approach might result in improved responses to prescription antidepressants and antipsychotics and a reduced incidence of adverse effects.

Methods and Strategies for Integration

An important opportunity for integrating biomedicine and Asian systems of medicine is at the level of outcomes assessment. For example, standardized symptom rating scales and biomedical tests such as blood chemistries and urinalysis are often useful when monitoring responses to Asian medical therapies. By the same token, pulse diagnosis in TCM, Tibetan medicine, and Ayurveda provide useful diagnostic information about energetic imbalances associated with disparate medical and psychiatric disorders and may provide a valuable adjunctive lens when added to conventional biomedical assessment.[18]

Most herbal medicines and other treatments used in Asian systems of medicine are less potent and less expensive than prescription medications used in biomedicine. When selecting the most appropriate treatment, different considerations apply depending on the type and severity of symptoms being addressed. The judicious biomedical or Asian medical practitioner will place the highest priority on the patient's safety and well-being. Other important considerations involved when determining the most appropriate treatment include each unique patient's history of response or lack thereof to previously tried conventional and CAM treatments, cost, and personal or cultural preferences. Individuals afflicted with severe depression, bipolar disorder, schizophrenia, or other severe mental health problems are at significant risk of self-harm or suicide. Many aspects of contemporary biomedicine can be used with benefit by individuals being treated with Asian medicine. An important strength of biomedicine is its systematic approach to diagnosis and prognosis. In contrast to Asian systems of medicine, which rely largely on highly subjective reports that reflect energetic balance, biomedicine emphasizes collecting information through history-taking and a systematic approach to differential diagnosis based on objective findings. This difference translates into greater diagnostic accuracy in biomedicine, which, in turn, often leads to more appropriate treatment recommendations and better outcomes.

Because pharmacologic treatments are generally more potent and in most cases work faster than Asian herbal medicines, it is appropriate to initially recommend prescription medications to patients complaining of severe psychiatric symptoms. When a patient reports symptoms and a history that suggest a severe, chronic, or life-threatening illness, it is appropriate to refer the patient for urgent medical evaluation by a conventionally trained Western physician, including a thorough medical examination to rule out possible unrecognized medical problems. When a patient who has severe symptoms fails to respond to appropriate biomedical treatment administered by a qualified clinician or the patient responds but elects to discontinue treatment because of adverse effects, it is appropriate to refer the patient to a qualified CAM practitioner for further evaluation and consideration of appropriate nonpharmacologic treatment options. When a patient who is seen by both an Asian medical practitioner and a physician or other conventionally trained practitioner is considering discontinuing a prescription medication, the patient should be referred to his physician to determine the most prudent course to take. In general, any questions regarding prescription medications should be referred to the patient's physician. By the same token, questions pertaining to Asian herbal formulas or other treatments should be referred to the patient's Asian medical practitioner.

Assuming a patient does not have a severe, life-threatening, or chronic condition and there is good evidence for the effectiveness and safety of a particular Asian medical therapy for his or her condition, it is both reasonable and appropriate to initially refer the patient to a qualified Asian medical practitioner if this approach is congruent with the patient's beliefs, values, and personal preferences. When a patient fails to respond or has a poor response after completing the prescribed course of an Asian medical treatment administered by a well-trained practitioner or when the patient has not adhered to the treatment regimen because of adverse effects, cost, or other issues, a consultation between the Asian medical practitioner and conventionally trained physician involved in the patient's care may yield valuable insights about further diagnostic and treatment considerations. Just as physicians and other conventionally trained practitioners may refer patients to Asian medical practitioners when they do not improve with treatment, it is appropriate and prudent for Asian medical practitioners to refer patients to physicians when patients do not respond to an appropriate Asian medical therapy administered by a well-trained Asian medical practitioner.

Integrative medicine takes into account the strengths and limitations of all systems of medicine in the context of each patient's unique needs, preferences, and resources. The result is an evidence-based treatment plan centered on a biomedical treatment, an Asian medical treatment, or a range of biomedical and CAM therapies. It is both reasonable and prudent to recommend an Asian medical treatment that is established as safe and efficacious for a particular mental health problem assuming the patient is not impaired by severe psychiatric symptoms or at risk of suicide. The choice of an Asian medical treatment over a biomedical treatment that is equally safe and effective makes sense when the biomedical treatment is expensive or has a higher risk of adverse effects. By the same token, it is prudent to consider switching therapy to a conventional prescription medication when an Asian medical treatment does not result in desired therapeutic results assuming the latter has been correctly administered by a well-trained clinician and the patient has adhered to the treatment regimen.

Select Asian medical diagnostic approaches and therapies can be safely combined with conventional biomedical approaches yielding greater diagnostic clarity and beneficial synergistic effects. For example, energetic pattern diagnosis, acupuncture, and Qigong (QG) can be safely used in conjunction with conventional psychiatric assessment, prescription medications, and hypnotherapy in the management of generalized anxiety disorder (GAD).[19] Because they rest on different mechanisms, acupuncture, moxibustion, and energetic massage (*tui na*) cannot *potentially* interact with Western prescription medications, and these modalities may be safely combined depending on the particular energetic imbalance or symptoms of each unique patient. Combining potent synthetic pharmaceuticals and Asian herbal medicines poses more complex challenges. When the safety and efficacy of a particular combination have not been clearly established from published case reports or research studies the prudent physician or Asian medical practitioner will advise against combining *any* Asian herbal medicine with *any* prescription medication. Because of the paucity of information about safe combinations of Asian medicinal herbals and pharmaceuticals when treating a patient who is taking a prescription medication, the Asian medical practitioner should recommend small initial doses of herbals while monitoring for toxic interactions. Combining a prescription medication and an Asian herbal formula is advisable only when there is strong evidence that the combination has beneficial synergistic effects and little risk of toxic interactions as well as after documenting the patient's informed consent about potential risks and benefits of the treatment regimen. The reader is referred to valuable resources that cover important issues pertaining to herb–drug interactions to keep in mind when considering combinations of Chinese herbal formulas and Western prescription medications.[20]

The following summary offers important considerations when approaching a patient complaining of a mental health problem from an integrative perspective.

Integrative Considerations When Treating Mentally Ill Patients

- When treating a person with a severe mental illness, always refer him or her for urgent evaluation by a conventionally trained physician. Refer patients who are suicidal or homicidal to the nearest emergency room *immediately.*
- For moderate symptoms, choose the most appropriate treatment after reviewing the research evidence for efficacy and safety. If two or more treatments have equivalent efficacy, cost considerations play an important role in treatment selection.
- When an Asian medical treatment and a biomedical treatment are equally effective, the Asian medical intervention may represent the more holistic treatment choice. In contrast, biomedical treatments are often more potent, more expensive, and have more adverse effects.
- When an Asian medical therapy has been tried without benefit, evidence-based biomedical treatments should be considered.
- When a patient has not responded to a biomedical treatment or reports severe adverse effects and there is comparable or stronger evidence for an Asian medical treatment, it is prudent to refer the patient to an Asian medical practitioner.
- When a patient has failed to respond or has adverse effects after trying an Asian or biomedical treatment, the Asian medical practitioner and the biomedical practitioner should consult on promising treatment options that have not been tried previously.
- Fully informed consent about the risks and benefits of treatment should be documented in the patient's medical record prior to starting any new Asian, biomedical, or combined treatment regimen.

Research and Future Directions

Research progress in biomedicine and Asian systems of medicine will ensure continued rapid growth in both healing traditions. Increasing acceptance of Asian systems of medicine in Western countries will result from research progress characterizing the mechanisms of action of herbal formulas at the level of neurotransmitters. This will eventually lead to evidence-based clinical guidelines for the evidence-based use of particular herbal formulas alone or in combination with Western pharmacologic therapies for depressed mood, anxiety, and other common mental health problems. In parallel with this trend, Asian medical practitioners will increasingly use Western biomedical treatments to augment the beneficial effects of Asian medical treatments for promoting wellness and treating mental health problems. These trends will result in a holistic or systems approach to diagnosing, treating, and preventing mental illness that encompasses the strengths of biomedicine and Asian medicine while avoiding the limitations of any particular healing tradition.[21]

Conclusion

The limitations and advantages of biomedicine and so-called CAM approaches including Asian medical therapies are stimulating rapid growth in integrative medicine globally. Ayurveda, Tibetan medicine, and TCM are highly evolved, coherent Asian systems of medicine that have been empirically validated and refined over millennia, are widely used in their parent cultures for maintaining wellness and treating illness, and are increasingly used in Western countries. Asian diagnostic methods may complement biomedical diagnostic methods by providing useful information that will clarify underlying pathology and aid in treatment planning. Emerging research findings support that Asian medical treatments including acupuncture and herbal formulas are generally well tolerated and that select herbal formulas used in Asian medicine consistently result in symptomatic improvement of depressed mood, anxiety, and schizophrenia. Additional studies are needed to further characterize the safety, efficacy, and optimal dosing considerations of specific herbal formulas and other Asian medical treatments of mental health problems.

Case Study

Adam is a 45-year-old married software engineer who has a stressful job at a start-up tech company. Beth, his spouse of 10 years, is also in the tech industry and was recently laid off from her company because of downsizing during an economic downturn. Adam and Beth have two children; one has a severe learning disorder and attends an expensive private school. Adam has been depressed and "tired all the time" for the past few months and admits to a drinking problem. He has had difficulty sleeping and concentrating at work as well as forgetting to finish important tasks. His appetite has been "low" for several weeks, and he has lost weight. Adam used to enjoy exercising but has not worked out for several weeks and feels "depleted" much of the time, tries to "just get through the day," and avoids social contact as much as possible.

(*Continued*)

(Continued)

Adam started to have a problem with depression about five years ago, which he believed was related to the "stress of life" at work and "the whole family thing." Adam and his spouse have been in couples' therapy "to try to help each other be more understanding about the stress in our lives" and "manage the kids better" but have grown apart in recent years. Beth's job loss has added more stress to the relationship. Adam previously tried acupuncture, "but it did not really make a difference" in the severity of depressed mood. He tried two antidepressants but with little benefit and recently discontinued the last one (an SSRI) because of sexual side effects. Although his experience with acupuncture was disappointing, Adam is interested in exploring other Asian healing approaches. He found out about a doctor of Tibetan medicine who practices in his city and is known for his expertise treating mental and emotional problems. While in the waiting room before his appointment, Adam listened to a recording of Tibetan "singing bowls" and entered into a deeply relaxed state. After inviting Adam to sit for a few minutes while closing his eyes, Dr. Lhundup gently held Adam's wrist and examined his pulse. Afterward, he asked Adam about his life history and confirmed the absence of serious medical problems. Adam disclosed his 5-year struggle with depressed mood, two failed trials on Western-style antidepressants, and his problems with adverse effects. Adam confirmed that he is not suicidal and has never attempted suicide. He denied previous or current symptoms of mania, panic attacks, psychosis, or other severe mental health problems. He told Dr. Lhundup that both parents are currently being treated for depressed mood, but there is no family history of bipolar disorder or other severe mental health problems. Adam talked about his work stress; marital problems; his drinking; and recent problems with appetite loss, physical inactivity, anxiety, and insomnia. After briefly describing the basic principles of Tibetan medicine to Adam, Dr. Lhundup suggested a simple daily mindfulness practice for stress reduction and improved sleep and dietary changes such as increased protein and "warm, oily" foods. He recommended avoiding cold, damp, or windy areas and encouraged Adam to engage in a daily spiritual practice and to cultivate friendships. An herbal formula with Aquilaria (aloeswood) as its principal ingredient is prescribed to nourish and rebalance the life-sustaining *rlung*. Dr. Lhundup also prescribed several weeks of Tibetan massage therapy (Ku Nye), addressing Adam's symptoms of anxiety and depressed mood after explaining that both problems are manifestations of excess *rlung*. He advised Adam about other approaches that he may recommend depending on his response to the initial treatment plan and briefly described specialized needling techniques used to regulate *rlung*: herbal baths for calming anxiety and promoting improved sleep, the therapeutic principles of moxa, and cupping. Dr. Lhundup gave Adam a packet containing the herbal medicine he had prescribed and mentioned possible adverse effects. They scheduled two return appointments to take place in 2 and 6 weeks.

Adam demonstrated typical mental symptoms of excess *rlung*, including difficulty concentrating, being forgetful, and feeling empty as well as having anxiety and insomnia. According to Tibetan medical theory, depressed mood, along with other mental health problems, is a manifestation of excess *rlung* (sometimes labeled wind in Western countries), the Nyepa that is associated with mind, and all aspects of consciousness. Imbalances in *rlung* may be caused by external factors such as diet, stress, medications or natural supplements, and seasonal changes as well as internal factors having to do with the mind, such as excess desire or attachment. In Tibetan medicine (Sowa-Rigpa), the human body, disease processes, and the interventions that constitute treatment comprise the five elements (metal, wood, water, fire, and earth). Each element plays a fundamental role in the universe, including the human body.

Each element is related to all other elements in a web of complex dynamic relationships. Different combinations of elements comprise the three Nyepas: (1) *rlung,* (2) *Tripa,* and (3) *Peken.* Harmony between the three Nyepas and the five elements manifests as a state of physical, emotional, and mental health. Accordingly, loss of harmony or proper balance between the five elements or the three Nyepas manifests as illness. In Adam's case, the core teachings of Tibetan medicine, which are closely tied to Tibetan Buddhist philosophy, offered an alternative understanding of healing. Tibetan medicine strives to diagnose and correctly treat imbalances between the elements through herbal formulas; changes in diet or lifestyle; acupuncture; and different somatic therapies, such as massage, cupping, and others.

DISCUSSION QUESTIONS

1. Traditional Asian healing approaches and Western "biomedicine" have different strengths and limitations. What are two strengths of Asian medicine and two strengths of Western medicine? Give an example of when an Asian medical approach would be the preferred approach in mental health care.
2. Western medicine and Asian traditional healing are grounded in different basic concepts and theories. Briefly describe one conceptual difference between the two paradigms and how that difference translates into different kinds of diagnostic procedures.
3. The concept of "harmony" is a useful metaphor when describing how Asian medicine and Western biomedicine view both the causes of illness and the conditions or factors that result in improved health. Discuss the relationship between harmony and a particular mental health problem from the viewpoint of Western medicine or a specific Asian healing tradition.
4. Integrative considerations are important when treating any client who complains of a mental health problem because many individuals who struggle with depression, anxiety, bipolar disorder, and other mental health problems may be taking a potent prescription medication and an herbal formula at the same time. What are potential safety issues that may result when this happens, and what are prudent steps to take when advising a client about responsible steps to follow when considering combining herbal formulas and prescription medications?

REFERENCES

1. Jonas, W. B., Eisenberg, D., Hufford, D., & Crawford, C. (2013). The evolution of complementary and alternative medicine (CAM) in the USA over the last 20 years. *Forsch Komplementmed, 20*(1), 65–72.

2. Tindle, H. A., Davis, R. B., Phillips, R. S., & Eisenberg, D. M. (2005). Trends in use of complementary and alternative medicine by US adults: 1997–2002. *Alternative Therapy Health Medicine*, *11*(1), 42–49.
3. Sussman, N. (2004). The "file-drawer" effect: Assessing efficacy and safety of antidepressants. *Primary Psychiatry*, *11*(7), 12.
4. Keitner, G. (2004). *Limits to the treatment of major depression.* APA Annual Meeting, New York City. (Abstract no. 34)
5. Kligler, B., Maizes, V., Schachter, S., Park, C. M., Gaudet, T., Benn, R., . . . Education Working Group, Consortium of Academic Health Centers for Integrative Medicine. (2004). Core competencies in integrative medicine for medical school curricula: A proposal. *Academic Medicine*, *79*(6), 521–531.
6. Jonas et al., The evolution of complementary and alternative medicine.
7. Astin, J. A., Marie, A, Pelletier, K., Hansen, E., & Haskell, W. L. (1998). A review of the incorporation of complementary and alternative medicine by mainstream physicians. *Archives of Internal Medicine*, *158*, 2303–2310.
8. Astin, J. (1998). Why patients use alternative medicine. *JAMA*, *279*(19), 1548–1553; Rees, L. (2001). Integrated medicine: Imbues orthodox medicine with the values of complementary medicine. *British Medical Journal*, *322*, 119–120.
9. Unützer, J., Klap, R., Sturm, R., Young, A. S., Marmon, T., Shatkin, J., & Wells, K. B. (2000). Mental disorders and the use of alternative medicine: Results from a national survey. *American Journal of Psychiatry*, *157*, 1851–1857.
10. Ibid.
11. Kessler, R. C., Soukup, J., Davis, R. B., Foster, D. F., Wilkey, S. A., Van Rompay, M. I., & Eisenberg, D. M. (2004). The use of complementary and alternative therapies to treat anxiety and depression in the United States. *American Journal of Psychiatry*, *158*, 289–294.
12. Shorter, E., & Segesser, K. (2013). Traditional Chinese medicine and Western psychopharmacology: Building bridges. *Phytotherapy Research*, *27*(12), 1739–1744.
13. Lam, T. P. (2001). Strengths and weaknesses of traditional Chinese medicine and Western medicine in the eyes of some Hong Kong Chinese. *Journal of Epidemiology and Community Health*, *55*, 762–765.
14. Ven Murthy, M. R., Ranjekar, P. K., Ramassamy, C., & Deshpande, M. (2010). Scientific basis for the use of Indian ayurvedic medicinal plants in the treatment of neurodegenerative disorders: Ashwagandha. *Central Nervous System Agents in Medicinal Chemistry*, *10*(3), 238–246.
15. Yoeli-Tlalim, R. (2010). Tibetan "wind" and "wind" illnesses: Towards a multicultural approach to health and illness. *Studies in History and Philosophy of Biological and Biomedical Sciences*, *41*(4), 318–324.
16. Jacobson, E. (2003). Life-wind illness in Tibetan medicine: Depression, generalized anxiety and panic attack. In M. Schrempf (Ed.), Soundings in Tibetan medicine: Anthropological and historical perspectives. *Proceedings of the Tenth International Association for Tibetan Studies*, Oxford, England.
17. Millard, C. (2013). Tibetan medicine and the classification and treatment of mental illness. *The Journal of Traditional Tibetan Medicine*, *5*, 8–15; Aung, S. K., Fay, H., & Hobbs, R. F. (2013). Traditional Chinese medicine as a basis for treating psychiatric disorders: A review of theory with illustrative cases. *Medical Acupuncture Journal*, *25*(6), 398–406; Pratikanti, S. (2007). Ayurvedic treatments. In J. Lake & D. Spiegel (Eds.), *Complementary and alternative treatments in mental health care* (pp. 225–272). Washington, DC: American Psychiatric Publishing.

18. Lu, A., Jiang, M., Zhang C, & Chan, K. (2012). An integrative approach of linking traditional Chinese medicine pattern classification and biomedicine diagnosis. *Journal of Ethnopharmacology*, *141*(2), 549–556.
19. Aung et al., Traditional Chinese medicine.
20. Chen, J. (2006). Recognition and prevention of herb-drug interactions, Part 1: Pharmacokinetic interactions, naturopathy digest. *Acupuncture Today*, *7*(11), 1. Retrieved from http://www.naturopathydigest.com/archives/2006/dec/chen.php; Thai, H. C. (2004). *Chinese and Western herbal medicine: A guide to potential risks and drug interactions.* Retrieved from https://ethnomed.org/clinical/pharmacy/herb-drug-interactions; Chen, J. K., & Chen, T. (2004). *Chinese medical herbology and pharmacology.* City of Industry, CA: Art of Medicine Press.
21. Shorter & Segesser, Traditional Chinese medicine.

SUGGESTED READINGS

Clifford, T. (1984). *Tibetan Buddhist medicine and psychiatry: The diamond healing.* York Beach, ME: Samuel Weiser Inc.

The volume represents an introduction to the arcane Tibetan art of healing. The author discusses the many components of Tibetan Buddhist medicine: its religious, philosophical and psychological foundations, its history and deities, its tantric and ritual aspects, and unusual methods of diagnosis and cure.

Flaws, B., & Lake, J. (2001). *Chinese medical psychiatry: A textbook and clinical manual.* Boulder, CO: Blue Poppy Press.

This book provides a comprehensive text on psychiatry, connecting Western and Eastern concepts in this field. It serves as a reference source for both Eastern and Western medical students as well as practitioners as it bridges many of the gaps between these two systems and motivates one to rethink ways of addressing mental disorders in an integrative manner.

Hammer, L. I. (2005). *Dragon rises, red bird flies: Psychology and Chinese medicine* (Rev. ed.). Seattle, WA: Eastland Press.

In this book, Hammer offers a new model for appreciating the traditional healer's effective and profound respect for individual integrity and energetic balance. Explaining, and moving beyond, the five-phase (element) system, he shows that this Eastern practice is as much a spiritual science as a physical one. Accessible to the layman, yet a resource for the professional in any healing art, this book examines the natural energy functions of the human organism as a key to mental, emotional, and spiritual health.

Kleinman, A. (1981). *Patients and healers in the context of culture: An exploration of the borderland between anthropology, medicine, and psychiatry.* Berkeley: University of California Press.

Kleinman, a psychiatrist trained in anthropology, reports on his studies of health care in Taiwan. He describes his observations of clinical interviews between various medical practitioners, folk healers, temple medicine men, and Chinese-style and Western-style physicians—and their patients. He stresses the importance of adopting the proper cultural perspective, making interpretations within that framework.

9 Integrating Mindfulness, Meditation, Buddhism, and Therapeutic Practices

Marco Mascarin

In the contemporary North American lexicon, *mindful* is often used as a descriptive prefix to any number of activities: mindful investing, mindful parenting, and mindful eating, to name a few. As a clinical term, *mindfulness* can describe evidence-based psychotherapeutic interventions, such as **mindfulness-based stress reduction** (MBSR) or mindfulness-based cognitive therapy (MBCT). As a 2,500-year-old Asian contemplative practice, mindfulness meditation is an integral component of the Buddhist path that promises liberation from existential suffering.

Over the past few decades, the secular and clinical applications of mindfulness have generated enormous and ever-growing interest. Mindfulness has been the subject of thousands of research papers; empirical measurement scales with associated psychometric studies; courses at universities; and programs in hospitals, prisons, and a variety of educational institutions. In a 2004 paper titled "Mindfulness: A Proposed Operational Definition," Bishop and colleagues described "the results of recent meetings held to establish a consensus on mindfulness and to conjointly develop a testable operational definition" (p. 230).[1] Bishop and his colleagues referred to earlier research, which broadly conceptualized mindfulness as "a kind of non-elaborative, non-judgmental, present-centered awareness in which each thought, feeling or sensation that arises in the attentional field is acknowledged and accepted as it is" (p. 232).[2] The authors then offered a number of operational definitions of mindfulness, one of them being as follows:

> We see mindfulness as a process of regulating attention to bring a quality of non-elaborative awareness to current experience and a quality of relating to one's experience within an orientation of curiosity, experiential openness and acceptance. (p. 234)[3]

What various applications of mindfulness hold in common is the cultivated practice of **metacognitive acuity**—that is, the honed capacity to observe events in awareness (i.e., thoughts, feelings, and sensations) without habituated reactivity. The shift from "enmeshment with" to "observation of" the contents of awareness suggests broad and promising applications in the field of mental health. Mindfulness as a praxis has a 2,500-year history as an integral component of Buddhism, with a prodigious corpus of accompanying and supportive literature (ethical precepts, philosophy, epistemology, teachings on cognition, perception, etc.) replete with working definitions; detailed instructions; phenomenological insights; and, perhaps most importantly, a comprehensive system of graduated practices. However, much of the contemporary mindfulness literature, from the 1980s and 1990s forward, has endeavored to furnish definitions of mindfulness without corroborating research into the aforementioned tradition, or with minimal reference to it.

This is indicative of a curious phenomenon in contemporary mindfulness research and pedagogy, with few exceptions: an absence of attention to the contextual Buddhist tradition out of which mindfulness has been extracted and out of which these contemporary protocols and clinical interventions have been developed.[4] Thus, much of the existing literature disavows mindfulness from the ethical; historical; cultural; and, perhaps most significantly, soteriological context in which it was initially introduced.

In response, this chapter will explore how mindfulness meditation is understood and practiced in a historical Buddhist context, focusing on how it was referenced by practitioners and described in authoritative texts, such as the *Maha-satipatthana Sutta*. It will also introduce the use of mindfulness as a modern psychotherapeutic tool, addressing how it is applied for use with various populations. The chapter will argue that mindfulness meditation was never intended to be used as an isolated, stand-alone practice, protocol, or intervention; rather, it is one component in a systematic approach to the alleviation of human suffering. When mindfulness meditation is misappropriated as an exclusive practice or clinical intervention unto itself, a potential disservice is done to the tradition and to students, psychotherapy clients, and the larger community interested in the cultivation of mental health and the alleviation of suffering.

Brief History of Buddhism and Mindfulness Meditation

Approximately 2,500 years ago in northern India, the historical Buddha ("Awakened One") known as *Shakyamuni* (teacher from the Shakya clan) introduced a detailed analysis of human suffering, (Pali: *dukkha*) both causative factors and cures, which was subsequently enshrined as the Four Noble Truths. The fourth of the noble truths presents an eightfold systematic approach to the alleviation of suffering, known to Buddhist practitioners as the Eightfold Path.

For pragmatic and pedagogical purposes, the Eightfold Path was later subdivided into three divisions, often referred to as the **three higher trainings**—wisdom (*paññakkhandha*), ethical conduct (*silakkhandha*), and mental development (*samadhikkhandha*). Mental development was further subdivided into right effort, right mindfulness, and right concentration, which are indispensable practices in the larger project of decreasing suffering. The prefix *right* suggested "perfect, appropriate, we might almost say fitting" (p. 53).[5] Mental development and, therefore, mindfulness practice(s) are crucial to liberation. Contemporary Buddhist scholar Alan Wallace articulated in a modern idiom a long-standing Buddhist insight into the centrality of mental development and transformation: "It is the afflictions of our own minds that lie at the root of our mental troubles, not the material world, not other people, not our bodies, not intangible spirits or demons, and not God" (p. 49).[6]

The term *mindfulness* is derived from the Pali word *sati* or in Sanskrit *smṛti* and translates as nonforgetfulness or recollection. The term is related to the verb *sarati*: "to remember or to keep in mind" and can be used in the context of recall or memory of past events, or remembering to engage in an activity in the future.[7] In the context of mindfulness meditation, it relates to present-focused attention, the "keeping in mind" of arising phenomena—that is, the object of one's meditation, such as the sensations related to breathing *(ānāpānasati)*.

The ***Maha-satipatthana Sutta***, the great aphorism or sermon on the foundation or establishment of mindfulness, contains the Buddha's instructions on the foundations of mindfulness and is regarded as the canonical Buddhist text that contains the most comprehensive teachings on mindfulness meditation techniques. "The word '*satipatthana*' is the name for an approach to meditation aimed at establishing *sati* or mindfulness."[8] A sample of the instructions on mindfulness of breathing, or *Ānāpānasati Sutta,* are as follows:

> Here (in this teaching), bhikkhus (monks), a bhikkhu having gone to the forest, or to the foot of a tree, or to an empty, solitary place; sits down cross-legged, keeping his body erect, and directs his mindfulness (towards the object of mindfulness). Then only with keen mindfulness he breathes in and only with keen mindfulness he breathes out. Breathing in a long breath, he knows, "I breathe in a long breath"; breathing out a long breath, he knows, "I breathe out a long breath"; breathing in a short breath, he knows, "I breathe in a short breath"; breathing out a short breath, he knows, "I breathe out a short breath," "Aware of the whole breath body, I shall breathe in," thus he trains himself; "Aware of the whole breath body, I shall breathe out," thus he trains himself. (p. 8)[9]

Right mindfulness is defined in the context of the Eightfold Path as "guided by right view, motivated by right intention, grounded in ethics, and to be cultivated in conjunction with right effort. Without right view or right intention, one could be practicing bare attention without its ever developing into right mindfulness" (p. 63).[10] Thus, mindfulness in its contemporary formulation, "paying attention in a particular way: on purpose, in the present moment, and non-judgmentally," misses the nuances and complexity of how the tradition intended mindfulness to be understood and practiced (p. 4).[11] What becomes apparent is that the operational definition of mindfulness as, "a process of regulating attention to bring a quality of non-elaborative awareness to current experience and a quality of relating to one's experience within an orientation of curiosity, experiential openness and acceptance" fails to address the need for accompanying wholesome mental factors and prescriptive ethical behavior aligned in a trajectory culminating in liberating wisdom (p. 234).[12]

What is evident from this cursory investigation of the tradition from which contemporary mindfulness has been extracted is that there is tremendous benefit from engaging 2,500 years of applied insight into the process of decreasing human suffering. More of this work needs to be done; at present, a conversation has commenced between Buddhist practitioners and clinicians, neuroscientists and seasoned meditators, and thus far, there is every reason to celebrate these collaborations as more of the tradition is explored and opportunities for shared research and integration arise. With such ongoing exchanges, perhaps mindfulness will come to be increasingly appreciated in the context it was intended: as one component of a vast host of practices and approaches aimed at the alleviation of suffering.

Inasmuch as mindfulness meditation is embedded in the Buddhist Eightfold Path and is an integral component of Buddhism's trajectory toward liberation, it is concerned with healing. The metaphor often used to describe Buddhism's Three Jewels of Buddha, Dharma, and Sangha is borrowed from medicine. The Buddha is the master physician dispensing the dharma teachings—the prescriptive antidote to suffering. The Sangha is the willing community of patients, gathered to practice the Buddha's medicine.

Tibetan medicine is unique because it is a healing tradition or medical modality that is inextricably bound and informed by Buddhist principles. Although Tibetan medicine identifies imbalance of the three humors—phlegm, bile, and wind—as the root of all disease, the three poisons—ignorance, anger, and desire—pose a greater risk. Kilty, translator of *The Mirror of Beryl: A Historical Introduction to Tibetan Medicine*, argued the following:

> With Buddhism as its spiritual philosophy, Tibetan medicine says that the true path to perfect and permanent health is Buddhist practice aimed at eliminating the three poisons, whereas following medical treatments can alleviate the suffering of illness only temporarily as long as the three poisons reside in the mind. (p. 9)[13]

Ultimate well-being is exemplified in the activities of a Buddha, who according to the tradition is one who has eradicated the three roots of suffering in their entirety and, as such, is able to confer on others the healing balm of the Dharma (teachings) and their antidotes to suffering. Mindfulness meditation practice done as part of the prescriptive program of the three higher trainings of wisdom, ethical conduct, and mental development is directly aimed at the transformation of the three poisons.

In a contemporary clinical context, the therapist's and client's ambitions may not be so lofty as to aim for the eradication of suffering. However, as will be examined later, there is an ever-growing body of evidence-based literature suggesting that a variety of mindfulness-based interventions have the potential to address a range of symptoms and concerns: for example, depression, post-traumatic stress disorder (PTSD), substance abuse, and eating disorders. We may come to learn that Buddhism's systemic approach to the alleviation of suffering may offer further insights and strategies for clinical work and complement or even enhance existing interventions.

Mindfulness Training and Development, Supervision, Accreditation, Licensure, and Certification

> We can make our minds so like still water that beings gather about us, that they may see, it may be, their own images, and so live for a moment with a clearer, perhaps even with a fiercer life because of our quiet.[14]

Mindfulness training for therapists is available in a number of settings, from universities and independent institutions to individualized instruction from seasoned teacher–practitioners. At present (2017) in North America, there is no national professional college overseeing training or licensure, nor is there required universal compliance to ethical standards for mindfulness teachers. However, those who have developed some of the mindfulness-based protocols have devised criteria to determine a clinician's preparedness to use the respective protocol(s) and, in so doing, have outlined appropriate guidelines for certification. At present, it is incumbent on those institutions that are training mindfulness teachers to establish their specific criteria for certification.

There are meditation or mindfulness communities that offer teacher training and create their own set of ethical guidelines to which future mindfulness teachers must adhere. Some draw inspiration from Buddhist lay precepts as an ethical foundation for teachers. As an example, Spirit Rock Meditation Center, a well-established organization founded by Jack Kornfield in Northern California, has developed a Teacher Code of Ethics based on the five Buddhist precepts.

The need for such guidelines is explained on the Spirit Rock website as follows:

> We acknowledge that without the support of monastic vows and Asian customs, we have a need for clear Western guidelines. In keeping with this understanding, and for the long-term benefit of ourselves and the community at large, we, as lay teachers, agree to uphold the five lay training precepts. Furthermore, we have specifically expanded the scope of these five precepts to make them explicitly appropriate to our role as teachers of the Dharma in our specific cultural setting.

The five precepts are as follows:

1. We undertake the precept of refraining from killing.
2. We undertake the precept of refraining from stealing.
3. We undertake the precept of refraining from false speech.
4. We undertake the precept of refraining from sexual misconduct.
5. We undertake the precept of refraining from intoxicants that cause heedlessness or loss of awareness.

As indicated, these precepts are presented with commentary that attempts to adapt them to the needs of Western teachers and students.

In 2010, having identified the need to create and maintain standards for teacher's education, the UK Network for Mindfulness-Based Teacher Training Organizations presented practice guidelines for those teaching mindfulness-based courses. These are presented as "Good Practice Guidelines for Trainers of Mindfulness-Based Teachers." Some of their guidelines are as follows:

- Have had full teaching responsibility for at least nine mindfulness-based courses over a minimum of 3 years.
- Have trained to be a trainer via an apprenticeship with a more experienced trainer and demonstrated a competency in training others.
- Be in a regular supervisory relationship in relation to teaching practice and its interface with personal mindfulness practice, and engage in peer relationships with other trainers.
- Attend annual retreats that facilitate practice at depth, some of which are at least 7 to 10 days in duration.
- Stay up to date with the current and developing evidence base for mindfulness-based interventions, with a particular emphasis on the training organization's area of expertise.

The list also suggests "skills, understandings, and attitudes" in a number of teaching-related skills and competencies.

Mindfulness Meditation and Collaboration With Western Medicine

> The faculty of bringing back a wandering attention over and over again is the very root of judgment, character, and will. No one is *compos sui* if he have it not. An education that should improve this faculty would be the education par excellence. (p. 424)[15]

Kabat-Zinn was introduced to the ideas and practices of Buddhist meditation during his undergraduate and graduate studies and was influenced by the teachings of Phillip Kapleau (1912–2004), an American Zen Buddhist *Roshi* (teacher) and author of numerous books. Kabat-Zinn's formal practice commenced with Korean Zen master Seung Sahn (1927–2004) and continued at the Cambridge Zen Center. As his immersion in formal meditation practice deepened, Kabat-Zinn was struck by the following insight: "This was unbelievably powerful stuff that no one was looking at from a scientific point" (p. 2).[16]

As a scientist, Kabat-Zinn had the inclination and prescience to document his work methodically, which initiated interest in the practical applications of mindfulness and related practices in a wide variety of settings and for the treatment of a host of mind–body conditions. Indeed, what Kabat-Zinn and other researchers found, and what has been corroborated by 2,500 years of Buddhist phenomenological research, is that the practice of placing one's attention on an experiential anchor in the present moment (i.e., body and breath) and allowing thoughts, feelings, and sensations to arise without engaging them, allows a person to exercise a greater range of choice when responding to internal narratives, desires, urges, addictive behaviors, and the vicissitudes of life in general. In Buddhism, this exercised capacity is an integral component of "mental development" as referenced previously. Professor Baer echoed these observations: "Sustained, nonjudgmental observation of anxiety-related sensations, without attempts to escape or avoid them, may lead to reductions in the emotional reactivity typically elicited by anxiety symptoms" (p. 128).[17]

As a protocol, Kabat-Zinn's MBSR program is typically introduced to students as an 8- to 10-week program for groups of up to 30 participants, who commit to meeting for 2 to 3 hours a week. Examples of mindfulness techniques introduced in MBSR training are the body scan (a participant directs their attention through the body, cultivating increased proprioception), walking meditation, hatha yoga, diaphragmatic breathing, and seated meditation.

Initially, Kabat-Zinn's students were those presenting with a variety of ailments. The MBSR program has since been utilized by a wider audience seeking the benefits of relaxation and mental clarity. On the precedent of Kabat-Zinn's research, psychotherapists and researchers have developed the next generation of mindfulness techniques as an array of promising interventions and protocols that have been described as a "growing range of purpose-built adaptations for specific client groups" (p. 61).[18] These adaptations include MBCT, acceptance and commitment therapy (ACT), and dialectical behavior therapy (DBT), which will be explored in greater detail.

The growing body of evidence-based literature on mindfulness suggests that mindfulness interventions may lead to reductions in a variety of problematic conditions, including pain, stress, anxiety, depressive relapse, and disordered eating. Kabat-Zinn's abilities to see the potential efficacy of applied mindfulness in clinical environments and to publish his research set the stage for mindfulness to become a widely used, evidence-based, clinical intervention. Importantly, Kabat-Zinn also recognized that any reference to Buddhism might dissuade some of those who would potentially benefit from the practices. The decision to refrain from overt references to Buddhism has arguably contributed to the inclusion of mindfulness in secular institutions. It has also had the consequence of stripping mindfulness of the ancillary practices and teachings that have augmented it for the past 2,500 years. Nevertheless, the importance and potential of Buddhist practices were not lost on Kabat-Zinn. He suggested that the way forward may be to engage Buddhism not as religious doctrine or dogma but as a framework for mindfulness and supportive practices as human existential investigations concerned with the alleviation of suffering.

> One might think of dharma as a sort of universal generative grammar (Chomsky, 1965) an innate set of empirically testable rules that govern and describe the generation of the inward, first-person experiences of suffering and happiness in human beings. In that sense, dharma is at its core truly universal, not exclusively Buddhist. (p. 145)[19]

However flawed the latter statement may be, it does at the very least suggest that Buddhism continues to remain in conversation with the new dispensation of mindfulness. Next are brief descriptions of the next generation of mindfulness-based interventions. Although designed for unique client populations presenting with specific concerns, the following protocols hold in common an emphasis on shifting a client's relationship with maladaptive patterns by cultivating present-moment acceptance of arising experience.

Mindfulness-Based Cognitive Therapy

This is an 8-week intervention for a group of up to 12 participants. MBCT is based largely on Kabat-Zinn's model of the MBSR program and is adapted for individuals who have suffered with repeated bouts of depression and are vulnerable to recurring episodes. The MBCT protocol incorporates elements of cognitive behavioral therapy (CBT) with mindfulness strategies designed to cultivate a detached or decentered relationship to one's cognitive processes, feelings, and sensations. In this context, decentering suggests a capacity to observe and identify one's thoughts and feelings as impermanent phenomena arising in awareness that do not necessarily correspond to reality. Some authors argue that the aforementioned decentered relationship to one's thoughts, which they also describe as "metacognitive insight," coupled with a nonjudgmental stance facilitated by mindfulness practice may allow individuals to recognize and decrease engagement with ruminative patterns associated with episodic depression.

Dialectical Behavior Therapy

This is a comprehensive psychosocial approach to the treatment of borderline personality disorder (BPD), developed by Linehan. The approach emphasizes the equilibrium between acceptance and change, which is one of the reasons that DBT uses the Hegelian term and principle of "dialectical" progress. DBT utilizes CBTs, interpersonal effectiveness skills, emotional regulation, distress tolerance, and mindfulness practices to address emotional regulation, which is viewed as the central area of dysfunction in a BPD diagnosis. DBT introduces mindfulness as "psychological and behavioral versions of meditation skills usually taught in Eastern spiritual practices" aimed at "observing, describing, participating, taking a nonjudgmental stance, focusing on one thing in the moment, being effective" (p. 114).[20] DBT offers clients a range of mindfulness exercises, operationalized as three mindfulness "what" skills—observing, describing, and spontaneous participation—and three mindfulness "how" skills—nonjudgmentally, one-mindfully, and effectively. Thus, in DBT, mindfulness is viewed more as a set of adaptive skills rather than a formal meditation practice.

Acceptance and Commitment Therapy

This has its theoretical roots in contemporary behavior analysis and mindfulness and acceptance processes. ACT's therapeutic strategies result from a behavioral analysis of a client's challenges and are tailored to their individual needs (e.g., skills training, psychoeducation, problem solving). ACT employs interventions consistent with other mindfulness and acceptance skills; these include "contact with the present moment" and "acceptance and cognitive defusion or deliteralization" (disidentification from thoughts). The practice of "observing the self" teaches participants to recognize a witness or observing self, capable of noting the arising of somatic sensations, cognitive processes, and affect without reactivity and as manifestations separate from the observer.

Relapse Prevention

This is a cognitive behavioral intervention used to assist individuals who are being treated for a variety of substance abuse concerns. Mindfulness techniques are introduced to aid in coping with urges related to chronic substance use, conceptualized as an inability to accept the present moment, as one searches continually for the next intoxication. A mindfulness tool utilized in relapse prevention (RP) is "urge surfing," which likens urges to mounting ocean waves growing gradually to a crescendo then decreasing in intensity. A client's education includes "riding" waves (affective and physiological) with open nonjudgmental awareness, without succumbing to the urges. Inherent in this practice is the insight that, despite their intensity, urges are subject to impermanence and, thus, will arise, peak, and dissipate. Within the RP protocol, mindfulness skills offer clients the opportunity to observe urges nonjudgmentally as they arise and subside, thereby increasing the window of tolerance and introducing a growing range of choice and adaptive strategies.

Research and Future Directions

The exponential growth of mindfulness and its applications in personal and professional contexts and in an ever-growing variety of settings can be attributed to a number of concurrent factors. Mindfulness provides both clinicians and their clients with a praxis that includes ongoing research; a body of growing literature; applicable theories; psychoeducation; accessible practice tools; and, in some instances, the option of psychometric evaluation. Mindfulness also draws upon Buddhism's 2,500 years of insight into the human psyche and reliable tools for the alleviation of suffering. As functional interventions, mindfulness practices are adaptable to clients' needs and, thereby, empower them to experience the results of ongoing practice wherein individuals can phenomenologically evaluate efficacy (e.g., improved affect regulation, increased resilience and flexibility, and enhancement of adaptive skills).

As has been suggested previously in this chapter, contemporary use of mindfulness by clinicians and researchers, while serving an ever-growing spectrum of the population, has yet to engage fully the Buddhist tradition from which mindfulness is derived. Although this disavowing of the Buddhist tradition was done strategically to gain legitimacy and access to secular institutions, it can be argued that there is potential benefit in exploring how these practices could serve populations struggling to cultivate and maintain mental, emotional, and spiritual well-being.

The ongoing dialogue with the Buddhist tradition promises that mindfulness, used strictly as a clinical intervention, will be called upon to consider questions related to the larger project of the transformation of both individual human beings and human communities and culture. Thus, the scope of consideration is at once behavioral, economic, environmental, and beyond. In other words, Buddhism's response to suffering is systemic and revolutionary, as the historical Buddha arguably intended the dharma to be.

The work ahead requires great sensitivity. The challenge is how to maintain the systemic integrity of Buddhism while introducing insights and tools from the tradition that do not require individuals to become Buddhist but, nevertheless, offer benefits from 2,500 years of accumulated wisdom.

Conclusion

A promising future that embraces both challenges and opportunities will necessarily be inspired by integration. Integration invites the practice of mindfulness into our daily lives "on and off the cushion" and insists on the incorporation of ancillary practices, compassion, and ethical conduct so that engaged systemic practice informs both personal and professional lives. This promises a cultural shift in which the behavioral consequences of applied or integrated mindfulness become shared and encouraged community values. It is integration as well that is desired in joint explorations of the human mind, the work consisting of the creation of novel and shared languages across disciplines. Organizations like the Mind and Life Institute, founded in 1990 and described as "building a scientific understanding of the mind to reduce suffering and promote well-being," or the Nalanda Institute for Contemplative Science, founded in 1998 and offering "programs combining mind science with mind-training skills, to end stress, nurture happiness, and cultivate lives of sustainable well-being, compassion, and altruism," are portends of a collaborative future. They are auguries of opportunities that include both collaboration and integration, that summon accessible antidotes to suffering, embedded in the fabric of daily life.

Case Study

Melissa is a 23-year-old client who had recently completed her undergraduate studies and was involved in an automobile accident. She was the lone driver in a rural location and suffered minor physical injuries. Melissa identified as an independent and resilient person; this was her first experience of a major trauma. Melissa presented with symptoms congruent with a post-traumatic stress disorder (PTSD) diagnosis (see the *Diagnostic and Statistical Manual of Mental Disorders* [*DSM–5*] criteria for Posttraumatic Stress Disorder 309.81). Melissa had direct exposure to a traumatic event, as described in Criterion A. She reported instances of hypervigilance throughout the day and at times had interrupted sleep that would negatively impact her daytime functioning. Memories from the accident occasionally intruded Melissa's experiences, described in Criterion B as recurring involuntary distressing memories of the inciting traumatic event. Additionally, Melissa had developed some avoidant behaviors as described in Criterion C of a PTSD diagnosis; although Melissa was able to drive on her own, she was reticent to do so at night, particularly in rural areas. Melissa described an ongoing experience in which her agency and autonomy felt compromised. Melissa had applied to graduate school and expressed a strong desire to "have my life back."

(*Continued*)

(Continued)

During our first few sessions, I learned more about Melissa's personal life and professional goals, and we began to establish a therapeutic alliance. We spoke about introducing mindfulness-based tools that she could use to address the following concerns: symptom management and reduction as well as affect regulation and resilience. The agreed upon treatment plan included psychoeducation about trauma symptomatology and warning signs to be tracked and highlighted. I explained that mindfulness-based interventions enhanced metacognitive acuity, which could assist Melissa in managing emotional dysregulation by being present to her thoughts, feelings, and sensations as they arise, without attempting to alter or change them. Some of the practices introduced to Melissa were nourishing breath and slow–mindful breathing, which are described in trauma therapist Dana Moore's training manual "Yoga in Psychotherapy of Traumatized Clients: A Clinician's Toolbox" as follows[21]:

Nourishing breath is an opportunity for a person to relate to their body in a positive way. Participants or clients are invited to send oxygen to nourish every cell of their body with mindful intention. This simple self-care exercise requires very little physical or mental effort on the part of the participant. Slow–mindful breathing is a self-regulation practice. Moore wrote that it "slows down the respiration rate and focuses attention on the breathing process. Reducing the rate of respiration reduces the heart rate making this exercise a powerful self-regulation tool." The two latter practices provided an opportunity for Melissa to develop a relationship with sensation and breath that was comforting and calming. As mindfulness practices, they introduced an experience of present moment awareness without the need to be reactive or fearful. Between session practices were as follows:

- *Body scan meditation*—This allowed Melissa to become familiar with and tolerant of a fuller range of somatic sensations. This began in clinic with a titrated introduction, so Melissa could determine her level of comfort. The body scan was also done before sleep, which assisted her in maintaining consistent rest.
- *Sitting and walking meditation and Qigong (QG) practices*—These practices coordinated mind, body, and breath with stillness and simple movements and increased Melissa's agency and self-determination.
- *Journal*—Melissa recorded her insights related to therapy and chronicled what transpired when she felt anxiety—namely, what was arising cognitively, somatically, and affectively. This brought her experience of anxiety into conscious awareness and required Melissa to note the details of how it manifested.
- *Thoughts are just thoughts practice*—Melissa endeavored to note thoughts as passing clouds in the sky of awareness—noting that the observer (Melissa) witnessed thoughts but was separate from them. Melissa reported that this had the effect of decreasing reactivity.

When we met for sessions, we would check in about the efficacy of the practices and then build on Melissa's growing capacity to tolerate more intense affect and accompanying sensations. After about five sessions, Melissa reported that there had been a significant decrease in intrusive thoughts and images, and when they did occur, she was able to apply a number of antidotes that she had learned. Melissa was having longer hours of uninterrupted sleep and felt more present and nourished during the day. Building on Melissa's growing capacity to be present with her feelings and sensations, I introduced a practice that psychologist Ronald Siegel referred to as "mindfulness of anxiety in the body." We approached this as a form of exposure therapy and spoke about the practice beforehand to determine what would be comfortable for Melissa. The session began with basic seated mindfulness with attention placed on the natural breath. I asked Melissa to imagine driving in the country at night and then to notice and track how anxiety manifested cognitively and somatically and to be aware of narrative(s), image(s), and any feelings that accompanied the experience. My instructions followed Siegel's suggestion to approach the phenomena arising in awareness with an inner stance of nonjudgmental interest and curiosity. Rather than indulge a narrative or explore meaning of arising sensations, one is directed to observe them moment to moment. Additionally, I encouraged Melissa to remain present to what was happening in her body rather than avoid or attempt to make sensations cease. The combination of therapy, a variety of tailored mindfulness interventions, and Melissa's motivation made for steady progress, and after 9 weeks, she felt that she "had her life back." Although there were occasional experiences of anxiety, Melissa was able to address them in the moment and felt she had tools that would provide her with skills and resiliency to move ahead with her personal and professional goals.

The success of Melissa's treatment was a combination of psychoeducation, therapeutic alliance, and mindfulness tools (aimed at forming a nonreactive relationship with traumatic memory). This mindfulness-based approach allowed Melissa to manage distress by cultivating acceptance and building tolerance toward a spectrum of anxiety-related symptoms. The learned tools (i.e., mindful movements, breath work, body scan) created a foundation in which Melissa built capacity to be increasingly comfortable with a wider range of sensations (distress tolerance), which then allowed us to initiate exposure therapy. "Exposure" was not intended as a reexperiencing of the trauma-inducing incident but as an opportunity to shift her relationship to thoughts, feelings, and sensations via a cultivated metacognitive awareness. As such, avoidance and resistance decreased as Melissa's window of tolerance grew. On the continuum to acceptance was Melissa's growing capacity to be present to what arose in the moment with decreased reactivity. The mindful-based interventions, while effective for the therapeutic process, were also useful as life tools to facilitate greater choice, creativity, and agency.

DISCUSSION QUESTIONS

1. What is the context and purpose of mindfulness meditation in a traditional Buddhist context?
2. Identify three different benefits of mindfulness that are potentially useful in clinical work.
3. How do secular, clinical, and traditional applications of mindfulness meditation compare and contrast?
4. How are the historical Buddha's teaching of the Four Noble Truths, which describe the causes and cessation of suffering, relevant for present-day psychotherapists?

REFERENCES

1. Bishop, S., Lau, M., Shapiro, S., Carlson, L., Anderson, N. D., Carmody, J., . . . Devins, G. (2004). Mindfulness: A proposed operational definition. *Clinical Psychology: Science & Practice*, *11*(3), 230–241.
2. Ibid.
3. Ibid.
4. Gethin, R. (2011). On some definitions of mindfulness. *Contemporary Buddhism*, *12*(1), 263–279.
5. Williams, P. (with Tribe, A.). (2000). *Buddhist thought: A complete introduction to the Indian tradition*. New York, NY: Routledge.
6. Wallace, B. A. (1998). *The bridge of quiescence: Experiencing Tibetan Buddhist meditation*. Peru, IL: Carus Publishing Company.
7. Bhikkhu, T. (Trans.). (2000). *Maha-satipatthana Sutta: The great frames of reference* (DN 22). Retrieved from http://www.accesstoinsight.org/tipitaka/dn/dn.22.0.than.html
8. Ibid.
9. Ibid.
10. Wallace, A. (2008, Spring). A mindful balance. *Tricycle: The Buddhist Review*.
11. Kabat-Zinn, J. (1994). *Wherever you go there you are*. London, England: Piatkus.
12. Bishop et al., Mindfulness.
13. Sangyé Gyatso, D. (2010). *Mirror of Beryl: A historical introduction to Tibetan medicine* (G. Kilty, Trans.). Boston, MA: Wisdom Publications.
14. Yeats, W. B. (1902). *The Celtic twilight*. London, England: A. H. Bullen.
15. James, W. (1950). *The principles of psychology* (Vol. 1). Queens, NY: Dover Publications (Original work published 1890)
16. Pintak, L. (1999, September). Jon Kabat-Zinn: The prescription is meditation. *Shambhala Sun*. Retrieved from www.shambhalasun.com/index.php?option=content&task=view&id=1859&Itemid=244&limit=1&limitstart=1
17. Baer, R. A. (2003). Mindfulness training as a clinical intervention: A conceptual and empirical review. *Clinical Psychology: Science and Practice*, *10*, 125–143.
18. Mace, C. (2008). *Mindfulness and mental health: Therapy, theory, and science*. London, England: Routledge.
19. Kabat-Zinn, J. (2003). Mindfulness-based interventions in context: Past, present, and future. *Clinical Psychology: Science & Practice*, *10*, 144–156.
20. Linehan, M. M. (1993). *Cognitive-behavioral treatment of borderline personality disorder*. New York, NY: Guilford Press.
21. Moore, Dana (2013). Yoga in Psychotherapy of Traumatized Clients: A Clinician's Toolbox. In B. van der Kolk & D. Moore (Eds), Frontiers of Trauma Treatment.

SUGGESTED READINGS

Chödrön, P. (2013). *How to meditate: A practical guide to making friends with your mind*. Louisville, CO: Sounds True.

This is an excellent book for those interested in beginning and maintaining a daily meditation practice. The book provides easy-to-follow, step-by-step instructions on the basics of meditation with practical insights and suggestions for skillfully relating with one's mind, emotions, and sense perceptions. The book presents approaches to obstacles that are at once practical and transformative.

Germer, C. K., Siegel, R. D., & Fulton, P. R. (2005). *Mindfulness and psychotherapy.* New York, NY: Guilford Press.

This book presents a comprehensive introduction to mindfulness as a clinical intervention from the perspective of seasoned practitioners. It is replete with reviews of research, case examples, and practices. Various mindfulness applications are explored for a variety of presenting symptoms. Mindfulness is also presented as a tool for the practicing psychotherapist to increase empathy and presence in the therapeutic relationship.

Gunaratana, H. (2001). *Eight mindful steps to happiness: Walking the path of the Buddha.* Boston, MA: Wisdom Publications.

The Buddha's Eightfold Path aimed at the cessation of suffering is presented in accessible language with key points highlighted at the end of each chapter. This is an important book for those who wish to understand the systemic context in which mindfulness was intended to be practiced.

Siegel, D. J. (2010). *Mindsight: The new science of personal transformation.* New York, NY: Bantam Books.

Siegel cites research and examples from his own practice to argue that we can learn to change the wiring and architecture of our brains. Compelling evidence suggests that human behavior is not hardwired and that we can use our mind to transform our brain and behaviors. Siegel's book is a groundbreaking contribution toward the integration of neuroscience and the practice of psychotherapy.

PART C

Asian Healing Traditions and Their Contemporary Formulations

10 Chinese Taoist Cognitive Psychotherapy

Yu-ping Cao, Jie Zeng, and Ya-lin Zhang

Introduction

Chinese Taoist cognitive psychotherapy (CTCP) is derived from Taoism, the ancient philosophy of Chinese culture, to cultivate mental health and well-being. CTCP manages to organize the core principles of Taoist principles in an organic way with respect to cultural roots as well as awareness of acceptability and adherence in clinical practice. It was first practiced in China in 1998 by psychotherapists Zhang and Young at the Hunan Medical University (in China) as therapeutic solutions in patients with mental illness such as depression, anxiety, and other neuroses.[1] It has evolved to be an efficient and effective way in treating Chinese patients.

In order to understand the essence of CTCP, one should first understand Taoism. The learning journey is like hiking into a mysterious cave for mountainous treasure. Taoism opens the gate to the secret of life, promotes the idea that human beings are an integral part of nature and the universe, and enables people to face fearlessly their problems with calmness and courage. Also, it behooves individuals to follow the natural order by returning to our original state of innocence. Therefore, its role in solace and guidance particularly during times of crisis is undeniable.

Brief History of Chinese Taoist Cognitive Psychotherapy

According to Laozi (or Lao-Tzu), the founder of Taoism, the Tao is the essence of the world—it is impossible to recognize, but it is also impossible to deny. He made a convincing and detailed case by considering the proposition that one should shut out from sight the things of desire in order to protect one's mind from disturbances. As stated in Taoism, "Man models himself after the earth; the earth models itself after heaven; the heaven models itself after Tao; and Tao models itself after nature."[2]

Taoism has a long history in China. In the 3rd century BC, during the time of the matriarchal dynastic tribes, early Taoist concepts such as the interconnectedness and unity of individuals, nature, and the universe were recorded. Laozi consolidated these teachings into a cohesive philosophical theory: Taoism.

Taoism could be regarded as a feminine counterpart to the masculine energy of Confucianism. Confucianism, which is based on the Northern Chinese culture and focuses on social hierarchies and collective responsibility, promotes a view of the individual as an active change agent with the key points of values of self-reliance, persistence, courageousness, assertiveness, moral development, Confucian self-cultivation, professional achievement, and man's control over nature, while Taoism emphasizes the easy enjoyment of life's pleasure, the development of a flexible personality, and conformity to natural laws. Actually, Chinese culture has been shaped, to a large extent, by philosophical influences of both Taoism and Confucianism; many other East Asian cultures have also been influenced by the imprint of the two philosophies. How could the ancient wisdom of Taoism leave its imprint on contemporary culture? Taoism is like the gentle bamboo or the grass in the field, or as soft as water. Yet its vitality is like its philosophy: The soft could beat the strong, and to retreat is to advance. Therefore, it moves along with the wind and the rain, surviving thousands of years. There appears to be many reasons for the increasing enthusiasm toward Taoism—especially in today's competitive society. Admittedly, **Confucian self-cultivation** for glorying one's country is seen as one of the main Confucian values that has contributed to social, economic, and psychological development, but individual and social improvements cannot always be handled in a smooth and linear fashion.

How can human beings achieve such enviable freedom from setbacks, challenges, and reversals during periods of unpredictable stress and strain? In Tao, the nameless is the origin of heaven and earth; the named is the mother of all things. Taoism urges individuals to empty their minds, feed their hunger, discourage their ambitions, and strengthen their frames so that people may be exempt from knowledge and desires. One shall not scheme and contend, and our energy will connect to the greater universe with stability and comfort, exempting us from the stresses and illness of everyday life, which comes to the final essence of Tao "may all live in peace."[3]

After observing the ways in which Taoist-based coping was organically invoked in psychotherapy sessions with Chinese culture background, Zhang and Young developed CTCP as a culturally grounded cognitive therapy.[4] Embracing the essence of Taoism, CTCP has been applied clinically for the treatment of patients with neurotic and psychosomatic disorders. Preliminary trials, qualitative or quantitative, have demonstrated superior effects of CTCP in hundreds of patients over time compared to medications alone.[5]

It's a long story: Zhang, a PhD candidate under the mentorship of Young, engaged in a journey of theory and technique of psychotherapy that could bear the imprint of Chinese social and cultural milieu, because they realized that "Western products" could sometimes be problematic for patient in eastern countries.[6] They found that the principle of Taoism, "living in harmony with the greater universe to ease the mind, loosen the stress, alleviate the pain, strengthen the body and stabilize the emotion," fitted well with the therapeutic goal of clients who were in need of psychotherapy. CTCP, through the 32-word mnemonic (discussed later) and representing the subtle wisdom and depth of Taoism, was used to develop an indigenous psychotherapy and a Chinese specific healing approach that offered a culturally grounded alternative to standard mental health interventions.

Cultural Representations of Illness and Wellness

The definition of wellness in mental health has strong ties with traditional culture in Taoism. Although it seems hard to understand doctrines such as "perfectly good is like water which benefits everything by giving without taking, therefore wellness in mind is for those advocates with virtue of noncontention," noncontention refers to being simple and plain, selfless by controlling or subduing one's desire or personal profit. One needs to keep in mind why the old master Laozi succeeded in passing the divine law down many generations. To be free from desire, one could understand the internal mystery of the infinite law and observe the external manifestations.

Mental weakness or mind illness in Taoism means insatiable desire, uncontrollable interference, inordinate contention, or excessive contentment. According to Taoism, the hardest thing in the world may be the weakest, the purified mental mirror may be blemished, the rare goods may tempt one to do bad acts, and the praise and blame would make one's mind go up and down. These are just a few examples of "weakness" according to Taoism. On a large scale, the visible scene, the audible sound, and the tangible touch are all sources of illness in daily life. With the emphasis of an easy enjoyment of life's pleasures, the development of a flexible personality, acceptance over action, and conformity to natural laws even during periods of stress and strain, peace, stability, and comfort could be regarded as wellness.

Current Ways in Which Chinese Taoist Cognitive Psychotherapy Is Practiced

The aim of CTCP is to regulate patients' negative affection, correct maladaptive behavior, and treat mental health problems by changing personal mode of thinking and style of coping with troubles in life through Taoist values. It takes extraordinary steps to save one's spirits with respect to nature. Therefore, one strips oneself of passion in order to see the secret of life; one regards life with passion in order to see its manifest forms.

In the clinical application, CTCP involves five steps, summarized as ABCDE—A: to find actual stress factors; B: to understand belief and value system; C: to analyze conflicts and coping styles; D: to imbue doctrine of Taoism; and E: to evaluate effect and reinforcement. It is like pumping the fresh water of the Tao wisdom into the therapy.[7]

1. A. *Actual stress factors*—In this initial assessment phase, the patient is helped to identify and analyze the actual stressors connected with their illness.

2. B. *Belief and value system*—Next, the patient's core beliefs and values are systematically analyzed with regard to their role in mediating the affective and behavioral impact of life stressors. The practitioner discusses how a change in value orientation can also produce a change in one's emotional and behavioral reaction to stressful events.

3. C. *Conflict and coping style*—After evaluating the patient's actual stressors and core values and beliefs, analysis proceeds to his or her psychological conflicts and coping style. Since it is virtually impossible for an individual's needs to be perfectly fulfilled, one either has to change the reality of one's circumstances or alter one's desires. If neither of these is feasible, psychological conflicts will inevitably arise and necessitate the use of coping strategies. The relative usefulness of these coping methods is evaluated in this stage of the treatment.

4. D. *Doctrine of Taoism—Direction and practice*—This is the therapeutic core of CTCP. In this stage, the patient is instructed in the 32-character Taoist formula and guided in applying its principles to reframe his or her psychological conflicts and approach to coping. The first eight characters, '*li er bu hai, wei er bu zheng*' (利而不害, 为而不争), are interpreted as benefiting without hurting others and acting without striving. The second set of eight characters, '*shao si gua yu, zhi zu zhi zhi*' (少私寡欲, 知足知止), emphasizes restricting selfish desires, learning to be content, and knowing how to let go. The third set of eight characters, '*zhi he chu xia, yi rou sheng gang*' (知和处下, 以柔胜刚), refers to the importance of humility and interpersonal harmony and using softness to defeat hardness. The final set of eight characters, '*qing jing wu wei, shun qi zi ran*' (清净无为, 顺其自然), is the central tenet of Taoism. It suggests that a person should cultivate tranquility, practice inaction, and align one's will with the laws of nature. The patient is helped to grasp as well as put the principles into practice in daily life. Patients are required to keep a journal in which they practice applying the doctrine in the context of their psychosocial difficulties.

5. E. *Effect evaluation and reinforcement*—In the final stage, the effectiveness of the treatment is evaluated with regard to symptom reduction and functional status as well the patient's subjective experience. Treatment gains are solidified through review of core treatment components and application of principles to current stressors.

Training and Development, Supervisions, Accreditation, Licensure, and Certification

Formal academic or professional training programs in counseling and clinical psychology had not yet become widespread in China until the last decade of the 20th century. For various reasons, academic programs in clinical or counseling psychology could not be established until the end of the Cultural Revolution.[8] Even in the past 10 years, considered as the "booming years" in the development of psychotherapy in Western countries, there were only 10 institutions reported having a graduate training program in clinical psychology or a related field (e.g., medical psychology) in mainland China—1 was in a university, 1 was in an academic institute, and 8 were in medical schools—according to the national survey conducted in the 1990s.[9]

Professional training, supervision, accreditation, licensure, and certification sprang up only at the end of 1990s. At that time, clinical and counseling psychology in mainland China began to emerge as distinct subspecialties. CTCP training was established at the same time, with various programs such as clinical use, psychological training, and professional education. Things have changed since the early 21st century: Several formal training programs in CTCP have been established and widely accepted in the field. The training courses were designed in accordance with the standards of other therapeutic trainings. Over the past 10 years, programs, courses, and public presentations have promulgated CTCP to become a recognized strategy in the field of psychotherapy in China, and its standard practice had spread all over the country. In 2014, the CTCP training program, as one of Chinese advanced continuous training programs, was launched in the Second Xiangya Hospital of Central South University attracting many of professionals' attention. The program is running under systematic supervision professionals conducting CTCP. All speakers for the training have at least 5 years of CTCP clinical experiences. And many of them have pursued continuing education in supervisory skills. Since then, a system for registering qualified supervisors has been developed, and criterion of specialized training and education has been established.

Although professional guidelines and requirements of CTCP for clinical use have been instituted since its first emergence, the actual counseling practice varies according to the reality in the past two decades. One possible explanation could be that insufficient therapists obtain formal supervision when facing an increasing need for supervision. Especially, the practice of psychotherapy and counseling is a relatively new phenomenon in China; training tends to focus more on theory and clinical technique and less on supervisory skills. Self-evaluation, self-learning, and peer supervision may serve as alternatives. Additionally, integration into the academic curriculum of programs in clinical psychology, medical psychology, education, and social work would lead to new paradigm in future CTCP training. Over time, these changes will elevate the quality of supervision in China and the standard of clinical practice in CTCP.

Strengths, Weaknesses, Opportunities, and Challenges

As a newly sprouted psychotherapy, the strengths, weaknesses, opportunities, and threats (SWOT) of CTCP in counseling and practicing all over China are still too early to be appraised.

A significant merit is that the emergence of CTCP fills the need for a modern Chinese indigenous psychotherapeutic worldview. For a long time, the dominant counseling and psychotherapy schools in China continued to be those originating in the West, such as cognitive behavioral therapy (CBT), psychoanalysis, person-centered therapy, family therapy, and so on.

Since China's unique cultural and philosophical traditions argue for a more contextually grounded approach to counseling and psychotherapy, CTCP has inspired adaptations and innovations in clinical theory and practice. It describes the essence of Tao, which creatively acts by the rule to benefit oneself and directly demonstrates the core "as being simple and plain, being selfless and desireless, being unlearned and unworried."[10]

Due to the culture-specific elements in counseling and psychotherapy, greater understanding of the universal and culture-specific elements of effective clinical practice could be accessible to both the practitioners and the clients. Since culture shapes one's thoughts, values, and behaviors, culturally grounded forms of counseling and psychotherapy in CTCP could be much more readily accepted and likely to be effective.

One obvious weakness is the growing demand for counseling and psychotherapy of CTCP services, agencies, or clinics, leading to an uneven quality of CTCP performance across mental health care facilities. Although access to training in CTCP has improved as a result of national and international collaborations, relatively few academic and professional books or training materials exist to provide further guidance or instruction to the practitioners. As a result of support from the Ministry of Science and Technology of the People's Republic of China in 2010, a 5-year plan had been launched under the leadership of Zhang and Cao to encourage the researching, teaching, and learning of different psychotherapies including CTCP. It could be anticipated that trained CTCP professionals would fill some gap of the need and supply in the near future.

From ancient times to the present era, the essence of Taoism has not faded away. Instead, it is deeply rooted in the Chinese social and cultural foundation. With the increases of stresses accompanied by a greater willingness to seek professional help in the competitive society and culture, CTCP has encountered a tipping point for becoming a superior choice for Chinese individuals. The growth of CTCP over the past 20 years has opened a window to show a nationality-specific psychotherapy for the peers in the West. Secondly, because the ideas and practices of CTCP served as sources of inspiration, wisdom, and guidance of life, the societal trends offered rich opportunities for the continued development of a model of CTCP practice. Officially, CTCP was brought into the psychological treatment norm by the National Health and Family Planning Commission of the People's Republic of China in 2013. That is to say, CTCP has been allowed to be practiced under an international framework. This is tailored to the needs of the Chinese cultural context in the Western world. It is very encouraging to the Chinese practitioners, whether they are from a rural village in Hunan or the bustling metropolis of Shanghai. The growth of recognition of CTCP is the result of renewed interest in traditional Chinese culture as well as the practical utility of CTCP.

However, it is also important to recognize that Chinese society is rapidly evolving, integrating and reformulating cultural influences from a variety of sources. Clearly, patients' expectations and preferences for counseling and therapy are also changing over from time to time, as evidenced by the psychotherapy surveys conducted by Gong and Li in 1997 and Qian in 2008.[11]

A number of important tasks remain. A standardized licensure and certification process for clinical and counseling psychologists in CTCP has yet to be realized. At present, more efforts need to be taken by the cooperation of different organizations, such as the Ministry of Labor and Social Security, the Ministry of Health, and the Chinese Psychological Society, to develop a standard training curriculum and qualified training, education, and supervision system. Hence, a modern model of therapeutic practice in CTCP will be contextually grounded and standardized with integration of different approaches as a standard, centralized system of training, licensure, and certification system of CTCP.

The second core challenge for CTCP will be cultivating a Chinese-centered approach to counseling practice in the midst of ample cross-cultural training opportunities and international research collaborations. It is of much interest to experts to mutually learn therapeutic techniques from each other. However, practitioners' bias toward Western models of practice has led to the relative neglect of traditional Chinese medicine (TCM) and traditional Chinese philosophy as sources of therapeutic ideas. Therefore, a key direction for the field is to define and consider the value of the culturally grounded approach of CTCP as an efficient and effective tool for counseling and psychotherapy.

Research and Future Direction

CTCP was initially proved to be applicable in the field of neurosis, such as anxiety, and was also used in Chinese immigrants with anxiety in New York.[12] Randomized controlled trials were also conducted to probe into the interventional effect of CTCP on type A behavior of patients with coronary heart disease (CHD).[13] Patients in the control group underwent mere drug treatment, and those in the psychotherapy group received both medication and CTCP. Comparison of scoring of the type A behavior questionnaire (TABQ) and mental detachment scale and incidence of type A behavior before and after therapy in patients displayed significant decrease of the scores of TABQ and higher scores of mental detachment. This will lead to increased therapeutic effect and improvement of the prognosis of CHD sufferers.

In the treatment of poststroke depression (PSD), researchers found the effects of CTCP together with fluoxetine (20 mg/d) to be better improvement of scores on the Hamilton Depression Rating Scale (HAM-D), Modified Edinburgh–Scandinavian Stroke Scale (MESSS), and activities of daily living (ADL) than conventional medication only, as well as with patients with generalized anxiety disorder (GAD).[14] To evaluate the curative effect of the combined CTCP with medication for hypertension, Wang, Zhang, Huang, Wang, and Long found the score of *N* in the Eysenck Personality Questionnaire (EPQ), the scores of somatization and anxiety factors, total score in Symptom Checklist-90 (SCL-90), and the total score of TABQ in the combined strategy group were all reduced with statistical significance compared with the other group with medication only.[15] In a study of CTCP, which focused on the treatment of depression in late life, the patients in the group with CTCP combined with mianserin showed a significantly higher response rate than those on mianserin only.[16] CTCP was also found to be somewhat effective in the prevention of cognitive impairment following cerebral infarction.[17]

Cognitive task analysis (CTA) is a qualitative approach that is being used by some researchers in China to explore cognitive processes occurring during psychotherapy sessions.[18] CTA focuses on the cognitive elements involved in the process of performing a task effectively. Such elements include mapping the sequence of thoughts when the operator completes the task and acquires the knowledge needed in order to increase task competence; alternatively, the analysis may also identify cognitive deficits that may impede task performance.

Conclusion

Since the birth of CTCP, its service has been improved significantly as a result of increased public demand and governmental support over the past

20 years. Leaders in the field are working to increase the professionalism, normalization, localization, and globalization of Chinese counseling and psychotherapy with promising results. As stated in Taoism, "cautious, like crossing a wintry stream; irresolute, like one facing danger all around; grave, like one acting as guest; self-effacing, like ice beginning to melt; genuine, like a piece of undressed wood; open-minded, like a valley, And mixing freely, like murky water," the future of CTCP is a mix of caution, resolution, graveness, self-effacement, genuineness, and open-mindedness to realize the Tao in a psychotherapeutic way.[19]

Case Study

Mao is a 42 year old Chinese male who is single. He works as a police officer in Shanghai. Mao presented with boredom, restlessness, uncontrollable anxiety, loss of appetite, and sleeplessness. He has been experiencing some or all of these symptoms for a little more than a year. He also indicated that he experiences excessive worries about his physical health and mental situation, which he said is affecting his life and work. During therapy, more associated symptoms were revealed, as follows: feeling restless or feeling keyed up or on edge, being easily fatigued, irritability, and having muscle tension. Mao self-reported that he is free of headache, hallucination, delusion, or emotional fluctuation.

Mao graduated as a police officer from the police academy with a bachelor's degree and was promoted to mid-level in his department a year before therapy began. He stated that he did not experience any obvious working stress or burden in this position. He lived alone in an urban area and reported himself as being a bachelor, with no recent sexual contacts or recreational drug use. He drank alcohol rarely but was a heavy smoker—about 20 cigarettes a day. His medical history included fatty liver and lumbar degenerative change. His family history revealed that no one in his family has mental illness. Mao presented to a psychiatric outpatient clinic in a tertiary care hospital. The physical examination was unremarkable. According to the *Diagnostic and Statistical Manual of Mental Disorders, Fifth Edition* (*DSM–5*), the patient had been diagnosed with unspecified anxiety disorder under the *Structured Clinical Interview for DSM-5 (SCID-5)*. His medications included escitalopram, citalopram, mirtazapine, trazodone, buspirone, alprazolam, and lorazepam in previous months without any complaints of adverse effects related to the medications; no obviously favorable turn was noticed. Mao asked for a combined therapy of both medication and psychotherapy. No significant negative taboo was observed for Chinese Taoist cognitive psychotherapy (CTCP).

Mao undertook CTCP through five stages:

1. *Actual stress factors* (60–90 min.)—In this initial assessment phase, Mao was helped to identify and analyze the actual stressors connected with his illness. He admitted excessive worries about possible poor performance at work, helpless life without a partner when he is older, potential financial disaster, or sudden loss in daily life.
2. *Belief and value system* (40–60 min.)—Next, Mao's core beliefs and values were systematically analyzed with regard to their roles in mediating the affective and

(*Continued*)

(Continued)

behavioral impact of his life stressors. The three most important things in Mao's life were (1) integrated family, (2) financial stability, and (3) respectable social status.

3. *Conflict and coping style* (40–60 min.)—After evaluating Mao's actual stressors and core values and beliefs, analysis proceeded to his psychological conflicts and coping style. Mao desired a harmony bond as family members usually show, though he was single for more than 10 years. He valued economic stability as a key aspect in his life; however, he was afraid to take any risk financially or at work. He pursued and desired an honored status in his social life, wanting to move up the social ladder, all the while hesitating to get into a fight because of some possible failure. Mao exhibited a tendency to use self-punishment, self-depression, and self-denial as coping styles. Since it is virtually impossible for an individual's needs to be perfectly fulfilled, Mao either had to change the reality of his circumstances or alter his desires. If neither of these is feasible, psychological conflicts will inadvertently arise and necessitate the use of coping strategies.

4. *Doctrine direction and practice* (100–120 min.)—*"Li er bu hai, wei er bu zheng"* (利而不害, 为而不争) attempted to help Mao to understand being a better person did not mean hurting others or sacrificing oneself, even without striving. *"Shao si gua yu, zhi zu zhi zhi"* (少私寡欲, 知足知止) emphasizes that he should not be too ambitious for unrealistic aims but learn to be content and know how to let go. *"Zhi he chu xia, yi rou sheng gang"* (知和处下, 以柔胜刚) refers to the importance of humility and interpersonal harmony and using softness to defeat hardness, especially when Mao planned to establish a relationship in personal life and work. *"Qing jing wu wei, shun qi zi ran"* (清净无为, 顺其自然) is the central tenet of Taoism. It smooths the feeling of Mao that once he does what he should, there is nothing to regret or to be afraid of or to be blamed for. Step 4 is repeated three times to reinforce the Taoist concepts.

5. *Effect evaluation and reinforcement* (45–60 min.)—After the combined usage of CTCP and sertraline (started at 50 mg/d), the psychiatric complaints were ameliorated. The effectiveness of the treatment was evaluated with regard to symptom reduction and functional status as well as the patient's subjective experience. Treatment gains were solidified through review of core treatment components and application of principles to current stressors.

Mao was well-educated with advocacy of Chinese traditional culture, which made him a suitable applicant for CTCP. He exhibited stresses that were derived from unrealistic beliefs toward reality, such as yearning for love but failing to express and accept love or desiring and wanting a better life but lacking enough stimulation or forces to engage with life. This created in him a conflicting coping style that resulted in him experiencing much compressed pressures, as well as exhausting himself into anxiety and depression. Cognition reconstruction from CTCP turned the original values into new ones. For example, Mao began to recognize the reality of his situation and tried a "let it go" principle to help him in his aim-making process toward a final achievement, thereby forming a positive loop. Here we can see that the relationship of the five steps in CTCP is not just a one-way street but more like gear and wheel, where the components influence each other at different time points and multifunctions in his inner world. Finally, CTCP helped Mao cultivate tranquility, practice inaction, and align his will with the laws of nature under the framework of Taoism.

DISCUSSION QUESTIONS

1. The essence of Tao is difficult to teach and understand for its classic Chinese writing style, but the performance of CTCP has proved to be teachable. Is it possible to replicate this by integrating traditional philosophical ideas with modern therapeutic techniques?
2. Is there any difference between Eastern Tao practitioners and Western ones?
3. CTCP is born of an integration of Eastern philosophical culture and Western psychotherapeutic framework; could it be seen as a representative of cultural mergence?
4. How could Western culture reform Taoism?

REFERENCES

1. Zhang, Y. L., & Young, D. (1998). The cognitive psychotherapy according to Taoism: A technical brief introduction. *Chinese Mental Health Journal*, *12*, 188–190. (in Chinese); Zhang, Y., Young, D., Lee, S., Zhang, H., Xiao, Z., Hao, W., . . . Zhang, Y. (2002). Chinese Taoist cognitive psychotherapy in the treatment of generalized anxiety disorder in contemporary China. *Transcultural Psychiatry*, *39*, 115–129.
2. Zhang & Young, The cognitive psychotherapy.
3. Ibid.
4. Ibid.
5. Zhang et al., Chinese Taoist cognitive psychotherapy.
6. Zhang, Q. H. (Ed.). (2003). *Dao De Jing*. Beijing, China: Times and Literature Publishing House; Tseng, W. S. (1999). Culture and psychotherapy: Review and practical guidelines. *Transcultural Psychiatry*, *36*, 131–179; Young, D. (1996). Chinese people's mind and Chinese specific psychotherapy. In W. S. Tseng (Ed.), *Chinese people's mind and therapy* (pp. 417–435). Taiwan: Gueiguan.
7. Zhang et al., Chinese Taoist cognitive psychotherapy.
8. Qian, M. (2002). Psychotherapy in Asia: China. In A. Pritz (Ed.), *Globalized psychotherapy* (pp. 465–479). Vienna, Austria: Facultas Verlags-und Buchhandels AG.
9. Chang, D. F., Tong, H., Shi, Q., & Zeng, Q. (2005). Letting a hundred flowers bloom: Counseling and psychotherapy in the People's Republic of China. *Journal of Mental Health Counseling*, *27*, 104–116; Gong, Y. X., & Li, Q. Z. (1997). The survey and analysis on current training of clinical psychology as a profession in China. *Chinese Journal of Clinical Psychology*, *5*(1), 1–7. (in Chinese)
10. Zhang & Young, The cognitive psychotherapy.
11. Gong & Li, The survey and analysis on current training; Qian, Psychotherapy in Asia.
12. Zhang et al., Chinese Taoist cognitive psychotherapy; Xiao, S. Y., Young, D. S., & Zhang, H. G. (1998). Taoist cognitive psychotherapy for neurotic patients:

A preliminary clinical trial [Suppl.]. *Journal of Psychiatry and Clinical Neurosciences*, *52*, S238–S241. (in Chinese); Chang D. F., Hung, T., Ng, N., Ling A., Chen, T., Cao, Y. P., & Zhang, Y. L. (in press). Taoist cognitive therapy: Treatment of generalized anxiety disorder in a Chinese immigrant woman. *Asian American Journal of Psychology*,

13. Zhu, J. F., Young, D. S., Xiao, S. Y., & Liu, S. X. (2005). The improvement of the coronary heart disease patients' A type behavior by Daoistic cognitive therapy. *Chinese Mental Health Journal*, *19*, 553–556. (in Chinese)
14. Wang, J. P., & Xu, J. (2005). Effects of Taoist cognitive psychotherapy in the treatment of post-stroke depression. *Chinese Journal of Behavioral Medical Science*, *14*(6), 490–421; Zhang, Y. L., Zhao, J. P., Yang, D. S., Lu, X. H., Zhang, X. J., & Cao, Y. P. (2000). A longitudinal study of monoamine neurotransmitters, neuroendocrine and immune parameter in the patients with generalized anxiety disorder. *Chinese Journal of Psychiatry*, *33*(14), 200–202.
15. Wang, G. Q., Zhang, Y. L., Huang, G. P., Wang, X. M., & Long, X. (2007). Randomly control study on nonage hypertension with the combined Tao cognition therapy with medication. *Chinese Journal of Clinical Psychology*, *15*(3), 326–328.
16. Yang, J. Q., Zhao, L. M., & Mai, X. L. (2005). A comparative study of Taoist cognitive psychotherapy from and mianserin in the treatment of depression in late life. *Journal of Nervous Mental Disease*, *31*(5), 333–335. (in Chinese)
17. Wang, Y. Q., Song,Y. C., & He, R. (2009). Effects of Taoistic cognitive psychotherapy on the prevention of cognitive impairment following cerebral infarction. *Nursing Journal*, *24*(1), 41–42.
18. Ai, X. Q., Cao, Y. P., & Zhang, Y. L. (2012). Clinical research methods of psychotherapy. *Chinese Mental Health Journal*, *20*(1), 125–128; Zhang, J., & Yang, Y. C. (2009). A self-analysis psychotherapy model and its qualitative research framework. *Medicine and Philosophy*, *6*, 49–51. (in Chinese)
19. Zhang & Young, The cognitive psychotherapy.

SUGGESTED READINGS

Liao, W. (2011). *Nine nights with the Taoist master: Deluxe study edition.* Oak Park, IL: Taichi Tao Productions.

The book illustrates the *Tao Te Ching* with stories making it understandable, fun, and interesting to read.

Wong, E. (Trans.). (1992). *Cultivating stillness: A Taoist manual for transforming body and mind.* Boston, MA: Shambhala Publications.

The book explains the alchemical symbolism of the text and the methods for cultivating internal stillness of body and mind.

Wong, E. (2011). *Taoism: An essential guide.* Boston, MA: Shambhala Publications.

The great depth and diversity of Taoist spirituality is introduced in a single, accessible manual in this book.

Zhao, Q. (2010). *Do nothing and do everything: An illustrated new Taoism.* St. Paul, MN: Paragon House.

This book is a near-perfect supplement for anyone who finds the unique tenets of traditional mountain-born Taoism appealing or relevant in their lives.

11 Acceptance and Commitment Therapy and Asian Thought

Kenneth Fung and Zhuo-Hong Zhu

Worldviews can vary widely among cultures with implications in the understanding of suffering, healing, and recovery. Compared to the West, Eastern values place more emphasis on acceptance, harmony, and indirect coping than mastery, control, and active coping strategies, with the former sometimes perceived as inferior coping due to cultural bias.[1] On the other hand, newer forms of evidence-based, **third-wave behavioral psychotherapies** have in common the explicit use of acceptance as well as mindfulness.[2] This includes dialectical behavior therapy (DBT) for borderline personality disorder (BPD), mindfulness-based cognitive therapy (MBCT) for chronic depression, and acceptance and commitment therapy (ACT), which is the focus of this chapter.

ACT is based on an underlying scientific philosophy, *functional* contextualism.[3] The root metaphor in contextualism is an "act in context," with the premise that any action cannot be separated from its context, including its history and environment. The truth criterion is "workability" in a pragmatic sense, with the stated analytic goal of being able to predict and influence events. From this perspective, typical psychological theories emphasize structure and mechanism, focusing on identifying "broken" or "defective" thoughts and feelings in need of repair or replacement. From a functional contextualist perspective, the aim of therapy is instead on influencing functioning through the manipulation of context.

Based on functional contextualism, relational frame theory (RFT) is a behavioral theory about human language and cognition, describing how cognition develops and becomes contextually controlled.[4] According to RFT, human language—that is, the use of symbols and hence cognition—develops from our unique capacity to relate events arbitrarily in a specific way called relational frames. There are several properties with this kind of relational responding: mutual entailment, combinatorial entailment, and transformation of stimulus functions. Mutual entailment describes the bidirectionality of stimulus relations (e.g., if A is greater than B, then B is less than A—in the class of "relation frame" of comparisons [of quantities]). Combinatorial entailment describes the relationships among more than two stimuli, which themselves are in mutual entailment (e.g., if A is greater than B and B is greater than C, then A is greater than C and C is less than A). Transformation of stimulus function is when the function of a stimulus in the relational network is altered based on the functions of another stimulus in the network and the derived relation between the two (e.g., if A is greater than B and B becomes anxiety-provoking, then A also becomes anxiety-provoking and even more so than B).

The arbitrary aspect of these relations has relevant implications for clinicians. We can be trained to know that a dime is greater than a nickel in terms of cash value in accordance to an arbitrary societal convention, even though a dime is physically smaller. Similarly, human suffering and psychological problems arise as a person becomes entrapped in an arbitrary verbally constructed world and function according to arbitrary constructed rules—from "I am of less value than others" to "death is better than life."

There are many different classes of relational frames. Deictic frames are one specific class that describes the relationship between you vs. I, here vs. there, and then vs. now—that is, it describes a relationship with reference to the speaker's perspective. This is critical for perspective taking, and it may be deficient in people with autistic disorder. Deictic frames give rise to a sense of self as perspective, as the "I-here-now"—that is, "self-as-context" described in the next section.

The Six Core ACT Processes

ACT is a clinical application of functional contextualism and RFT, developed and refined from an earlier form of behavioral intervention called *comprehensive distancing* in the 1980s.[5] The core ACT principles had been outlined in its current form since the publication of the original text in 1999. It consists of six core interrelated therapeutic processes that the therapists work with clients to enhance: (1) cognitive defusion, (2) acceptance, (3) contact with the present moment, (4) self-as-context, (5) values, and (6) committed action.[6]

Cognitive Defusion

Cognitive defusion is the process of relating to thoughts as thoughts rather than to their literal cognitive content. This is in contrast with *fusion*, which occurs when symbols (e.g., thoughts) and their literal meaning function as a fused unit to elicit the clients' responses as if they are indeed the same. A variety of techniques, such as cognitive defusion exercises, facilitate clients to gain the capacity to defuse. For example, rather than being "fused" with the meaning of the thought "I am inadequate," one increases the capacity to observe this internal experience as a thought when consciously labeling it—that is, "I am having the thought 'I am inadequate' right now." Another example of a defusion exercise is singing the same phrase "I am inadequate" repeatedly in a high-pitched voice, thereby changing how the client is relating to and experiencing the thought. These techniques are not used to promote insight, as in dynamic therapy, or to prove that the clients' thoughts are erroneous, as in cognitive therapy. In fact, most cognitive defusion exercises work on any type of thoughts regardless of whether they are true (e.g., "the sky is blue") or not (e.g., "the sky is green"). Cognitive defusion is especially helpful with rigid rules. For example, fusion with the rule "I must listen to what my in-laws say" may lead to psychological distress regardless of what the client does, as the client may feel forced to do something against his or her will if the rule is followed and guilty if the rule is not followed. Further, even if an opposite rule is then formulated into "I will *not* listen to what my in-laws say," the in-laws' behavior will nevertheless remain a salient influence on the client.

Acceptance

Acceptance describes the process of being open and willing to experience internal private events such as thoughts, feelings, emotions, and sensations rather than attempting to avoid, control, or suppress them. From an ACT perspective, a lot of suffering and what has been described as psychopathology stems from experiential avoidance. This is most evident in the case of anxiety. Worrying about having anxiety can heighten anxiety; avoidance of feared stimuli, such as phobic objects or internal sensations, can further lead to increased fear of the avoided stimuli. Thus, acceptance from an ACT perspective is not "giving up," but rather, the willingness to experience and "let go" of the need to control, change, or avoid aversive unavoidable internal experiences.

Contact With the Present Moment

Contact with the present moment allows us to focus on our experience in the here and now, rather than letting our minds trap us in past memories, which may be filled with regret, sorrow, or anger, or the constructed future, which may be filled with anxiety, dread, or uncertainty. For clients who have experienced significant trauma, past events may continue to affect their functioning for years, from how they engage in relationships to how they make decisions in their daily lives. Under closer examination, all of us frequently think about the immediate past or future in our day-to-day functioning. Whether we are walking, eating, or taking transit, our minds are often busy reviewing what happened earlier in the day, planning tasks up ahead, or musing about various associated thoughts. Training our minds to deliberately focus on and observe the present moment allows us to better attend to the task at hand and fully appreciate our current context. This may be facilitated by formal mindfulness meditation or deliberately bringing our attention and presence to our various activities throughout the day. Reconnecting with the present allows us to be more alive and at peace, as we loosen our bondage to the past or imagined future.

Self-as-Context

Self-as-context, also called the observer-self or transcendent self, is a sense of self to be distinguished from "self-as-content." Often, we define ourselves using psychological concepts such as our gender, cultural identities, family roles, professional identities, and personality traits. In a way, our selves become "fused" with these concepts, which leads to rigidity. For example, a person may refuse to go to a social event because they see themselves as inherently shy. Further, when an aspect of these self-concepts are lost or become uncertain, people may experience "losing" their sense of self, such as losing a loved one or a job. Self-as-context facilitates the patient to get in contact with a sense of self as the context in which these psychological events unfold. While we *have* feelings, thoughts, roles, traits, illness, and a physical body, we are not any one of these concepts or things. In mental health, rather than saying "he is a schizophrenic," the more accurate and acceptable way of expressing this is "he has an illness we call schizophrenia." In this example, we are separating the personhood from the illness. Further, self-as-context can take on an enduring quality as a sense of perspective—that is, *I* have always been *I* (and not you) throughout all conscious experiences in time and space.

Values

Values refer to life directions that are freely chosen by an individual, giving a sense of meaning, purpose, and vitality. They can describe the qualities of actions that an individual strives toward—for example, loving, kind, and compassionate. Values are distinguished from goals as the latter can be attained. For example, being a loving, caring parent is an endless endeavor and does not end with completing a set number of concrete goals or tasks, like changing a certain number of diapers or cooking a certain number of meals. Values may be expressed in different domains of life, such as family, work, relationships, spirituality, and self-care. While ACT undermines the role of internal rules, thoughts, and reasons for determining behaviors, it seeks to increase values as the main verbal constructs to guide one's behaviors.

Committed Action

Committed action refers to the persistent behaviors in pursuing one's values, even in the face of internal barriers or external obstacles. In many ways, this is the ultimate objective of ACT—to facilitate clients' capacity to engage in actions that give their life a sense of meaning. This process is intricately related to the other ACT processes. The commitment to values is expressed through action, and "staying the course" is often facilitated by the process of defusion and acceptance. As committed action becomes an objective of therapy, this allows a shift in emphasis from outcome to process. For instance, it is the committed action of learning itself that provides intrinsic meaning and vitality rather than high grades or a certificate on a wall.

Contexts and Current Ways in Which ACT Is Practiced

As ACT is based on a transdiagnostic process-based model, it has been widely applied in different contexts.[7] In the mental health field, ACT has been used to treat diverse psychopathologies from depression and anxiety disorders to psychotic disorders. It has also been applied in the treatment of substance abuse and chronic pain. In non–mental-health-related populations, ACT has been used to facilitate positive changes in attitudes and behaviors, such as reducing stigma, promoting health management (e.g., epilepsy and diabetes), and decreasing burnouts.

ACT is often practiced as a form of individual psychotherapy between a therapist and a client. With its emphasis on functional change, metaphors, experiential exercises, and mindfulness practices are often integratively used instead of cognitive restructuring or dynamic interpretation. Therapists are encouraged to embody the model, and self-disclosure may be judiciously used. ACT can also be applied in a group format, incorporating group therapy principles and psychodrama techniques. The length of the intervention varies, from single sessions to multiple sessions to open-ended interventions. Like many therapies, a large number of self-help books are available to address various clinical problems. Most recently, emerging mobile applications are used to deliver ACT and help users track their progress.

Relationship Between Buddhism and ACT

While ACT is derived from functional contextualism and RFT, there is similarity between some of the philosophy and theoretical orientation behind ACT and traditional Asian thought, especially Buddhism.[8]

The origin of Buddhism, a nontheistic religion from Asia, stems mainly from the teachings of Siddhartha Gautama, a prince of the Shakya clan. Although his father attempted to give him a sheltered life, he eventually came across an old man, a sick man, a corpse, and an ascetic, and these encounters deeply impacted on him. He strove to find a way to overcome the suffering caused by aging, sickness, and death by becoming an ascetic. Through his experiences, he found that neither a life of luxury nor a life of harsh asceticism and self-mortification was helpful. Rather, he discovered the Middle Way, a path of moderation, which led to his enlightenment in becoming the Buddha, the "Awakened One."

From Gautama's teachings, there are two derived Buddhist traditions historically, which may be grouped as the Pali and Sanskrit traditions, with three main established canons compiled over the centuries in Pali, Chinese, and Tibetan.[9] The two current major branches of Buddhism are Theravada, "the school of the Elders," following the Pali tradition and being practiced in Sri Lanka and Southeast Asia, and Mahayana, "The Great Vehicle," following the Sanskrit tradition and being practiced in East Asia. Vajrayana, practiced in Tibet, Mongolia, and some parts of China and Russia, is sometimes considered a separate branch or as a part of the Mahayana Sanskrit tradition. Each of the various schools and traditions has their own canons, practices, and interpretations of Buddhist concepts. For the scope of this discussion, some of the common fundamental doctrines are highlighted, acknowledging that this is not an exhaustive comparative analysis.

One of the key teachings of Buddhism is the Four Noble Truths (*catvāri āryasatyāni*四聖諦): (1) *duḥkha*苦 (Sanskrit and corresponding Chinese terms are used in this chapter) there is suffering; (2) the origin of *duḥkha* can be known, and it is caused by ignorance (*moha/avidyā* 痴), desire or attachment (*rāga* 貪), and aversion (*dveṣa* 嗔); (3) the cessation of *duḥkha* is possible; and (4) the cessation of *duḥkha* is through the Eightfold Path.[10] The Eightfold Path (*āryāṣṭāṅgamārga*八正道) can be grouped into three clusters: *wisdom* (*prajñā*慧)—(1) right view (*samyag-dṛṣṭi*正見) and (2) right intention (*samyak-saṃkalpa* 正思維); *ethical conduct* (*śīla*戒)—(3) right speech (*samyag-vāc* 正語), (4) right action (*samyak-karmānta*正業), and (5) right livelihood (*samyag-ājīva*正命); and *concentration of the mind* (*samādhi*定)—(6) right effort (*samyag-vyāyāma*正精進), (7) right mindfulness (*samyak-smṛti*正念), and (8) right concentration (*samyak-samādhi*正定).[11] Through ethical conduct, proper concentration of the mind, and attainment of wisdom, ignorance can be dispelled, leading to enlightenment and freedom from suffering in this lifetime and ultimately from the cycles of death and rebirth, or *saṃsāra*輪迴.

The Dharma Seals are key concepts in Buddhism that are important to the understanding of the Four Noble Truths. They also provide a means to evaluate if a teaching or a person is true and adherent to the core Buddhist tenets. In some traditions, there are three Dharma Seals: (1) *impermanence*—that all phenomena change, arising and disintegrating; (2) *emptiness/nonself*—that there is no entity or self that is truly permanent and independent; and

(3) *nirvana*—that extinction of ignorance can ultimately lead to peace and liberation from the cycle of *saṃsāra*.[12] In some schools, there are four Dharma Seals; the additional seal, a corollary of the first, is that all polluted (or constituted) phenomena are unsatisfactory.[13]

In comparing Buddhism and ACT, there is an overall correspondence from a broad perspective. Philosophically, both similarly emphasize pragmatism, prioritizing what is workable. In practice, both emphasize experiential learning over intellectualized understanding alone. Further, there are commonalities in their approach toward understanding human suffering.

Grounded in RFT and functional contextualism, ACT views language and the capacity for cognition and internalized rules as essential for daily functioning and yet our source of suffering, dysfunction, and psychopathology. Arising from our fusion with thoughts, suffering is seen as an inevitable part of life, consistent with the first two of the Four Noble Truths. In ACT, the "letting go" of our attachment is facilitated by core processes of defusion—seeing thoughts as thoughts; acceptance—willingness to accept what is experienced; present moment—staying in contact with the here and now; and self-as-context—letting go of self-concepts. These four processes, including the incorporation of mindfulness practice in ACT, are consistent with the Eightfold Path.[14] Clarification of our values and aligning and sustaining committed action to our (wholesome) values are consistent with the ethical conduct of the Eightfold Path. Clinically, increased compassion can emerge through the core ACT processes just as the practice of Buddhism cultivates compassion.

There are many different systems to catalog and characterize mental factors in Buddhism. In one of the Mahayana traditions, there are six root unwholesome mental factors: (1) *Rāga*貪—"attachment or desire"; (2) *Pratigha*嗔—"anger or aversion"; (3) *Avidyā*痴—"ignorance or delusion"; (4) *Māna*慢—"pride/conceit"; (5) *Vicikitsā* 疑—"doubt"; and (6) *Dṛiṣṭi* 見—"wrong view or belief." There is some similarity between these factors and the model of psychopathology in ACT: attachment to the past or future, experiential avoidance, fusion, inaction, lack of values clarity, and attachment to conceptualized self. The most discrepant pairing would be *Māna*. Pride is not specifically identified or singled out in ACT; pride is generally considered a much more negative emotion in Asian than in Western cultures.[15]

Similarly, the six transcendent perfections (*paramitas*, 波羅蜜), virtues to be cultivated in Buddhism, appear to have partial correspondence with the core ACT processes:[16]

- Present moment with *Dhyāna pāramitā 禪定波羅蜜* ("concentration, contemplation")
- Acceptance with *Kṣānti (kshanti) pāramitā 忍辱波羅蜜* ("forbearance, acceptance")
- Defusion with *Śīla pāramitā 持戒波羅蜜* ("discipline, proper conduct")
- Values with *Dāna pāramitā 布施波羅蜜* ("generosity, giving of self")

- Committed action with *Vīrya pāramitā* 精進波羅蜜 ("diligence, energy, effort")
- Self-as-context with *Prajñā pāramitā* 般若波羅蜜 ("wisdom, insight")

The most apparent discrepancy is with defusion, except in the sense that through defusion, our actions are no longer bounded by fused unworkable rules or unwholesome thoughts, allowing proper conduct to be guided by our values. Similar to the case with pride, generosity is not specifically identified in ACT, which leaves values to be freely self-determined.

As evident, there are both similarities and differences between basic Buddhist tenets and the ACT model. This is unsurprising given that their aim and scope differ. While both aim to decrease human suffering, Buddhism aims to promote spiritual growth, cessation of suffering, and enlightenment that is not bound to this lifetime. To address the latter, many different Buddhist schools evolving through the centuries have rich, intricate, and detailed elaborations beyond the scope of this chapter. While Buddhism can be more prescriptive and include explicit moralistic values, the values in ACT are emphasized as individualistic choices and freely chosen, reflecting the stance of psychotherapy, which attempts to avoid the imposition of the therapist's values on the client.

Looking specifically at the three Dharma Seals, ACT does not address issues related to nirvana or karma. It also does not emphasize impermanence in its deep sense, although it promotes defusion, flexibility, and adaptation to change. Finally, while ACT undermines the conceptualized self, it increases an enduring sense of *self-as-context,* which may seem contradictory to the Buddhist nonself.

However, the Buddhist *nonself* is actually complex, and its relationship with ACT's self-as-context may not be incompatible.[17] In Buddhism, a dualistic approach to whether there is or is not a self is seen as limiting and flawed.[18] A "self" can be acknowledged for functioning in conventional reality, just as self-as-context is functionally used in therapy. In the ultimate reality, the "no-self" in Buddhism can be understood through the concepts of *impermanence*, that everything fluctuates and changes, and *emptiness*, that nothing is actually an independent and essential entity separable from others.[19] Thus, a concept of *interbeing* is one approach toward understanding the no-self, where nonself elements can be found in the self.[20]

In ACT, rather than ontologically asserting an existence of a metaphysical self, the self-as-context is actually a psychological concept used for therapeutic aims and merely a verbal construct created from deictic frames in RFT. Further, in RFT, "the other" may be constructed as the other-as-context (vs. other-as-content).[21] In this case, other-as-context will be perceived as a purely conscious transcendent person in the here and now, effectively linked to the self-as-context in the here and now, thereby creating the "self-other-as-context" or "transcendent self-other." This is similar to the concept of interbeing or the concept of interdependent-self in Asian psychology taken a step further, where the "we" (vs. "I") are perceived from a transcendent perspective. ACT has yet to develop clinical techniques to facilitate contact with this conjoined "self-other-as-context."

Strategies for Integration

While no-self and *interbeing* have rarely been used clinically, ACT has incorporated various forms of mindfulness practices. Further, other Buddhist concepts may be fruitfully used to further the understanding of ACT. One pragmatic approach that I had successfully employed was to colead "ACT–Buddhism" groups with Buddhist monks for Cambodian Buddhist clients. In each session, related ACT and Buddhist concepts were presented. The collaboration enabled me as a non-Buddhist to focus on ACT experiential exercises and metaphors while the monk incorporated Dharma talks, poetry, and traditional stories. The concept of rebirth, karma, and past lives facilitated clients to look at acceptance from a spiritual perspective. In the role of a respected spiritual leader, the monk could be more prescriptive than a more neutral stance of a therapist. The success of the groups was in part due to the openness of the group members who were Buddhists. In addition, individual sessions before and after the group helped ensure that the clients made informed choices about joining the group and did not feel values were being imposed on them.

In addition to Buddhism, ACT is congruent with other aspects of Asian thought. Asian cultures and philosophies are not monolithic or homogeneous, but rather, they are complex, heterogeneous, and ever evolving. The origin of Buddhism itself reflects elements of mixed ancient religious traditions, including the diametrically opposing ancient *Indus Valley religion*, which emphasized renunciation, meditation, and asceticism, and *Aryan religion*, which included priesthood and various Aryan gods that were incorporated into Buddhist scriptures.[22] In East Asia, Buddhism had been further adapted and integrated into Chinese culture, philosophy, religion, literature, and art.[23] Chinese philosophy and culture is a syncretic product of Confucianism, Buddhism, and Taoism, with the three doctrines mutually influencing one another through the years.[24] Thus, other aspects of Asian cultures may also be integrated and utilized with the ACT model.

In Asian culture, acceptance and the related concepts of tolerance and forbearance are seen as positive ways of coping. In a collectivistic culture, social harmony is promoted while interpersonal conflict is avoided through tolerance of one's thoughts and feelings.[25] Tolerance of internal experiences is often extended to dealing with external problems and obstacles. In this context, the belief in fate and karma further promotes acceptance. From a psychological perspective, this is sometimes conceptualized as Asians having higher external and lower internal locus of control compared to Caucasians. In Asian culture, accepting and tolerating, rather than fighting back, are often seen as strengths, virtues, or healthy coping mechanisms. This is embedded in the concept of endorsing "softness" over "hardness" in approaching conflicts, and many such idioms may be utilized in therapy. For example, in Taoism, 柔弱勝剛強 means "it is thus that the soft overcomes the hard, and the weak, the strong" and 強大處下, 柔弱處上 means "truly, the hard and mighty are cast down; the soft and weak set on high."[26] Confucius had been quoted as saying 小不忍、則亂大謀, which means "want of forbearance in small matters confounds great plans."[27] There are also commonly used idioms, such as 逆来順受, which means "when adversity comes, bear it with acceptance" and 退一步海闊天空, which means "if you take a step back (i.e., backing down in a conflict), you will see that the sea is wide and the sky is boundless."

However, there is a subtle difference between acceptance and forbearance. Forbearance, although highly valued as a discipline and virtue, can imply a sense of suffering. Acceptance through mindfulness, on the other hand, can lead to a decreased sense of struggle or suffering. A brief vignette illustrates this. In therapy with a Chinese client, a middle-age woman felt stuck in having to "tolerate" a lot because of her stormy marriage and noncaring family. We discussed acceptance as a shift from forbearance (忍) toward mindfulness (念) as we studied the difference in Chinese ideographic characters—shifting from a knife over one's heart to having the present moment over one's heart. This motivated her to explore the use of mindfulness in her own life.

Acceptance does not mean resignation over external circumstances that can be changed, as committed action may be required to bring about changes in the service of values. In ACT, there is an emphasis on an individual's values. If a value is chosen merely to meet social expectations, it is usually not regarded as the person's "true" value. One common technique is to ask whether the value is still important to the person if no one else would ever find out about it. However, in Asian and other collectivistic cultures, cultural values and what others think often play an integral role in guiding one's behaviors.[28] Thus, when using ACT with Asians, both cultural and individual values may need to be identified and worked through depending on the therapeutic goals of the individual, which may be culturally congruent or countercultural.[29]

In fact, the self as an autonomous being that can choose and commit to abstract values is grounded in modern Western thought. In Asian cultures, the *self* and *values* are harder to separate from their context. In Chinese, literal translations of *values* and *commitment* are fraught with difficulty; words that convey principles, virtues, or literal translation of values fail to fully convey the sense and scope of values in English. To facilitate a discussion on values, it may be easier to discuss what a meaningful life means with the values embedded in their natural context—for example, "having loving relationship with my family" or "being able to produce and contribute at the workplace" versus the abstract value of being "loving" and "productive." From a Western perspective, one can commit to a value of compassion as an abstract quality and express this in a multitude of contexts, flexibly applied to many situations. In Chinese, it is unusual to make a commitment to an abstract quality in the absence of its context. The closest method may be to attach these qualities to the person's character—being a compassionate person, being a *junzi*君子 (upright person). While this works pragmatically, one may need to address the potentially conflicting concept of self-as-context in a nuanced way, highlighting the choice in values versus rigid self-concepts.

Conclusion

Based on RFT and rooted in functional contextualism, ACT is a versatile transdiagnostic psychotherapy. One of its strengths is that it is principle driven and experientially delivered, and its core processes can be flexibly adapted to suit each individual patient's needs. It is also largely congruent with traditional Asian thought and culture. Nevertheless, its application in non-Western populations may still need cultural adaptation, as it is framed from a Western perspective and potentially constrained by its particular cultural worldview. Through this review, the discrepancies between ACT and Buddhism highlight potential opportunities in which ACT or other therapies can be further developed. The challenge of translating core concepts of Buddhism that are missing in ACT, including impermanence, nonself, and interbeing, into therapeutic techniques may ultimately prove to be both beneficial and consistent with RFT. The careful incorporation of cultural values in ACT can make this therapy even more suitable for diverse cultures. As Western psychotherapy continues to evolve, the influence of Asian wisdom and philosophy may continue to help advance and enrich the way psychotherapy is developed and practiced, and the quest toward alleviation of human suffering may best be addressed through thoughtful collective efforts across boundaries.

Case Study

Mr. Lee was a 24-year-old single Chinese Canadian man who emigrated from Hong Kong to Canada 6 years prior to presentation. He was living with his mother and studied music at a local university as a part-time student.

Mr. Lee had an 8-year history of body dysmorphic disorder and panic disorder. This had been increasingly severe, and he had been having trouble completing his studies at school. Mr. Lee had failed to respond adequately to antidepressants and several courses of cognitive behavioral therapy (CBT) in the past. He was a pianist prodigy and had undergone specialized training in Hong Kong and the United States. He described having many days when he was unable to leave the house when he thought that his face "looked strange." He had cancelled a number of piano performances at the last minute, and his social life was severely limited, spending most of his time at home, practicing piano, and playing computer games. His parents divorced when he was very young, and his mother was exasperated and worried about his future. She complained that she had given up a lot to help him succeed.

(*Continued*)

(Continued)

Mr. Lee hesitantly agreed to participate in an ACT group in Chinese. He initially had great doubts whether he would be able to complete the group. With the therapist's encouragement, he was able to attend all but one session. He made remarkable improvement as the group progressed. In one of the pivotal sessions, a group exercise on acceptance was conducted with participants sitting in a circle. A single chair was placed in the center of the circle representing psychological pain—"the chair of pain." Participants took turns describing their unique attempts to cope with their own psychological pain. They then took their own chair, representing their coping strategy, and piled it on top or placed it near the center chair to cover up the chair of pain. This physicalized reflective exercise demonstrated the futility of coping strategies to eliminate pain, since the addition of more chairs to the center could never obliterate the center chair of pain. The process only added to the clutter, and the participants lost their own chair to sit on in the process. The participants were then invited to take back their own chair and re-form the circle and then contemplate on just allowing the chair of pain to be in the center as a model of acceptance. This session proved to be the turning point for Mr. Lee. He disclosed his symptoms to the other group participants about his beliefs of "being ugly." He also became regretful about how his avoidant behaviors affected other spheres in his life, including his long-distance relationship with his girlfriend in Hong Kong. He said that he never dared to fully invest in the relationship given his disorder. His disclosure moved the group. Several older women in the group became very nurturing toward him. His group disclosure, the supportive group process, and sessions on values and committed action consolidated his gains as he became much more active both in the group and outside the group. When he completed the group, he had dramatically improved. There were only very few occasions when he could not go out, as he was able to observe his self-denigrating thoughts whenever they arose, which still occurred from time to time. He became more actively engaged in his relationship with his girlfriend and his studies at school. He was more open to committing to opportunities to perform, and he actively pursued volunteer opportunities in the Chinese community.

Although the client had previous individual psychotherapy, he was able to make important breakthroughs in the ACT group, and this appeared to be related both to the therapeutic effects of group therapy in general and the use of the ACT model in particular. As one of the client's main presenting problems was social avoidance, group therapy offered him an opportunity to confront his social fears in a controlled therapeutic setting. For the client, there was an element of behavioral exposure as he learned that he could persist in attending a therapy group with his anxiety abating with time. He was feeling less isolated as he identified with and learned from others who shared their struggle with anxiety and depression. He experienced disconfirmation of his expectations of being harshly judged, as others were very supportive of him, which lessened his sense of shame. Finally, the unique role he played in the group helped him find new confidence. Being a younger man in a predominately older female group, he was able to help others understand subtle ACT concepts while being explicitly appreciated and gently nurtured by other group members, something that he missed in his relationship with his mother. Unlike his previous therapies, which focused on disputing his negative self-perception and exploring his past, the use of ACT, especially the "Chair Sculpture of Suffering" exercise, helped him step back and reflect on the overall function and consequence of his belief system and avoidant pattern of behavioral responses.[30] The shift from a content-focused to a contextual functional approach loosened his preoccupation with his negative thoughts and accompanying narrative, as he gradually relinquished attempts to avoid, dispute, and rationalize these thoughts. He gave up his original assumptions that insight into the cause of his negative perception would liberate him from any more negative thoughts or self-doubt and that he would need to experience more self-confidence to move forward. These shifts, in addition to becoming deeply in touch with his values, helped him realize and confront other avoidant areas of his life. Rather than approaching human relationships with the focus on his need for approval and fear of rejection, he allowed these thoughts and emotions to be there in the background while authentically connecting with others in the present moment, guided by his values. This helped him connect with his own family and girlfriend and broadened his desire to connect with others through voluntary work.

DISCUSSION QUESTIONS

1. In psychotherapy, one of the key tenets is for therapists not to impose their own values on their clients. For instance, this marks one of the differences between Buddhist teachings and the practice of acceptance and commitment therapy (ACT), as seen in the latter's emphasis on individual chosen values. In practice, how can a therapist ensure this, and is this possible? Is the concept of individual chosen values itself "value free"? When the clients' values are in conflict with the therapist, how can this be handled?

2. In mindfulness-based therapies such as ACT, what are the underlying values and assumptions? Discuss whether therapists using mindfulness-based practice, including ACT practitioners, must have an active mindfulness practice and share a particular worldview.

3. Discuss the boundary and interface between psychotherapy and spirituality and between psychotherapy and philosophy. In view of this, how does the practitioner's personal spirituality and philosophical outlook influence the practice of therapy? For example, how do the beliefs in various spiritual traditions affect a therapist's approach to self-as-context or the transcendent self? How do beliefs in functional contextualism, a form of behaviorism, influence the practice of ACT?

4. What are the ethical and practical implications of incorporating Asian and other cultural values, traditions, and practices such as ACT in psychotherapy? For the developers and researchers, what is the role of acknowledging the origins and source of the therapeutic model and techniques (e.g., the historical source of the practice of mindfulness)? For the practitioners, what are the related implications regarding disclosure and application of therapy (e.g., some religions forbid certain kinds of practices if they appear to derive from another religion)?

REFERENCES

1. Hall, G. C., Hong, J. J., Zane, N. W., & Meyer, O. L. (2011). Culturally competent treatments for Asian Americans: The relevance of mindfulness and acceptance-based psychotherapies. *Clinical Psychology: Science and Practice, 18*(3), 215–231.
2. Hayes, S. C., Follette, V. M., & Linehan, M. (2004). *Mindfulness and acceptance: Expanding the cognitive-behavioral tradition.* New York, NY: Guilford Press.
3. Hayes, S. C., Strosahl, K., & Wilson, K. G. (2012). *Acceptance and commitment therapy: The process and practice of mindful change.* New York, NY: Guilford Press.
4. Ibid.
5. Hayes et al., *Mindfulness and acceptance.*
6. Hayes et al., *Mindfulness and acceptance*; Hayes et al., *Acceptance and commitment therapy*; Fung, K. (2015). Acceptance and commitment therapy: Western adoption of Buddhist tenets? *Transcultural Psychiatry, 52*(4), 561–576.
7. Ruiz, F. (2010). A review of acceptance and commitment therapy (ACT) empirical evidence: Correlational, experimental psychopathology, component and outcome studies. *International Journal of Psychology and Psychological Therapy, 10*(1), 125–162.
8. Fung, Acceptance and commitment therapy; Hayes, S. C. (2002). Buddhism and acceptance and commitment therapy. *Cognitive and Behavioral Practice, 9*(1), 58–66.
9. Dalai Lama. (2014). *XIV B-D-R-M, Chodron T. Buddhism.* New York, NY: Simon and Schuster.
10. Santina, P. D. (1984). *Fundamentals of Buddhism.* Singapore: Sri Lankaramaya Buddhist Temple.
11. Ibid.
12. Nhất Hạnh, T. (2006). *Understanding our mind.* Berkeley, CA: Parallax Press.
13. Dalai Lama, *XIV B-D-R-M.*
14. Fung, Acceptance and commitment therapy; Hayes, Buddhism and acceptance and commitment therapy.
15. Lo, H.-T., & Fung, K. P. (2003). Culturally competent psychotherapy. *Canadian Journal of Psychiatry Revue Canadienne de Psychiatrie, 48*(3), 161–170; Ryder, A. G., Dere, J., Yang, J., & Fung, K. P. (2012). Personality disorders in Asians. In E. C. Chang (Ed.), *Handbook of adult psychopathology in Asians* (pp. 357–390). New York, NY: Oxford University Press.
16. Dalai Lama, *XIV B-D-R-M*; Sheng-yen. (2002). *The six paramitas.* Elmhurst, NY: Dharma Drum Publications.
17. Fung, Acceptance and commitment therapy.
18. Nhất Hạnh, T. (2010). *Beyond the self: Teachings on the Middle Way.* Berkeley, CA: Parallax Press.
19. Dalai Lama, XIV B-D-R-M; Nhất Hạnh, *Understanding our mind.*
20. Nhất Hạnh, *Understanding our mind*; Nhất Haảnh, *Beyond the self.*
21. Stewart, I., & McHugh, L. (2013). Perspective taking. In T. B. Kashdan & J. Ciarrochi (Eds.), *Mindfulness, acceptance, and positive psychology.* Oakland, CA: New Harbinger Publications.
22. Santina, *Fundamentals of Buddhism.*
23. Guang, X. (2013). Buddhist impact on Chinese culture. *Asian Philosophy, 23*(4), 305–322.
24. Ryder et al., Personality disorders; Guang, Buddhist impact; Hang, L. (2011). Traditional Confucianism and its contemporary relevance. *Asian Philosophy, 21*(4), 437–445.
25. Hall et al., Culturally competent treatments; Lo & Fung, Culturally competent psychotherapy; Ryder et al., Personality disorders.
26. Waley, A. (2005). *The way and its power.* New York, NY: Routledge.

27. Confucius. (2013). *The analects* (The revised James Legge translation). Prague, Czech Republic: e-artnow.
28. Fung, Acceptance and commitment therapy; Lo & Fung, Culturally competent psychotherapy; Ryder et al., Personality disorders.
29. Lo & Fung, Culturally competent psychotherapy; Fung, K. P., & Lo, T. (2012). Culturally competent practice and management of mental health in primary care. In A. Khenti, J. C. Sapag, S. Mohamoud, & A. V. Ravindran (Eds.), *Collaborative mental health.* Toronto, Canada: Centre for Addiction and Mental Health; Fung, K. P., & Wong, J. (2014). *ACT to reduce stigma of mental illness: A group intervention training manual on acceptance and commitment therapy.* Unpublished manuscript, University of Toronto and Ryerson University, Canada.
30. Fung, K. P., & Zurowski, M. (2016). Chair sculpture of suffering exercise. In A. Peterkin & P. Brett-McLean (Eds.), *Keeping reflection fresh: Top educators share their innovations in health professional education.* Kent, OH: Kent State University Press.

SUGGESTED READINGS

Aronson, H. B. (2004). *Buddhist practice on Western ground: Reconciling Eastern ideals and Western psychology.* Boston, MA: Shambhala Publishers.

This book addresses some of the important differences between Buddhism and Western psychology. In particular, Chapter 7: "Ego, Ego on the Wall: What Is Ego After All?" addresses the issue of no-self. Many other important ideas are explored, including the understanding of attachment and nonattachment.

Hayes, S. C., Strosahl, K., & Wilson, K. G. (2012). *Acceptance and commitment therapy: The process and practice of mindful change* (2nd ed.). New York, NY: Guilford Press.

This is the second edition of the original definitive 1999 text by the pioneers of ACT. The philosophy, theory, and hexaflex model of the six therapeutic processes central to the model are described in detail in the text.

Masuda, A. (2013). *Mindfulness and acceptance in multicultural competency.* Oakland, CA: New Harbinger Publications.

The book discusses the use of mindfulness-based therapies in the context of sociocultural diversity. It looks at the culturally competent application and adaptation of ACT, DBT, and MBCT. It also examines the potential application of mindfulness-based therapies to address diversity issues such as prejudice and stigma.

Nhất Hạnh, T. (2006). *Understanding our mind.* Berkeley, CA: Parallax Press.

Written by Zen Master Thich Nhất Haành, the book discusses the basic teachings of Buddhism that are of relevance to psychological functioning from a Buddhist perspective. It is based on the 50 verses on the nature of consciousness from the 5th-century Buddhist master Vasubandhu.

12 Japanese Contemplative Practice of Naikan

Chikako Ozawa-de Silva and Yoshihiko Miki

Naikan (also known as Naikan therapy or the Naikan method) is a Japanese indigenous introspective healing practice that has been derived from Japanese Mahayana Buddhism and established as a secular form of therapeutic self-cultivation. Naikan is hard to classify, as it lies at the border of psychotherapy and spirituality. Some call Naikan a "pre-religious practice" as it does not require any religious belief or knowledge but often leads to powerful experiences of self-transformation.[1] In Japanese, *nai* means inside and *kan* means looking, so Naikan literally means "introspection" or "inner-looking." As the name indicates, Naikan is a discursive and analytical method of structured self-reflection that helps people gain new insights into themselves, their relationships, and the causes of their problems.

Through Naikan, individuals dwell on their past acts and experiences in relationships with people who were close to them by reflecting on these questions: What did I receive from this person? What did I give back to this person? What trouble did I cause this person? These are called Naikan's "three themes," and for 1 week, individuals reexamine their past by using these questions. The three themes prompt individuals to reorient their usual "I"-centered perspectives (e.g., I did this; this person did this to me) to more "other"-centered perspectives (e.g., from this person's perspective, what I did was nothing but trouble). Normally people are accustomed to relating to the world and other people from their own perspectives rather than trying to put themselves in other people's shoes and seeing the situation from other people's perspectives. As a result, Naikan clients discover that even one's own self-history is not an objective fact but a subjective construction of the past through subjective interpretations. Naikan allows clients to shed light on their past and rewrite their life history. This rather simple method over the period of a week leads clients to recognize the interdependence of their lives through recalling the tremendous affection, kindness, and support they received from others and even from strangers. Many individuals end Naikan with increased feelings of gratitude, a sense of being loved and accepted by others, and a strong sense of connectedness with others.[2] Self-transformation occurs through cognitive and conceptual shifts, and many clients experience relief from psychological and physical problems. Mindfulness-based meditations have gained popularity internationally, and Naikan can be seen as a mindfulness practice directed toward compassion, in which people recall kindness and compassion as a means for healing.[3]

The identity of Naikan has been long debated. Scholars and practitioners of Naikan have sought to determine whether it is a form of psychotherapy, religious practice, or secular practice.[4] For that reason, Naikan is sometimes called Naikan psychotherapy, Naikan therapy, the Naikan method, or simply Naikan. Yoshimoto Ishin (1916–1988), the founder of Naikan, intentionally made Naikan secular so that it would be open to anyone regardless of religious affiliation, and he used to say "Naikan is Naikan," refusing to let Naikan be narrowly defined.[5]

Naikan attracts a wide variety of people for a wide range of reasons. Since Naikan is not strictly psychotherapy (unless offered at hospitals) and has a strong element of self-cultivation and self-searching, many individuals who are interested in personal growth, spiritual growth, and self-examination as well as solving personal problems visit Naikan centers. Counselors who are familiar with Naikan may also refer people who have diagnosed psychiatric conditions such as depression, anxiety disorders, anorexia, alcoholism, and psychosomatic disorders.[6]

This chapter shows the history of Naikan and its development over time; the relationship between Buddhism and Naikan, especially in relation to Naikan's understandings of the causes of illness and healing; how Naikan is currently practiced and perceived; how and why Naikan's notions of efficacy are difficult to assess within a standard biomedical framework; and future directions for Naikan.

Brief History of Naikan

Naikan was developed by the Buddhist practitioner and businessman Yoshimoto in the 1940s. In 1953, Yoshimoto retired from his business at the age of 38 and started the first Naikan center. He adapted Naikan from *mishirabe,* a meditation practice of the Japanese Mahayana Buddhist school of *Jōdo Shinshū* (True Pure Land School, or Shin Buddhism). ***Mishirabe*** literally means "self-examination," and it involves severe and ascetic bodily engagement such as fasting and deprivation of sleep until one achieves spiritual awakening. When Yoshimoto achieved such a state through *mishirabe,* he realized that his lifetime mission was to spread this practice to as many people as possible so that they could also experience the utter joy and happiness he experienced through this.[7] Yoshimoto modified *mishirabe* to make it less severe and more accessible and also removed its religious aspects so that it would be accessible to anyone regardless of religious belief.

There have been three waves in the history of Naikan's development. In the first wave, Naikan was introduced as a reform technique in prisons, in the second it was introduced into schools, and in the third it was introduced as a psychotherapy, especially for addiction, at hospitals. True to his Shin Buddhist belief that "even the good man can attain salvation, let alone the sinner," Yoshimoto started to teach Naikan in prison once he was appointed as a prison chaplain at the Nara Juvenile Prison. Its confined spaces and isolation turned out to be ideal for Naikan. During the early 1960s, Naikan was widely spread among reformatories and institutions for juvenile delinquents. Also in the 1960s, Naikan began to reach education institutions such as junior high and high schools. Eventually, Naikan began to be recognized more widely in medicine—and even in the training sections of companies.[8]

Around the same time, Yoshimoto gave many lectures at universities and at the Japan Defense Agency. He was invited five times to appear on NHK, the Japan Broadcasting Corporation (Japan's equivalent of the BBC in the United Kingdom), between 1978 and 1982. The number of Naikan clients increased rapidly after 1975, and his Nara Naikan center attracted over 1,000 clients per year until his death in 1987. Other Naikan centers have been opened since the 1970s by those who experienced Naikan under Yoshimoto's guidance. Even though the medical and psychological approach to Naikan has been dominant, a new trend to move Naikan away from medicalization toward spirituality has also been taking place.[9] Since Yoshimoto opened his Naikan center in 1953, Naikan has been practiced predominantly at Naikan centers, and its practice has not changed much to this day. Besides Naikan centers, Naikan is nowadays practiced at schools, hospitals, juvenile training schools, and prisons. Today there are over 40 Naikan centers in Japan. Naikan has also been gradually spreading outside of Japan, and there are now Naikan centers in Austria, Germany, the United States, and China.

Perhaps because Naikan is open to everyone and not limited to particular conditions or symptoms, it attracts people from a wide range of ages, occupations, and reasons for coming. Clients range from their early teens to their 80s. Overall, the ratio of men to women has been even in the past decade. In terms of occupations, *salarymen* (office workers and company employees) and civil servants form the majority of clients, followed by teachers, nurses, physicians, company managers, and homemakers. There are also college students, professional psychologists, and non-Japanese clients.[10]

During his life, Yoshimoto's charismatic appeal drew large numbers of Naikan clients to his and other Naikan centers.[11] After his death, the consensus is that the total number of Naikan clients has been in gradual decline. Nevertheless, it is not easy to generalize about this trend. For example, one popular Naikan center that measured its data over the past decade showed a steady number of Naikan clients over the past 10 years, with no sign of either increase on decrease.

In the past decade, there has also been a slight shift in the demographics of Naikan clients. Firstly, there has been a decrease among young clients.

Many Naikan centers nowadays attract people in their 30s to 60s.[12] Naikan also attracts people who have recently retired, who employ Naikan as a means to reflect on their life and think about their future. The increasing levels of unemployment among people in their 40s and 50s due to Japan's long-term economic recession may be one factor in the recent increase of Naikan clients among this generation. Secondly, Naikan has been attracting more women, and this seems to be a continuous trend over the last several decades. According to the record at Yoshimito's Naikan center between January and June 1966, the ratio of men to women was 4:1. In recent years, Naikan centers tend to attract women and men at a 1:1 ratio overall, although there is slight variation among individual centers. The speculation among some Naikan practitioners is that this is because women who in the past were unable to leave their house and abandon their domestic chores for a week are now more independent and able to take the time off to do Naikan. Thirdly, in recent years an increasing number of clients with depression have begun to visit Naikan centers.

Healing Traditions and Cultural Representations of Illness and Wellness

Naikan practitioners often cite Yoshimoto's famous dictum that "Naikan is Naikan," meaning that he refused to classify Naikan as merely a psychotherapy. It is therefore hard to put Naikan into any particular categorical box. This is magnified by Japanese traditional views on mental illness and wellness, which differ from biomedical views. It is to be noted that psychotherapy in general has had very little impact in Japan until recently. This is not due to a lack of familiarity with Western forms of psychotherapies including psychoanalysis. Japanese anthropologist Ohnuki-Tierney noted this interesting fact, writing that "it has been pointed out that Freudian psychoanalysis has never been widely accepted, despite the fact that the Japanese have eagerly adopted many Western technological and intellectual innovations" (p. 84).[13]

Mental illness is especially widely open to interpretation and cultural influence. In Japan, one of the central concepts in understanding both psychological and physical illness is the idea of *ki* (more commonly known as *chi* or *qi* in Chinese).[14] *Ki* has broad meanings. It can refer to vital energy, life force, consciousness, state of mind, and the mind's function. *Ki* could also be explained as a kind of wind-like energy that is both physical and connected to the mind. In this form, it is the central vital force of living beings according to traditional Chinese medicine (TCM) and traditional Japanese medicine.[15]

"Illness is from *ki*" is a common traditional saying in Japan. It is widely believed that one's state of mind affects both physical and psychological health. Again, *ki* as mind needs to be understood primarily within Buddhist concepts and not in the Western psychological understanding of mind. It is commonly accepted in Japan that mental and emotional states (including what we often call chemical imbalances, as they are imbalances of *ki*) affect one's health. Nowadays it has been more accepted in North America that the mind and body are closely connected and that mental states such as stress can cause serious mental and physical illness, but this notion has always been a part of Japanese traditional cultural understandings of illness and well-being.[16]

There are many expressions that show how *ki* is considered vital in understandings of health and illness in Japan. The following are only a few examples: "*Ki* dances": One is excited; "*Ki* sinks": One is depressed; "It rubs my *ki*": It is annoying; "To have small *ki*": To be timid; "To have long *ki*": To be patient; "To lose *ki*": To faint; "*Ki* has changed": To be insane.

Japanese notions of illness, whether mental or physical, hold that illness stems from an imbalance of *ki* within the mind and body. Therefore, the mind and body are considered as a single interactive entity, the "bodymind." If one part is affected with a pathological condition, then that will produce a pathological condition in the other. Further, we call certain aspects of our experience "physical" and others "mental"—but this is a matter of a convention and not a fact.[17] Perhaps for these reasons, practices of spiritual training such as the martial arts (MA; e.g., Aikido) and meditation, which aim for self-cultivation and strengthening the spirit by diminishing one's inflated ego through physical engagement, have been widely practiced in Japanese tradition. The mind is often not treated separately from the body in these Japanese practices.

Naikan shares many aspects with these traditional Japanese practices that work on one's mind through engaging the body. Even though Naikan does not require a strict cross-legged posture or straightening one's back, sitting behind a 3 foot by 3 foot screened space for 14 to 16 hours a day for 1 week involves significant physical engagement. The person who practices Naikan has to be still for an entire week in order to guide her or his mind inward.

Even though Naikan is mostly known for freeing people from mental pain, Naikan clients commonly find that their chronic backaches, knee pains, and even low blood pressure improve during their 1-week Naikan, even when these problems were not the primary reasons for visiting the Naikan center. It is also common for many post-Naikan clients to become more creative, and they often draw paintings or compose poems after one week of Naikan.[18]

Naikan Training and Development, Accreditation, Licensure, and Certification

Currently, there is no specific institute for Naikan training and no certification system to become a Naikan practitioner at a Naikan center. Yoshimoto was against the institutionalization of Naikan and also not interested in creating any kind of licensure system—nor was he interested in theorizing

Naikan. Traditionally, Naikan practitioners in training undergo intense 1-week Naikan at least once (in most cases several times) and, after that, they often assist Naikan under the guidance of an experienced Naikan practitioner. Many Naikan practitioners who are currently active have had Naikan under Yoshimoto's Naikan center, and many received guidance from Yoshimoto. The relationship between client and practitioner seems most similar to the "master and disciple" relationship in traditional Japanese spiritual training. Novice Naikan practitioners often spend some time at the senior Naikan practitioners' Naikan centers and learn from observing how they conduct Naikan, how they respond to questions from Naikan clients, and the way they carry themselves.

When Naikan is applied in clinical settings, medical professionals who conduct Naikan as psychotherapy must be qualified under the regulations set by the Japan Naikan Medical Association. They need to have 1 week of Naikan experience, to have experience working as a counselor at certain institutions for more than 3 years, and to be members of the association for more than 5 years prior to their application in order to be qualified to be certified as psychotherapists by the Japan Naikan Medical Association. There has been increasing pressure for Naikan practitioners at Naikan centers to be certified and a potential certification system has been discussed and may materialize within a few years.

Current Ways in Which Naikan is Practiced

An individual who does Naikan is called a ***Naikan-sha***—literally "a person who does Naikan." A Naikan practitioner is called a ***mensetsu-sha***, meaning "a person who interviews." *Mensetsu-sha* are also *Naikan-sha* as they also do Naikan, so there is no hierarchy that resembles that between doctor and patient in Naikan. For this chapter, we will retain the convention of using the terms *client* and *practitioner* for clarity, but these terms could be misleading if they are not understood within this context.

A typical weeklong Naikan session takes place at a Naikan center, which is usually the house of the Naikan practitioner. Naikan clients sit behind their screens in a small 3 foot by 3 foot square space formed by the two sides of a Japanese paper screen and the two walls of the corner of the room. They are not allowed to talk except during the 3- to 5-minute *mensetsu* interviews, which occur every 2 hours when the practitioner visits them. They cannot read, watch TV, check their e-mail, or make phone calls for the entire week. Three meals are served to them, and they eat behind the screen where they are seated. The only time Naikan clients leave their isolated space is to use the bathroom or take a bath in the evening. Each day, from early morning until night, for 14 to 16 hours, the clients review and reflect on their lives from the perspectives of others in their lives, usually starting and ending the week with their mothers. The mother is considered crucial in Naikan due to the fact that for many people mothers are the primary caretakers from their birth. Naikan practitioners often suggest to those who have difficult relationships with their mothers that they should start their Naikan with someone who took care of them, like their grandparents.

This self-reflection process is interrupted every 2 hours by a *mensetsu*, or interview, during which clients report on their self-examination thus far to the practitioner. The method of recollection is clearly defined: Clients must keep to **Naikan's three themes**: (1) what the client received from that person, (2) what he or she gave back to that person, and (3) what trouble he or she caused that person. Practitioners usually do not explain how these three themes should be interpreted. They do not say, for example, what it means to "receive something" from another person or how "trouble" should be defined. In fact, part of the Naikan process is a deepening of the client's understanding regarding the meaning of these three themes over time. There is no fourth theme of what trouble the other person caused the client, as Naikan holds that people are already experts at remembering troubles caused by others without spending a week at the Naikan center. People only tend to forget or fail to register troubles they caused others.

Two additional themes can be used in Naikan, namely "calculating how much one's parents spent while raising one" and recollecting incidents of "stealing and lying." For those who have difficulties remembering the kindness they received from others, calculating the expense their parents spent for them including food, education, and medical expenses as well as all other allowances often helps them to see vividly how much kindness they received. Almost all Naikan clients are shocked by the enormous amount of expense their parents have spent on them.[19] This topic is intimately connected to the first Naikan question: What did I receive from this person? Another theme, that of stealing and lying, can also be very powerful. Stealing does not just mean shoplifting, for example, but includes not returning a book one borrowed, cheating at exams, and taking a train ride without buying a ticket. Lying is something most individuals can recall easily, and when they do so without excuses and self-justifications, they are often shocked by how frequently they lied to people who were close to them.[20] It is believed in Naikan that individuals, operating from an I-centered perspective, often lie for their own convenience without even thinking this could cause trouble for others. This practice gives individuals a chance to think more about the misdeeds they committed and the negative effects they had on others. This theme is closely connected to the third Naikan question: What trouble did I cause this person?

In 1978, the Japan Naikan Association (*Nihon Naikan Gakkai*) was established with the purpose of theorizing and developing the Naikan method for its future survival after Yoshimoto's death. This association holds annual conferences in which attendees share Naikan experiences and exchange ideas about alternative Naikan methods. These alternative methods include "3-day Naikan," Naikan done through journaling for those who cannot do 1-week Naikan, and other Naikan variations. Naikan sessions abroad are quite similar to Naikan in Japan, but there are slight modifications. Often, slightly larger spaces are used and walking about the premises is permitted.

There is hardly anything that could be considered as collaboration with Western medicine at Naikan centers, but some clients are referred by their clinical counselors and psychiatrists who know Naikan. In addition, Naikan practitioners sometimes refer their clients to nearby hospitals that offer Naikan when they believe that the clients will benefit from medical attention and assistance. Naikan at hospitals could be considered a collaboration with Western medicine in the sense that hospitals offer Naikan along with the necessary medication and supervision by medical professionals. There, Naikan is used for very specific purposes: to treat psychiatric disorders such as drug and alcohol addiction—for example, depression and psychosomatic illness.

Research and Future Directions

In the 1960s, several psychiatrists such as Dr. Takemoto saw the potential benefit of Naikan as a psychotherapy and treatment for addictions such as alcoholism, *pachinko* ("gambling") addiction, and drug addictions, and they reported and published their research findings.[21] A number of medically oriented books were published by psychologists, including *Naikan Therapy* (*Naikan Ryōhō*, 1972) and *Zen-like Therapy: The Naikan Method* (*Zen-teki Ryōhō: Naikan hō*, 1972).[22]

Most scholarship on Naikan is published in Japanese, but a few scholars, including David Reynolds and Ozawa-de Silva, have conducted ethnographic research on Naikan in English.[23] Some Japanese scholarship has been translated into English, including work by the prolific Naikan scholar Murase.[24] In terms of supervision, there is no institutionalized supervision. All supervisions are on a volunteer basis and are carried out by senior Naikan practitioners when novice practitioners are working with them at their Naikan centers.

The future direction of Naikan has been a frequent topic of debate among Naikan practitioners and members of the Japan Naikan Association (*Nihon Naikan Gakkai*) over the past several decades.[25] The Naikan community is divided as to whether Naikan should remain a self-cultivation practice irreducible to psychotherapy or whether Naikan should be widely promoted as a psychotherapy in order to gain more credibility within medicine. Although some medical research has been conducted suggesting Naikan may be effective in clinical and nonclinical settings, there is a lack of research published in prominent scientific and medical journals as well as a lack of theoretical models that would explain Naikan's efficacy in a medical framework.[26] These two factors inhibit medical institutions from introducing Naikan in a more widespread way.

Another challenge that remains is whether Naikan needs to be offered in more accessible forms. Practitioners have long debated whether to offer 3-day

Naikan instead of 1-week Naikan, and many Naikan practitioners do offer the shorter version. Since the death of Yoshimoto, practitioners have also debated the essence of Naikan. Consequently, there has been hesitation in introducing any variations that differ from Yoshimoto's original Naikan method.

Conclusion

Despite the fact that Naikan is widely considered effective in clinical settings for treating psychiatric disorders such as addiction, depression, eating disorders, and psychosomatic illnesses, Naikan's use in clinical settings has not been growing as steadily as it could be. One of the hurdles to its growth in that context might be the incompatibility between Naikan's internal therapeutic mechanism and Western clinical psychology. Naikan's concept of the cause of illness (i.e., mental suffering) and its alleviation is firmly based on Buddhist philosophy and not aligned with the biomedical approach to mental illness. This presents challenges when conveying Naikan and its psychotherapeutic effectiveness within a biomedical framework.

As opposed to the biomedical view that symptoms should be removed, Naikan does not focus on individuals' symptoms themselves. Naikan considers an excessively I-centered ordinary perspective to be a fundamental distorted cognition that is the root cause of all suffering and even illness. Once Naikan clients change their views on themselves and others through Naikan by focusing on the kindness and support they have been receiving from others in their life, they realize the interdependent nature of their existence and their gratitude toward others increases.

Recent scientific studies of mind in cognitive psychology and contemplative meditation research have found a strong correlation between certain mental states such as gratitude, compassion, a sense of connectedness and belongingness, and mental well-being.[27] These mental states are commonly shared outcomes of Naikan practice.[28] Naikan might benefit from the number of contemplative studies that have been gaining increasing attention and the increasing number of researchers who are now studying the correlation between these mental states and positive mental health. If Naikan is further validated by scientific research, there may be more chance of a successful intersection between Naikan and the practices of clinical and counseling psychology.

Case Study

The client was a female airline stewardess who was 28 years old when she visited one of the Naikan centers in Japan. She had been married for 4 years and had been suffering from "anxiety neurosis" for 3 years when she came to the Naikan center on the advice of her psychiatrist. The client was convinced that the cause of her illness was her mother who did not

(Continued)

(Continued)

take care of her properly. The client struggled with Naikan's first and third questions, remembering kindness and support she received from her mother and troubles she caused her mother, due to her strong resentment against her mother. As a result, she treated these questions as opportunities to complain about how terrible her mother had been. The client's strong resentment against her mother was preventing her from being able to follow Naikan's three questions and make progress.

The client was diagnosed with anxiety neurosis 3 years before she came to the Naikan center. She came to realize that her environment as a child had been a partial cause of her illness. She disliked her mother even as a small child. The client felt strongly that she became ill because of her mother. The client spent the first three days doing Naikan in relation to her mother. Her strong resentment against her mother caused great difficulty for her to report anything about what she received from her mother or about the troubles she caused her mother. The practitioner suggested that the client should make a list of her problems with her mother. After the client made a list of 48 complaints, the practitioner asked the client to read through the list by reversing her descriptions of the complaints (e.g., she read "my mother did not cook three meals a day" as "my mother cooked three meals a day all the time"). Once she read the reversed version of her list, she was utterly shocked to realize that her expectations toward her mother were unrealistically demanding. On the fourth day, the practitioner advised the client to do Naikan in relation to her father, with whom she had no emotional problems. As she was able to recall the kindness, support, and affection she received from her father, she ended the day feeling great gratitude toward him and knowing that he loved her very much. Perhaps the combination of the client's new insight about her unrealistic expectations toward her mother and her realization of the love and kindness she received from her father led to her hostile feelings being replaced with warm, happy feelings by the end of the fifth day. On the sixth and seventh days, Naikan led her to experience powerful self-transformation. She realized all the affection she had been receiving from her mother despite her shortcomings and her tendency to focus on what she did not receive rather than what she received from her mother. She was filled with joy, the sense of being loved at the end of Naikan.

This is a case of someone whose understanding and perception of a significant other, her mother, changed dramatically during a 1-week session of Naikan. The client began with a negative image of her mother and ended her week of Naikan with a very positive image. She used to think the cause of her illness was her irresponsible mother, but toward the end of Naikan she reported that it was not her mother's fault. She stated that because she always paid attention to the things her mother did not do, she grew in anger and dissatisfaction and consequently built up stress and became sick. Many individuals blame external factors and others such as family for their suffering and illness. In Naikan, in accordance with Buddhist philosophy, the I-centered perspective, inflating one's importance over others due to the lack of understanding of the interdependent nature of human existence, is the cause of individuals' suffering. Through 1 week of Naikan, clients often change their views of significant others. As a consequence of doing so, they change their views of themselves. Once this client realized the interdependence of her existence through remembering the kindness and affection she had received from her mother, she was filled with an increased sense of gratitude, being loved, and inner security. When she ended her week of Naikan, she said, "I gained security and, since I am certain of the affection I've received now, I think I can finally live in the present."

DISCUSSION QUESTIONS

1. What is distinctive about the notion of "healing" within Naikan? What is the difference between the biomedical notion of a "cure" and Naikan's "healing"?
2. Why are Naikan's three themes or questions essential for its practice? What kind of insights do clients gain through remembering their past according to these three questions, and why are these insights healing?
3. Why is an I-centered ordinary perspective considered to cause illness and suffering in Naikan and Buddhist philosophy? What are the benefits of shifting from such a perspective to an other-centered perspective according to Naikan?
4. What are the main challenges for Naikan to have a more successful connection with counseling psychology? Why is Naikan so difficult to theorize within the biomedical framework?

REFERENCES

1. Yanagita, K. (1997). *Ai no Shinri Ryōhō Naikan: Yorokobi to Yasuragi no Sekai [Psychotherapy of love: The world of joy and calmness]*. Tokyo, Japan: Inabashobō.
2. Ozawa-de Silva, C. (2006). *Psychotherapy and religion in Japan: The Japanese introspection practice of Naikan*. London, England: Routledge.
3. Ozawa-de Silva, C. (2015). Mindfulness of the kindness of others: The contemplative practice of Naikan in cultural context. *Transcultural Psychiatry*, *52*(4), 1–19.
4. Ozawa-de Silva, *Psychotherapy and religion in Japan*.
5. Yoshimoto, I. (1997). *Naikanhō [The Naikan method]*. Tokyo, Japan: Shunjusha.
6. Ozawa-de Silva, *Psychotherapy and religion in Japan*.
7. Ozawa-de Silva, Mindfulness of the kindness.
8. Ibid.
9. Ozawa-de Silva, *Psychotherapy and religion in Japan*.
10. Miki, Y. (2015, June). Unpublished data collected from Naikan centers in Japan.
11. Ozawa-de Silva, Mindfulness of the kindness.
12. Miki, Unpublished data.
13. Ohnuki-Tierney, E. (1984). *Illness and culture in contemporary Japan*. Cambridge, England: Cambridge University Press.
14. Yuasa, Y. (1993). *The body, self-cultivation, and ki-energy*. New York: State University of New York Press.
15. Ozawa-de Silva, C. (2002). Beyond the body/mind? Japanese contemporary thinkers on alternative sociologies of the body. *Body & Society*, *8*(2), 21–38.
16. Kabat-Zinn, J. (1990). *Full catastrophe living*. New York, NY: Delta Trade Paperbacks.
17. Yuasa, *The body*; Ozawa-de Silva, Beyond the body/mind?; Ichikawa, H. (1991). *Seishin to Shiteno Shintai [The body as spirit]*. Tokyo, Japan: Keiso Shobo.
18. Ozawa-de Silva, *Psychotherapy and religion*; Ozawa-de Silva, C. (2007). Demystifying Japanese therapy: An analysis of Naikan and the Ajase complex through Buddhist thought. *Ethos*, *35*(4), 411–446.

19. Miki, Y. (2015). *The book about encountering your heart's treasure.* Nara City, Nara: Weissman Press.
20. Yoshimoto, *Naikanhō.*
21. Takemoto, T. (1984). Arukoru Kanja ni taisuru Naikan Ryōhō no Yukosei [The efficacy of Naikan for treating alcoholism]. *Gendai no Esupuri: Meisō no Seishinryōhō: Naikan Ryōhō no Riron to Jissai [Meditational Psychotherapy: The Naikan Method's Theory and Practice], 202,* 75–85; Kawahara, R. (1996). *Naikan Ryōhō [Naikan Therapy]*. Tokyo, Japan: Shinkō Igaku Shuppan.
22. Okumura, N., Sato, K., & Yamamoto, H. (Eds.). (1972). *Naikan Ryōhō [Naikan therapy]*. Tokyo, Japan: Igaku Shoin; Sato; K. (Ed.). (1972). *Zen-teki Ryōhō: Naikan ho [Zen-like therapy: The Naikan method]*. Tokyo, Japan: Bunkodo.
23. Ozawa-de Silva, *Psychotherapy and religion*; Ohnuki-Tierney, *Illness and culture.*
24. Murase, T. (1982). Sunao: A central value in Japanese psychotherapy. In A. J. Marsella & G. M. White (Eds.), *Cultural conceptions of mental health and therapy* (pp. 317–329). Dordrecht, Netherlands: D. Reidel.
25. Ozawa-de Silva, *Psychotherapy and religion.*
26. Jimu, K. (2010). Nihon Naikan Igaku Gakkai Nintei Ishi, Nintei Shinri Ryōhō Shi to Seido Kisoku [Japan Naikan Medical Association certified doctor, certified psychotherapists regulations]. *Naikan Igaku [Naikan Medicine], 12*(1), 66–69.
27. Pace, T. W. W., Negi, L. T., Adame, D. D., Cole, S. P., Sivilli, T. I., Brown, T. D., . . . Raison, C. L. (2009). Effect of compassion meditation on neuroendocrine, innate immune and behavioral responses to psychosocial stress. *Psychoneuroendocrinology, 34*(1), 87–98; Ozawa-de Silva, B., Dodson-Lavelle, B., Raison, C. L., & Negi, L. T. (2012). Compassion and ethics: Scientific and practical approaches to the cultivation for compassion as a foundation for ethical subjectivity and well-being. *The Journal of Healthcare, Sciences, and the Humanities*, *2*(1), 145–161.
28. Ozawa-de Silva, *Psychotherapy and religion*; Ozawa-de Silva, Mindfulness of the kindness; Ohnuki-Tierney, *Illness and culture.*

SUGGESTED READINGS

Krech, G. (2002). *Naikan: Gratitude, grace, and the Japanese art of self-reflection.* Berkeley, CA: Stone Bridge Press.

This is perhaps the best English book on Naikan that is most accessible to general readers and to those who are interested in the practice component of Naikan. This book provides an overview of what Naikan is, its focus on gratitude and self-reflection, and instructions that convey how to practice Naikan at home. The author is a leading Naikan practitioner outside of Japan and the director of the ToDo Institute, a U.S.-based organization that offers several Japanese alternative healing practices.

Miki, Y. (2015). *The book about encountering your heart's treasure.* Nara City, Nara: Weissman Press.

This is a handy booklet on Naikan. It is very short but contains a concise introduction to Naikan with extensive case histories. Written by a Japanese psychologist who is also a Naikan practitioner, this book is well suited to those who are in counseling and interested in incorporating some components of indigenous psychotherapy. Detailed descriptions of Naikan clients' Naikan experience offer a good sense of what it is like to go through a 1-week session of Naikan.

Ozawa-de Silva, C. (2006). *Psychotherapy and religion in Japan: The Japanese introspection practice of Naikan.* New York, NY: Routledge.

This is a highly valuable book to general readers with an interest in indigenous healing practice, meditation, contemplative studies, and anthropology. As this book explores how Naikan lies on the border of psychotherapy and spirituality and provides an important analysis of a non-Western psychotherapeutic method that works on the levels of both body and mind, it is helpful to those who are interested in the interconnection and infusion of indigenous healing practice and Western psychotherapy.

Reynolds, D. (1982). *Quiet therapies: Japanese pathways to personal growth.* Honolulu: University of Hawaii Press.

This is a highly valuable book for those who are interested in the interconnection between indigenous healing practices and Western psychotherapy and especially those who are in psychology and counseling. It offers a comprehensive introduction to numerous indigenous healing practices with many examples, methods, and case histories. It is very accessible to a general audience and is a good introduction to numerous indigenous healing practices, including Naikan.

13 Morita Therapy

Charles P. Chen

Morita therapy is a method of psychotherapy rooted in Eastern philosophies of life and health.[1] Beginning in the 1950s, this Eastern-influenced counseling modality received considerable attention from Western psychotherapy and counseling professionals.[2] Of particular interest was its approach in treating what is now commonly known as **social anxiety**.[3] Many counselors and psychologists are tasked with helping clients cope with emotional difficulties in social relationships.[4] These difficulties often result in feelings of anxiety, which negatively affect clients by inhibiting full participation and enjoyment in life. Following traditional Eastern philosophies, Morita therapy contends that anxious feelings are a normal part of the human experience and are thus impossible to eliminate.[5]

The goal of Morita therapy is to allow individuals to experience life alongside negative feelings, with the anxiety being accepted and integrated into daily living. It is expected that anxiety will become "a normal companion" in one's life, and therefore, its negative influence will be diminished, allowing the individual to live a satisfying life.[6] Traditional Morita therapy was an inpatient program that required a lengthy residential stay.[7] Clients progressed through four stages at which certain objectives of the therapeutic intervention were achieved.[8] Since its integration into the Western world, Morita therapy has become more flexible and open to changes.[9] Its theoretical base has expanded, and its progressive design is now considered a method of cognitive and behavioral therapy with Eastern philosophical roots.[10] Over time, interest in applying Morita therapy has grown even further. As a result, academic research and literature on Morita therapy has increased, with respect to the therapy's theory and clinical application.[11] In fact, it is now considered one of the few influential Eastern approaches in the Western world, especially in North America.[12]

This chapter provides a brief overview of the history of traditional Morita therapy and the ways it is currently practiced in the West. It begins with an overview of the healing traditions and cultural representations of illness and wellness, illustrating the main tenets of Morita therapy from a healing tradition perspective. Based on that, the potential application of Morita's traditional philosophies in clinical practice is further explored in the following section, which focuses on the current ways in which Morita therapy is practiced. Lastly, the chapter concludes with a discussion on Morita therapy's strengths and weaknesses along with future directions and research.

Brief History of Morita Therapy

Morita therapy was founded by Japanese psychiatrist Shoma Morita (1874–1938) in the early 1920s.[13] Like other contemporary mental health professionals at the time, Morita practiced and studied psychoanalytical theory.[14] However, Morita felt that in order to more effectively address ***shinkeishitsu***, a Japanese term describing nervousness and anxiety, a new treatment approach was needed.[15] This conclusion was based on Morita's clinical observations and interventions with patients over the course of 20 years. He was also influenced by his own personal affliction with nervousness and anxiety that had not been alleviated by any other psychotherapy treatment at the time. As Morita developed his therapy, he conducted residential treatment trials at his home on several of his patients. This residential treatment method later became a standard clinical intervention format in other settings, such as hospitals, therapeutic residences, and treatment centers.[16]

The original Morita therapy required a 4- to 6-week stay in a hospital or a residential treatment facility to ensure adherence to the traditional intervention protocol.[17] The intervention process includes the client's progression through four phases or stages; certain therapeutic tasks must be completed in order for the client to proceed to the next stage.[18] The central goal of these phases is to have the client capable of normalizing feelings of anxiety through engagement in active and productive daily life experiences.[19] Thus, the intervention techniques involve behavioral modification and cognitive reappraisal, as Morita often stressed the importance of working and changing practical elements in clients' lives.[20] He emphasized taking action as a means of producing change, since action-taking is an active learning process. As such, Morita therapy has a strong cognitive behavioral background.[21] However, it is important to note that Morita therapy's holistic view of health considers therapeutic change to be more than cognitions and behaviors; attention is also paid to the influence of the natural environment on an individual's well-being.[22] A part of the four stages of Morita therapy includes interacting with nature through daily tasks as well as trusting one's own natural state without judgment, thus allowing for active responding toward what needs to be attended to without overintellectualizing a situation.[23]

As Morita therapy grew in popularity, it became a dominant psychotherapy practice across Japan.[24] Many Japanese scholars and practitioners applied Morita therapy in their clinical practice and built upon the initial model, expanding its theoretical base. Eventually, it grew into a much more flexible intervention strategy that could be applied to nonresidential treatment interventions in group and individual counseling. Its influence on the Western world peaked during the 1970s and 1980s, where it became one of the few well-recognized and well-respected Eastern psychotherapies, particularly in North America.[25]

Healing Traditions and Cultural Representations of Illness and Wellness

Traditionally, Western psychological modalities regarded anxiety as an unwanted reaction, with the goal of reducing or eliminating symptoms.[26] Eastern philosophies, on the other hand, have contended that anxiety is a normal part of the human experience and therefore impossible to eliminate. Morita therapy differs from other modalities in its stage-like process along with its conception of health as holistic. The purpose of Morita therapy is to integrate anxiety into the individual's life.[27] It is believed that harmony between the individual and the anxious emotions will reduce the negative impact of the anxiety. Over time, and with practice, the individual's capacity to tolerate anxiety and discomfort will increase and will eventually allow for productive functioning. The client is encouraged to obey his or her own nature, to adopt an accepting attitude toward life experiences, and to connect with the natural environment.[28]

Central to Morita therapy is the notion of connectedness to nature. Psychological and physical environments are intertwined and present in our world, and attempts to control this natural process are seen as futile and even detrimental. For example, the second phase of Morita intervention requires the client to concentrate on light activities, such as weeding or observing animals or plants. These activities enable the client to learn to foster connections with natural life experiences. It allows the client to become a part of the universe and all living creatures. Morita's principle of obedience to nature reinforces the importance of accepting all living experiences. It is with this attitude that the client enables him- or herself to become a part of the world and its natural flow. By attending to action and nature and regarding the self as a connected entity with the universe, it is assumed that anxiety will be reduced.

Further evidence of the role Eastern philosophies play in Morita therapy are the common principles it shares with Zen Buddhism.[29] In Buddhism, one of the more effective ways one can deal with reality is to accept it. Since the existence of difficulties in life will always be present, it is the *perception* of such issues that leads to either healthy or unhealthy coping. Accepting the presence of an issue is the first step toward making a change. It should be noted that acceptance is an active process and not a passive one. Morita therapy, which deals with social anxiety, views social anxiety as a natural part of life. The next step is to make productive use of energy by accepting the issue, rather than to invest energy to fight or deny the issue.

The Chinese concept of *yin* and *yang* is also a foundational principle of Morita therapy.[30] Morita philosophy views life as whole, balanced entity that is made up of these interdependent energy forces: *yin* and *yang*. These complementary forces coexist in the universe, and one cannot exist without the other. This "bilateral worldview" reflects seemingly opposing human experiences, such as positive–negative, peaceful–violent, sufficient–inadequate, and so forth. However, both "opposites" coexist in human life, even though one may appear at times more dominant over the other. Therapy aims to utilize the perceived negative side, the anxiety feelings, as the complement for the growth of the positive side, which is personal development and improvement.

Morita Therapy: Training and Development, Accreditation, Licensure, and Certification

Morita therapy requires certain counselor characteristics.[31] The responsibility rests on both the client and the counselor to accept anxiety as it is and not as a symptom to be treated. If the counselor believes that anxiety must be changed or reduced, based upon his or her experience, values, or therapeutic orientation, then it would be assumed that the counselor's bias would inadvertently lead to the need to control feelings of anxiety as part of the therapeutic process. This might encourage the client to believe that anxiety is abnormal in nature and must be eliminated. Thus, for Morita therapy to be effective, the counselor should be eclectic by nature and flexible in conceptualizing anxiety symptoms. In addition, the counselor should be comfortable with experiencing anxiety in his or her own life in order to help clients with their anxiety. Role modeling of acceptance of anxiety is the key to success in Morita therapy. Counselors are encouraged to examine their own attitudes and theoretical preferences in terms of emotional acceptance, control, and confrontation during therapy.[32]

Two organizations involved in the training and development of Morita therapy include the Japanese Society for Morita Therapy (JSMT) and the International Committee for Morita Therapy (ICMT). The JSMT provides certification and training in order to become a Morita therapist. The ICMT oversees the development and accreditation of Morita therapy as well as promoting and hosting international conferences and educational workshops.

Current Ways in Which Morita Therapy Is Practiced

Traditional Morita therapy is composed of four stages that are action-oriented. The main objective in each phase is to normalize anxiety through active participation in life activities. Each phase has concrete behavioral goals, and clients must complete one stage before progressing to the next.[33] This section will describe the phases in detail.[34]

Phase One: Absolute Bed Rest

This phase lasts between 4 to 7 days and requires complete bed rest, aside from very basic activities of daily living (ADL), such as meals and hygiene. The client is forbidden from engaging in any social interaction. The counselor asks the client to experience agony rather than avoid it. This is done to intensify the negative feelings, which will reduce and simplify the inner psychic conflicts. The intense bed rest helps the client recover from the inner conflict, which in turn will spontaneously motivate the client to get up and take action. It is at this point that the counselor checks with the client whether the client is able to follow the therapy's procedures. If it is deemed an unfit modality for the client, then therapy is terminated.

Phase Two: Light Work

In this phase, the client is instructed to pursue light activities for a period of 3 to 7 days. Socialization is still not permitted at this stage. Sleep time is reduced to a regular 7 to 8 hours, with the majority of waking hours spent outdoors. Intense physical activity is prohibited, and the client is encouraged to spend time on light activities such as observing nature, weeding, or gathering leaves. The client is also asked to keep a diary to record his or her experiences throughout the day. The counselor provides three lectures to the client that focus on explaining the process of the therapy and the recovery period. The counselor uses the diary as a reference source to the client's feelings, thoughts, and physical state. These lectures direct the client's attention to facts rather than to ascribed meaning of said facts, while also drawing attention to behavior and action. This means that the client is directed to view events from an objective point of view, one that is void of personal interpretation. The primary goal of this phase is to transition the client from absolute bed rest to engagement in light activities. The client engages in action, and as a result, his or her thoughts are attenuated to life tasks that are devoid of psychic conflict. The amount of work the client puts forth in this phase is of utmost importance, as this stage is the foundation for proceeding stages of the intervention.

Phase Three: Life Chores

The third phase of chores lasts between 7 and 20 days. In this phase, the client is assigned daily tasks such as kitchen work, room cleaning, and other activities, based on the client's interests. This phase can be considered an extension of the previous phase and is tailored to each client's interests and abilities, along with a varying range of activities, intensity of work, and duration of time. Through this work, the client develops a sense of patience and contentment with the work itself. Happiness and satisfaction also grows, when the client discovers capacity and agency for being involved in daily tasks. The client becomes more confident about his or her ability to live a fulfilling and meaningful life, as this phase progresses.

Phase Four: Real-Life Experience

The last phase of the intervention lasts for 10 days. This phase is a transition period back to "real life." It expands on the learning that took place in previous phases and encourages the client to practice with patience the newly developed appreciation for daily activities. The client is entrusted with diverse tasks—even ones that are outside of one's personal desire or interest. Socialization is gradually introduced to the client, who is now able to experience life as dynamic, multifaceted, and complex. The central focus of this phase is to prepare the client to go back to living life with a new and positive outlook on life, one that encompasses inconvenient feelings along with satisfaction and happiness. As Morita therapy focuses on changing those conditions under which clients can feel free to express their inner character, continued awareness to one's growth allows the client to resume a healthy and productive life.

One of Morita therapy's central tenets is obedience to nature, and this principle can be practiced within counseling to help the client view anxiety as a natural part of the human experience.[35] Through the various phases, the client is encouraged to become aware of feelings of anxiety while also accepting the presence of such discomfort. This productive process aims to develop coping mechanisms as a natural response to negative experiences. As the client becomes more comfortable with the idea of coexisting with anxiety, the negative impact of the anxiety will slowly decline. Morita therapy does not aim to eliminate anxiety per se—its overreaching goal is to reduce the negative impact anxiety might have on the individual so that clients are equipped to live a productive life. The lack of preoccupation with one's anxiety will also make available cognitive resources that were previously invested in suppressing or fighting feelings of anxiety and inner conflict. This will return attention to daily activities as well as opportunities to achieve life goals. Thus, as clients realize they can live a full life without eliminating negative feelings, they will be less affected by said emotions. A *yin* and *yang* philosophy can be applied to help clients explore and perceive anxiety symptoms in a different light.[36] For example, a client who is bothered by anxiety is often preoccupied with the feeling itself and is less inclined to explore the issue from all viewpoints. The counselor's role, then, is to help the client view the situation in a more holistic manner, from both sides of the coin—as *yin* and *yang*. The client is to develop a tolerance for more flexible and dynamic cognitive appraisal of the world.

The client will view life experiences as a whole and learn to accept dichotomies as common phenomena.

Emerging interest in mindfulness in Western psychotherapy has paved the way for the integration of Morita therapy into current practice.[37] Mindfulness can be defined as the awareness that results from paying close attention to the present moment.[38] Mindfulness practice, similar to Morita therapy, is rooted in Eastern philosophies of the mind–body connection and balance. Mindfulness is a part of Buddhist Zen practice and ideology.[39] Morita therapy and mindfulness both aim to harness the individual's inner strength to improve their abilities to respond and withstand life changes with acceptance and harmony. Both view psychological balance as not eliminating symptoms and problems but rather enabling individuals to accept change and embrace the full spectrum of human living.[40]

Based on the ways Morita therapy is currently practiced, there are a number of suggested cognitive and behavioral activities that can be incorporated into the counseling process for social anxiety.[41]

Acknowledgment of Anxiety Feelings

Acknowledging the presence of anxiety is the first step toward change, as it provides the client with the opportunity to reflect on his or her feelings without any judgment or criticism. The client is encouraged to share anxiety-provoking events and associated feelings in counseling sessions. Together, the client and counselor explore specific antecedents and situations that may lead to experiencing anxiety. The counselor's role is to guide the client to consider the event itself first, without the client's original interpretation of it. This will clarify the connection between possible triggers and resulting anxiety. Moreover, it will allow clients to experience anxiety in the here and now as they reexperience the event through recollection of details. This is assumed to increase the tolerance the client might have toward anxiety.

Acceptance and Implementing Action

The next step, once anxiety feelings are acknowledged, is to assist the client in developing healthy coping mechanisms. The client comes to realize that although individuals have limited control on external events, they do have control and choice as to how they react and cope with a situation. The individual can choose to become preoccupied with the emotions or choose to accept them while taking proactive and constructive action. As the client focuses on action and does not dwell on the emotion, the negative feelings become a normal part of living and therefore less important and intense. To facilitate acceptance, anxiety feelings are normalized within therapy sessions and viewed as a natural part of human life, rather than as abnormal symptoms that need to be eliminated.

The counselor achieves this by asking the client to put aside the presenting problem and focus on other similar experiences in daily life. The client is encouraged to discuss anxiety feelings in other contexts that are separate from the presenting issue, such as an unexpected traffic jam, a very tight work schedule, and so on. This process provides the client with evidence that anxiety feelings are a common phenomenon in life and that in most situations he or she is able to overcome these experiences and go on with living. The client and counselor then explore together coping mechanisms that were effective with dealing with similar issues in the past, and the client comes to realize that such coping skills are transferable in dealing with the presenting issue. Lastly, to promote action, the client and counselor work together on the client's will and readiness to act as well as the client's specific action plans. Morita therapy intervention calls for flexibility and keeping an open mind, as action plans might necessitate change and adaptation since they are implemented in various contexts. Overall, clients can better cope with anxiety as they implement acceptance and a proactive action-taking.

Research and Future Directions

Research on the efficacy of Morita therapy on social anxiety along with other symptoms may shed light on the fit of Morita within contemporary therapy and the ways it can aid the therapy process. Clearly, there is a need to broaden the scope of disorders that can benefit from Morita therapy principles from the original *shinkeishitsu* to other anxiety-related disorders.[42] Another potential area of exploration would be to investigate change reinforcers and methods of maintaining progress after Morita intervention is complete. The questions that follow are only a few possible intriguing questions that will shed light on the value that Morita therapy might add to currently practiced therapy modalities: In what counseling frameworks can Morita principles add therapeutic value? How can improvement on post-Morita intervention be measured? How can change be maintained over time?

As with any other treatment modality, it is important to note Morita therapy's limitations when practiced in Western settings. Limitations include the long inpatient stay at treatment facilities and the stage model of Morita therapy that may seem rigid and inflexible when adopted in a Western therapeutic setting. Even though it is still practiced in this form, very few individuals have the time and resources to engage in such a lengthy and static process. To ameliorate these challenges, current Morita therapy has been adapted for use in outpatient practice, such as individual therapy and group work as well as psychoeducational interventions.[43] Another limitation to note is Morita's narrow focus on behavioral intervention. There is room for the integration of other modalities and aspects of change, such as affect regulation and additional cognitive work to strengthen the effect of the behavioral change.

With these limitations in mind, there are some overreaching principles of Morita therapy that can be adapted to a variety of contexts and modalities. The *yin* and *yang* concept and the bilateral worldview can contribute to cognitive and behavioral change. As previously discussed, clients are encouraged to view anxiety from a different perspective to gain a comprehensive understanding of the issue, thus accepting the *yin* and *yang* coexistence in life. The process of rationally exploring different viewpoints within a counseling framework can be beneficial in the treatment of issues other than anxiety. Attributions of life events are thus challenged, explored, and reinterpreted—therein lay the potential to use Morita therapy principles but to expand on its original scope.[44]

The Western world has begun to develop and accept Eastern philosophies, such as mindfulness, into contemporary and recognized clinical practices.[45] As Morita therapy has also progressed and become more flexible, there exists the opportunity to utilize Morita principles in research and in therapy. It is apparent that mindfulness and Morita therapy share common grounds. Parallels can be drawn from Morita phases to mindfulness practice. For example, the first phase of traditional Morita therapy involves merely noticing and experiencing anxiety in its truest form while on bed rest. No judgment is associated with the awareness of the agony of the conflicting inner psychic forces. The following phases of light activities and chores require the client to pay attention to the activities that he or she engages in and, again, with an accepting tone. The client pays attention to the work itself and not the meaning associated with it, as is often practiced in mindfulness. As interest in mindfulness practice grows and develops within Western practice, there is an apparent need and interest to enrich current practices with Eastern approaches, such as Morita therapy, within clinical frameworks.

Conclusion

Morita therapy, an Eastern psychotherapy model, provides a unique outlook on treatment of anxiety.[46] Even though Morita therapy has received growing interest from the West, it is still not widely known. The original Morita intervention had prescribed and rigid phases, but its implementation in Western countries has been broader and more flexible. Morita therapy principles can be used to guide clients during interventions.[47] It provides fresh insight into framing issues and aids clients to view issues from different lenses, thereby finding new ways to live a more positive and productive life. Moreover, Morita tenets can be used as a conceptual foundation for other therapy strategies within an eclectic intervention framework. Morita principles promote acceptance of anxiety as a natural part of living, and the focus of helping is on the formation of a holistic conceptualization of anxiety. The counseling work focuses on acknowledgment of feelings and action for change, rather than attempts to reduce or eliminate anxiety as a whole.[48] As the Western world begins to adopt Eastern-based counseling interventions, such as mindfulness, there is an opportunity to explore and integrate Morita perspectives into current counseling practice. At this point in time, Morita therapy in Western practice can be viewed as an overreaching therapeutic orientation alongside other commonly practiced interventions.

Case Study

Marie is a 22-year-old female who lives at home with her parents and her younger sister. She graduated from college several months ago and recently started a new job at a local news agency. The news agency is a fast-paced environment, and Marie is constantly working to meet deadlines. In her free time, Marie enjoys going to the movies, reading, and cycling. She also enjoys spending time with her two close friends whom she has known since childhood.

Upon starting her new job, Marie found herself feeling very anxious and overwhelmed. As the weeks went by, Marie's anxiety became increasingly more intense. She was particularly anxious around others, especially her new colleagues and in anticipation of team meetings. Marie began to avoid interacting with her colleagues and would try to steer clear of group conversations and gatherings. Marie was often intensely worried that she would embarrass herself or that those around her would think negatively of her. She was aware that her feelings might be irrational; however, she could not escape her feelings of dread and anxiety. Marie noticed how relieved she would feel when she could avoid social settings and would often make excuses in order not to have to be involved. As of late, her family has noticed her becoming increasingly withdrawn, especially on weekends where she opts to stay at home more often than usual.

Marie recalls meeting all milestones at their appropriate age and does not recall any significant events or traumas growing up. However, Marie remembers being somewhat shy and introverted as a child. She often felt uncomfortable and out of place in social settings and relied on her friends for interaction and comfort. However, she noted getting along well with her peers and having a small group of friends. Academically, Marie recalls doing well in school and not having any significant difficulties. She excelled in writing assignments and did quite well in math and science. However, she disliked presentations and would shy away from speaking in front of large groups of people. Marie recounted that she would participate in class only if she were very confident in her answer and often chose to take a back seat in class discussions. Marie enjoyed working from home and avoided going to libraries as she found that the presence of others made it harder for her to concentrate.

Through residential treatment using Morita therapy, Marie completed four phases: (1) absolute bed rest, (2) light work, (3) life chores, and (4) real-life experience. In the first phase, Marie committed to absolute bed rest and avoided all social interaction and other activities. The therapist encouraged Marie to experience her anxiety as it was and not to resist or avoid the unwanted feelings. Through this phase, Marie began to gain awareness of contradictory thinking and negative feelings that had previously intensified in her mind. In the second phase, light work was encouraged, and a majority of Marie's time was spent outdoors. Marie was directed to concentrate on activities such as observing animals or plants, or completing garden work like weeding or gathering fallen leaves. This began the adjustment toward taking action in spite of anxious symptoms. Socialization was still avoided, and sleep time was reduced to a regular 7 to 8 hours. At a cognitive level, the therapist worked with Marie to explore her feelings, thoughts, and physical state. Attempts to provide new perspectives that were void of personal interpretation were made. In the third phase, Marie continued to build on and incorporate daily tasks into her life. The goal for Marie was to normalize her anxiety through active participation in life activities, beginning with light work and progressing into more active chores. By increasing her behavior into more constructive activities, Marie felt more confident about living a productive life. In the fourth phase, Marie began the transition period back to "real life" and practiced with patience her newly developed appreciation for daily activities. Socialization was gradually introduced, and the main focus was to prepare Marie to go back to living life with a new and positive outlook on life and one that encompasses inconvenient feelings along with satisfaction and happiness.

Using Morita therapy, Marie was encouraged to view her anxious feelings as acceptable and normal. She learned to acknowledge the presence of her anxiety and to not resist the unwanted feelings. The more Marie attempted to suppress or escape her feelings of anxiety, the more disruptive it was to her functioning. Often attempting to control or eliminate unwanted symptoms results in a continued fixation and preoccupation on the feelings one is trying to avoid. Through Morita therapy, Marie was presented with the opportunity to let her thoughts and feelings come and go and to accept her anxious feelings as they arose. Alongside this acceptance, Marie focused on taking action, beginning with light activities and progressing into tasks that were important or necessary in her life. With the help of her therapist, Marie explored what it means to live a meaningful, purposeful, and constructive life. Eventually, her negative emotions reduced as greater harmony between her anxious feelings and current state was achieved. Marie also developed more tolerance toward her anxious feelings, further allowing her to continue to live a productive life.

DISCUSSION QUESTIONS

1. Morita therapy places emphasis on being in nature and interacting with the natural world. What do you think are some of the benefits one can attain from engaging with nature? Consider the last time you were outdoors and interacting with the natural environment. Do you think it affected you positively? If so, why?

2. What does living a life with meaning and purpose look like to you? How important do you think this principle is in order to manage anxiety? What factors do you think make it more challenging for you to live a life of meaning and purpose?

3. Think about a time when you may have felt anxious or nervous. Describe the situation as well as the feelings and thoughts that may have arisen. How intense were your feelings? How long did those feelings last? Considering Morita therapy's principle of acceptance and not resisting anxiety, how could you incorporate these principles? Do you think it would have made a difference?

4. Think about an activity you have recently engaged in today and preferably one you did by yourself (i.e., brushing your teeth, commuting to your place of work). Try to remember an activity that is recent in time. Notice if you were in fact present and engaged in the activity or if your mind was elsewhere and preoccupied with the future or the past. How do you think you can become more present in the moment as you engage in these activities?

REFERENCES

1. Chen, C. P. (1996). Positive living with anxiety: A Morita perspective of human agency. *Counselling Psychology Quarterly*, *9*(1), 5–14.
2. Chen, C. P. (2010). Morita therapy and its counseling implications for social anxiety. *Counselling Psychology Quarterly*, *23*(1), 67–82.
3. Chen, C. P. (2005). Morita therapy: A philosophy of yin/yang co-existence. In R. Moodley & W. West (Eds.), *Integrating traditional healing practices into counseling and psychotherapy.* Thousand Oaks, CA: Sage; Chen, Morita therapy and its counseling implications; Ishiyama, F. I. (1991). A Japanese reframing technique for brief social anxiety treatment: An exploratory study of cognitive and therapeutic effects of Morita therapy. *Journal of Cognitive Psychotherapy*, *5*(1), 55–70.
4. Chen, Morita therapy and its counseling implications.
5. Chen, Positive living with anxiety; Chen, Morita therapy: A philosophy; Chen, Morita therapy and its counseling implications.
6. Chen, Morita therapy and its counseling implications.
7. Goto, K. (1988). Shinkeishitsu treatment by Morita therapy in its original form. *International Bulletin of Morita Therapy*, *1*(2), 37–42.
8. Chen, Morita therapy: A philosophy; Chen, Morita therapy and its counseling implications.
9. Chen, Morita therapy and its counseling implications.
10. Chen, Positive living with anxiety; Chen, Morita therapy: A philosophy.
11. Chen, C. P. (1998). A holistic approach to worklife dynamics: Morita-philosophy-based career counselling. *Counselling Psychology Quarterly*, *11*(3), 239–256; Chen, C. P. (2003, March). Morita therapy intervention for work-related anxiety. Paper presented at the Fifth Interdisciplinary Conference on Occupational Stress and Health—Work, Stress, and Health: New Challenges in a Changing Workplace (American Psychological Association), Toronto, Canada; Donahue, P. A. (1988). Practical application of basic Morita concepts in fostering productive living: A trainee's account. *International Bulletin of Morita Therapy*, *1*(1), 26–30.
12. Chen, Morita therapy: A philosophy; Ishiyama, F. I. (2003). A bending willow tree: A Japanese (Morita therapy) model of human nature and client change. *Canadian Journal of Counselling and Psychotherapy*, *37*(3), 216–231; Walsh, R. (2000). Asian psychotherapies. In R. Corsini & D. Wedding (Eds.), *Current psychotherapies* (6th ed., pp. 407–444). Itasca, IL: F. E. Peacock Publishers.
13. Chen, Morita therapy and its counseling implications; Reynolds, D. K. (1976). *Morita psychotherapy*. Berkeley: University of California Press.
14. Walsh, R. (2000). Asian psychotherapies. In R. Corsini & D. Wedding (Eds.), *Current psychotherapies* (6th ed., pp. 407–444). Itasca, IL: F. E. Peacock Publishers.
15. Chen, Morita therapy: A philosophy; Chen, Morita therapy and its counseling implications.
16. Chen, Morita therapy: A philosophy.

17. Goto, Shinkeishitsu treatment.
18. Chen, Morita therapy and its counseling implications.
19. Ibid.
20. Chen, Morita therapy: A philosophy; Chen, Morita therapy and its counseling implications; Matesz, D. (1990). Morita and Buddhism: On the nature of suffering. *International Bulletin of Morita Therapy*, *3*(1), 14–25.
21. Chen, Positive living with anxiety.
22. Chen, Positive living with anxiety; Chen, Morita therapy: A philosophy; Chen, Morita therapy and its counseling implications.
23. Chen, Morita therapy: A philosophy.
24. Chen, Positive living with anxiety; Chen, Morita therapy: A philosophy.
25. Chen, Positive living with anxiety; Ishiyama, A bending willow tree; Walsh, Asian psychotherapies.
26. Chen, Positive living with anxiety.
27. Chen, Positive living with anxiety; Chen, Morita therapy: A philosophy; Chen, Morita therapy and its counseling implications.
28. Chen, Morita therapy: A philosophy.
29. Chen, Morita therapy and its counseling implications; Matesz, Morita and Buddhism.
30. Chen, Morita therapy: A philosophy.
31. Chen, Positive living with anxiety; Ishiyama, F. I. (1990). Japanese perspective on client inaction and procrastination: Morita therapy. *International Journal for the Advancement of Counselling*, *13*(2), 119–128.
32. Ishiyama, Japanese perspective.
33. Morita, S. (1974). Shinkeishitsu-no Hontai-to ryoho (Nature and treatment of nervosity). In *Shoma Morita collected works* (pp. 279–442). Tokyo, Japan: Hakuyosha. (Original work published 1928)
34. Chen, Morita therapy and its counseling implications.
35. Ibid.
36. Chen, Morita therapy: A philosophy.
37. Kabat-Zinn, J. (1990). *Full catastrophe living: Using the wisdom of your body and mind to face stress, pain, and illness.* New York, NY: Dell Publishing; Kabat-Zinn, J. (2003). Mindfulness-based interventions in context: Past, present, and future. *Clinical Psychology: Science and Practice*, *10*, 144–156; Segal, Z. V., Williams, J. B., & Teasdale, J. D. (2002). *Mindfulness-based cognitive therapy for depression.* New York, NY: Guilford Press.
38. Segal et al., *Mindfulness-based cognitive therapy.*
39. Chen, Morita therapy and its counseling implications; Segal et al., *Mindfulness-based cognitive therapy.*
40. Segal et al., *Mindfulness-based cognitive therapy.*
41. Chen, Morita therapy and its counseling implications.
42. Chen, Morita therapy: A philosophy.
43. Chen, Morita therapy and its counseling implications.
44. Ishiyama, A Japanese reframing technique.
45. Kabat-Zinn, *Full catastrophe living*; Kabat-Zinn, Mindfulness-based interventions; Segal et al., *Mindfulness-based cognitive therapy.*
46. Chen, Positive living with anxiety; Chen, Morita therapy: A philosophy; Chen, Morita therapy and its counseling implications.
47. Chen, Positive living with anxiety.
48. Chen, Morita therapy and its counseling implications.

SUGGESTED READINGS

Corsini, R., & Wedding, D. (Eds.). (2008). *Current psychotherapies* (6th ed.). Itasca, IL: F. E. Peacock Publishers.

This book provides a comprehensive overview of counseling and psychotherapy. It covers the prominent systems of psychotherapy and the main theoretical orientations with each chapter written by a leading proponent of one of the systems. It includes a chapter covering multicultural theories of psychotherapies and effectively incorporates case studies and examples throughout.

Moodley, R., & West, W. (Eds.). (2005). *Integrating traditional healing practices into counseling and psychotherapy* (pp. 221–232). Thousand Oaks, CA: Sage.

This book explores alternative health care and the integration of traditional healing into multicultural counseling and psychotherapy. It analyzes traditional healing practices of various racial, ethnic, and religious groups. It explores alternative health care movements including Morita therapy, paganism, New Age spirituality, Transcendental Meditation, and new religious movements.

Ogawa, B. (2007). *A river to live by: The 12 life principles of Morita therapy.* Bloomington, IN: Xlibris Corporation.

In this book, Dr. Ogawa shares principles of Morita therapy necessary to enhance well-being in everyday living. Dr. Ogawa effectively illustrates and describes 12 principles of Morita therapy as dependent components of successful living. The use of river analogy as a symbol of movement toward well-being is also incorporated as an effective metaphor to guide readers.

Reynolds, D. K. (1989). *Flowing bridges, quiet waters: Japanese psychotherapies, Morita and Naikan.* Albany: State University of New York Press.

This book was one of the first to discuss Japanese psychotherapies, including Morita therapy. It offers a look at transforming and implementing Japanese methods into approachable and useful techniques to be used in the West.

14 Reiki Therapy

Martha P. Novoa and Emily Kedar

Reiki (霊気), originated in Japan, is a holistic therapy that facilitates balance among mind, body, and spirit, and as a healing energy modality to correct energetic imbalances and restore the self to natural vitality and health, Reiki therapy is now rapidly growing in the West.[1] Reiki is the Japanese word for "universal life energy." The term is an Anglicism of two Japanese characters that combine to signify "conscious energy": *rei* (霊), meaning "spirit, consciousness, essence of creation"; and *ki* (氣), meaning "power" or "energy."[2] Reiki healing takes place through the energy field, a dynamic bioelectric magnetic field that surrounds all living beings. Within this paradigm, illness originates in the energy field before physical symptoms appear. Reiki works at the energetic root of illness by addressing energetic imbalances in this client's energy field.

In order to understand and practice Reiki, the therapist must be able to approach healing from a paradigm that differs significantly from the dominant Western biomedical model of illness and wellness. The practice of Reiki is based on the belief that when Reiki energy is channeled through a practitioner and passed to a client, the client's spirit is healed, which in turn heals the physical body. The therapist facilitates the flow of Reiki by placing his hands on or above the fully clothed client, 1 to 2 inches away from the body with ordered placement of the palms over determined locations.[3] This transference of healing energy is not based on an empirically proven scientific theory, as spiritual healing, but is subjective, individual, and experiential. The technique is neither symptom nor pathology specific but rather is based on transmitting universal life force through the practitioner into the energy field of the client. **Universal life force** is thought to have its own consciousness and wisdom and works to restore health at the root energetic level.[4]

Although spiritual and energetic healing can be at odds with the biomedical model, Reiki complements the Western approach to mental health in significant ways. As all mainstream psychotherapeutic models, Reiki aims to increase the client's awareness, both of his subjective and individual experience, as well as the governing paradigms that influence his life.[5] Reiki is a low risk, nondirective, and noninvasive therapeutic intervention. It often has an immediate calming effect. Because of these characteristics, it is offered in many hospitals across North and South America, the United Kingdom, and continental Europe as an adjunct to mainstream treatments to treat physical illness and facilitate well-being.[6] Newborn babies, end-of-life patients, cancer patients, and fibromyalgia patients are the most common recipients of Reiki in hospital settings.[7]

This chapter explores the history and current uses of Reiki therapy, as well as its relationship with the Western biomedical model of health. We discuss training, accreditation, licensure, and certification as well as contemporary practice including existing research and relationship with Western medicine. Implications of strengths and weaknesses in Reiki therapy and future directions for counseling practice are also discussed.

Brief History of Reiki Therapy

The traditional Reiki story starts with its founder Mikao Usui, a Japanese Buddhist monk, in 1922.[8] In his quest for enlightenment, Usui fasted and meditated on Mount Kurama for 21 days. On the last day, he had an enlightenment experience, during which spiritual light entered the top of his head. Coming down the mountain, Usui tripped on a rock, cut his toe, and instinctively gripped the wound with his hands. To his surprise, the cut healed. In this moment, Usui realized the purpose of the energy that had come through him. Usui developed and systematized the method now known as "Usui Reiki."[9] Usui, or Usui Sensei, established the Usui Reiki Ryoho Gakkai, a study institute where Reiki was taught openly to those interested in learning. The Usui method included three levels: (1) Shoden, (2) Okuden, and (3) **Shinpiden.**[10] His philosophy was that everyone has the ability to practice Reiki and that the system is effective for both physical and psychological imbalance. He believed that Reiki energy brings the body to a place where the energy of divine light penetrates the individual's energy field, integrating him with the oneness of the divine and thereby freeing him from any ailment.[11] Usui Sensei had provided the highest level of attunement to 20 Reiki practitioners when Usui passed away in 1926. During his lifetime, Reiki Ryoho was adopted by the Japanese navy and taught to its personnel because of its effectiveness and convenience on warships. Among Usui's successors was navy captain medical doctor Chujiro Hayashi. After the death of Usui, Dr. Hayashi broke away from the Reiki Ryoho Gakkai and created the Hayashi Reiki Institute. Hayashi developed his own style of Reiki while traveling and promoting Reiki in Japan. He was later invited to teach in Hawaii between 1937 and 1938. His primary students were Japanese-Hawaiians, and among them was Mrs. Hawayo Takata.[12] Takata is a controversial character in the history of traditional Reiki. However, she is acknowledged as the person who brought and spread Reiki to the West.[13]

Once Reiki reached the West, changes in the technique began to be evident. New Reiki techniques, approaches, and energetic symbols were developed. Due to the significant difference between the Eastern and Western paradigms of healing and illness, Reiki was interpreted and practiced in a new way once it reached the Americas. Traditional Reiki healing involves a silencing of the rational mind and egoic thought in order to surrender to the guidance and wisdom of the consciousness of Reiki energy itself. A key existential point in traditional Reiki is that healing is universal, impersonal, and available to all living beings. In the more individualistic Descartian environment of the West, the approach to Reiki began to rely more on the will and importance of the practitioner as well as rational explanations of illness. Disagreements emerged about the source and meaning of the healing energy used in Reiki, and new names were given to different methods that emerged. These new methods include The Radiance Technique, Karuna Reiki, Raku Kei, Tibetan Reiki, Reiki Jin Kei Do, and Seichim. Many others have followed these initial Western evolutions of Reiki.[14] However, it is necessary to understand that Reiki is bound to lineage. Although universal life force is available to all beings, practicing healing through Reiki requires that the practitioner be attuned by a healer who has himself been attuned. In this way, Reiki is passed on through lineage. Since Reiki is profoundly intuitive, it is expected that the methods will change over time, even giving rise to completely new methods of healing, such as the ones just listed. If practitioners are trained and attuned by a Reiki master, then their practice is considered a descendant of Usui Reiki.

How Reiki Therapy Works

Japanese medical tradition speaks of the concept of *ki*, which can be defined as the life force present in all living things.[15] *Ki* is a form of energy vibration binding energy to matter; it surrounds and interpenetrates the body providing a balanced and harmonious flow of the body and its organs and, secondly, the body and its environment. This is known in the West as the subtle energy body or system.[16] When the flow of *ki* is interrupted by disturbances in the environment, body, or mind, the individual shows signs of distress that manifest as pain or illness. *Ki* is also believed to carry our thoughts, intentions, and emotions. Our thoughts and actions affect the presence of *ki* in the body. According to traditional Japanese medicine, all disruptions or interruptions of *ki* cause illness.

Reiki can be described as *ki* guided by the universe, the divine, or a higher power to restore balance in the body system. It is important to note that Reiki is not a religious practice. There are no deities, gods, or structured belief systems that govern its practice. Instead, Reiki exists as an understanding that the universe is created out of energy. This energy contains its own consciousness and wisdom and can be channeled through a practitioner with the intention of healing. The practice requires an open heart and a willingness to set aside the belief that we rationally understand how life works, in favor of allowing ourselves to be guided by nature, intuition, and the flow of life.

Traditional Usui Reiki is practiced in different ways depending on what level of training the practitioner has received. After the first attunement, the practitioner invites the energy to flow through him and out of his hands. He does not direct the course of this energy or the placement of his hands in his client's energy field. The quality of treatment depends a great deal on the practitioner's intentions and ability to cede control to the consciousness of Reiki energy itself. Often, the hands will be drawn to places on the body that need healing or places in the energy field that are out of balance without the practitioner having any prior knowledge of the client's physiological or psychological history. As the hands move through the energetic field of the client, imbalances are restored and blocks are released, restoring the natural state of health and vitality to the client.

Reiki and the Biomedical Model

In the Western paradigm of health, illness is diagnosed and treated according to symptomatology and pathology. Health is considered as restored when symptoms of pathology are significantly reduced. In the field of psychology, mental health is determined by an absence of *Diagnostic and Statistical Manual of Mental Disorders, Fifth Edition (DSM–5)* diagnostic criteria rather than a presence of positive emotional and mental states or quality of life (QOL). In this way, the Western paradigm of illness and health focuses almost exclusively on what is "wrong" with clients and ignores the complex and interdependent relationship between parts of the self as well as the self and his environment. The current Western system of treatment rarely takes the whole person into account, ignoring social and spiritual determinants of health, and is determined in great part by a Cartesian mode of inquiry that divides the self into sickness and health and favors empirical evidence of efficacy over individual, subjective experiences of health and healing. Due to this framework, energetic healing and spiritual experiences that cannot be reduced to logic or adequately explained by a scientific model are often overlooked and dismissed—for example, traditional and indigenous practices of healing and all forms of spiritually based recovery, including Reiki.

Reiki works within a different contextual framework from the biomedical model. In Reiki, health emerges from energetic balance. Reiki works on the subtle energetic field of an individual to restore balance. It does not need a diagnosis or a client history to be effective, as Reiki is both impersonal and profoundly intimate. Anyone can practice and receive Reiki therapy. There is no need for narrative or causal explanation about pathology, trauma, or history unless the client chooses to share with the practitioner. Despite this aspect of impersonality and anonymity, the practice itself is intimate, as both client and healer share in a moment of focused presence.

Reiki healing is an effective way to nourish the spirit of an individual and promote wholeness. It cannot, however, serve as a diagnostic tool or treatment in the same way that a meticulously designed questionnaire or a carefully researched pill can. Even though an individual who receives Reiki can experience reduced rates of stress and anxiety and can experience shifts on a deep, energetic level, the mystery surrounding Reiki's methods have had limiting effects on its role in medicine and psychology.

Currently, Reiki is used in some hospital settings across the Americas and Europe as an adjunct to mainstream treatments. It is most often used in combination with standard medical techniques to soothe newborns and end-of-life patients as well as to increase the QOL of cancer and fibromyalgia patients. The fact that its uses are limited to these patient populations speaks less to its efficacy and more to the unwillingness of the medical profession to adopt a modality with no accreditation, licensure, or conclusive research results. These facets of Reiki will be discussed later on in the chapter.

Reiki is holistic, spiritual, and subjective in nature. It does not take symptomatology, pathology, and diagnosis into account. Health and illness are not approached as diametric opposites. The individual is seen through the lens of a dynamic energetic field that moves in and out of balance. Reiki is used to guide the client's energy back to its natural state of balance and vitality. This framework does not conform to the biomedical model of treatment, as healing through Reiki happens first on an energetic, spiritual, and immaterial level. A person does not have to be sick to benefit from Reiki. Spirit, the divine, and the energy of the universe cannot be divided from Reiki. These concepts are often omitted from mainstream healing, medicine, and counseling.

Although Reiki is still seen as an alternative therapy, its use in hospital and clinical settings is increasing, suggesting an increased recognition of the need for spirituality within clinical settings.

Reiki Therapy Training and Development, Supervision, Accreditation, Licensure, and Certification

Currently, Reiki therapy is not subject to licensure or accreditation. Certificates are provided by a teacher who had attained the Reiki master or teacher level. Standards of training are currently nonexistent. Reiki may be practiced without supervision by any person after receiving the first attunement, or Level 1. Thus, the quality of the treatment can be compromised by the competence, intention, and experience of the practitioner.[17] Reiki's unstructured and open training is the result of Usui's insistence that Reiki energy is free to all beings to use in order to benefit the world. This philosophy has aided in Reiki's spread throughout the Western world but has compromised Reiki's credibility, as the West requires quality control in professions in order to take these professions seriously.

Different sources indicate several levels of learning necessary to become a Reiki practitioner. However, there are three traditional levels of Usui Reiki: Levels 1, 2, and 3. In the first level, the practitioner is taught what Reiki energy is and how to channel it through their body. In the second level, the practitioner receives symbols that are drawn in the energetic field with the hands. These symbols call in energy in specific ways. In the third level of training, practitioners receive the master symbol that allows them to teach and attune others. Each level receives a specific energetic attunement. Each level can be learned over the course of one weekend, and the new techniques must be practiced daily for a specific amount of time in order to anchor the energetic change in the practitioner's field. There are no tests during training. Time is instead allotted to exercises that increase the practitioner's awareness of the subtle energy field and clinical practice in which students work on each other. All levels receive a class manual.[18]

The first step to become a Reiki practitioner is to receive an attunement or initiation. Each level requires a different attunement. The process of attunement is what differentiates Reiki from other energetic healing hand modalities, such as craniosacral healing and crystal therapy. Reiki energy is passed from Reiki master to student, opening energy centers in the student and allowing the healing light, divine life force, or *ki* to come through the practitioner into the recipient. The process of attunement sets Reiki apart from other healing modalities.[19] The Reiki practitioner acts as a hollow bamboo, allowing the universal life force energy to pass through with ease, without trying to direct it. The divine life force is believed to have a knowledge or consciousness of its own and will direct the energy where it is most needed. Herein lies the beauty and simplicity of the Reiki technique.

Reiki Level 1, or Basic Level or Shoden

After the first attunement, the new practitioner will be able to provide Reiki to himself or others who are physically present. Training takes 1 day and includes the first attunement and a review of the history of Reiki—what it is, how it works, its principles, ethical behavior, demonstration, and practice in how to give a Reiki treatment to yourself and others. At the discretion of the teacher, some Japanese techniques such as **Byosen scanning**, Gassho meditation, and the first Reiki symbol may also be taught.[20]

Reiki Level 2, or Okuden

On the second attunement, the Reiki practitioner will learn three **Reiki symbols** and how to apply them during the session. Training takes 1 day and includes the second attunement and a description of the second-level symbols—how to draw them, their meaning, and how and when to use these symbols as well as distance healing training. Students learn to provide Reiki to people who are not physically present. Students are encouraged to feel the differences between the symbols when applied to the energetic field. Other techniques or exercises are optional, chosen at the teacher's discretion.[21]

Reiki Level 3, or Master Level or Shinpiden (Teacher Level)

After the third attunement, the Reiki practitioner will be able to give attunements and teach all three levels of Reiki. Training may be done in 1 day. It includes learning the master or teacher symbol, how to use it in a session, and demonstration and practice of attunements for each level along with the meaning and responsibilities of becoming a Reiki teacher.[22] Reiki depends a great deal on trust. The practitioner's ability to trust the energy he is receiving and the client's trust in the practitioner strongly affect the healing outcome of Reiki.

Research and Future Directions

Reiki therapy research is limited, and findings are conflicted. Mental health professionals are currently bound to evidence-based interventions; however, individuals are more frequently seeking out Reiki as part of their treatment and self-care, regardless of inconclusive research and lack of coverage. This is a strong indication of the need to incorporate spirituality and energy healing practices in counseling and psychotherapy.

Reiki research has been limited to a small number of exploratory studies, most of which include a small number of subject–participants. It is important to remember that Western research methods are grounded in the biomedical model and that the outcomes of these studies are based on pathology-driven results. Because Reiki works from a different theoretical framework, these results may not adequately correlate with the experience of those receiving Reiki.[23]

Empirical research suggests that Reiki may be an effective intervention for a variety of problems listed in the *DSM–5* such as anxiety, stress and depression, fatigue, memory, mild cognitive impairment, and sleep disturbances.[24] Additionally, research on Reiki has proposed its effectiveness on a number of physiological states, associated with different physical conditions including heart rate, blood pressure, and cortisol levels as well as anxiety, stress, depression, fatigue, and pain.[25]

However, some empirical reports also suggest that Reiki did not affect stress and anxiety in women undergoing breast biopsy; did not reduce physiological symptoms of stress and anxiety on healthy college students; did not improve heart rate or blood pressure in older adults; did not improve symptoms of depression, anxiety, or well-being in patients treated for prostate cancer with EBRx; and did not improve symptoms of secondary traumatic stress.[26]

As stated earlier in this chapter, using standard research methodology to measure Reiki's efficacy is challenging. As the process of healing is invisible, a great deal depends on self-report. Furthermore, the competence and credibility of the practitioners are vital to outcome, and since there is currently no standardization or regulatory college for Reiki healers, measuring and ensuring quality of treatment has yet to be adequately considered. For these studies, data have been collected using validated instruments and standard physiological and psychological measurements.[27] Some studies use random assignment with control and comparison groups and the statistical methods chosen appear to have been appropriate. However, there still remain many limitations and methodological flaws that need to be addressed in future Reiki research. Research on Reiki calls for the standardization of the Reiki protocol; careful attention to the selection of the practitioners; treatment frequency; and number of treatments as well as residual Reiki effects, population and sample, control procedures, and confounding treatments.[28] None of the studies reported harmful effects of Reiki treatment. The general conclusion in the scientific community is that Reiki as an intervention has the potential to be effective in some situations. However, since the studies have not been replicated and many outlying factors have yet to be taken into consideration, there is a lack of consistent empirical evidence to support Reiki's efficacy.

The lack of standardized training, professional certification, and licensure for Reiki practice minimizes reliable access to the mental health profession. Mental health professionals are bound by ethical standards and licensure in order to protect and provide safe and effective services and referrals to clients. Although Reiki is widely accepted as completely safe, its lack of standardization makes it difficult to practice within the confines of professional licensure. The lack of accreditation and licensure, as well as the lack of consistency in research findings, are other challenges facing Reiki's future place in accepted healing practices in the West. Because of these unknowns, insurance providers are often hesitant to include coverage for this modality.

The greatest barrier to the acceptance of Reiki therapy into the mainstream health care system is the lack of consistent empirical evidence in research. Our current medical model requires validation with contemporary scientific models. Proponents of Reiki therapy believe that the nature of the technique may require a different way of knowing. Reiki did not emerge from the Western paradigm of the biomedical model. It is grounded in a paradigm that holds spiritual principles of faith, trust, and divine consciousness at its center. This does not mean that it is ineffective but rather that its nature is in conflict with the dominant Western model of health, illness, and treatment. Proponents suggest that the scientific model constrains the mechanisms and effectiveness of the technique. Although it is a challenging task, it is in the best interest for the future of the practice that efforts be made to illustrate Reiki's effectiveness.

Conclusion

Reiki is a noninvasive, nonharmful, and nonpathologically driven healing modality. A Reiki treatment provides a safe container for healing and the careful attention of a compassionate, skilled, and spiritually inclined practitioner. It has an immediate gentle and calming effect, with potential transformational results. Although there is currently no conclusive research and minimal coverage offered in North America, more and more individuals seeking solace and healing are receiving Reiki to deepen their well-being and come into balance. Reiki can increase a client's awareness of his own energetic field and restore deep energetic blocks and imbalances. It is a simple, gentle technique with profound effects. Counseling can be very challenging. There is discomfort in confronting maladaptive coping; deeply held beliefs; and fears, traumas, and anxieties. It is important work, but it can be draining and painful. Reiki can offer nourishment to bolster counseling clients as they undertake the transformative experience of psychotherapy. Bringing Reiki into counseling practice signifies many important shifts for the mental health community, toward a healing model that is more true to the human experience. Reiki offers the reality that we are deeply connected through mechanisms we do not need to understand but simply need to celebrate. Reiki cedes that universal life force, divine love, the great unknown, or any name one chooses for the energetic mystery of life is real, is important, and is inextricably connected to our individual lives.

Case Study

Mr. Everett was a 28-year-old single White male who arrived on time for the appointment and demonstrated a pleasant demeanor. He was of average height and weight and appropriately dressed. Mr. Everett was pursuing postdoctoral studies at the time of the appointment.

Mr. Everett presented with a major depressive episode and generalized anxiety characterized by occasional panic attacks, poor sleep, and a decrease in appetite. He stated, "I feel desperate to just feel normal and have someone to do things with. I am not eating. My friends stay busy and never call me." Mr. Everett presented as a kind and sensitive person who continued to struggle with symptoms of depression and anxiety despite his effort to seek treatment.

Mr. Everett had sought help for his problem from a community psychiatrist and therapist for the past 3 years, but his symptoms returned after termination of treatment. He reported two serious romantic relationships. The first relationship lasted 5 years and ended abruptly.

(*Continued*)

(Continued)

His partner requested that all her gifts be returned. His second relationship started well, but it quickly deteriorated after they moved in together, reportedly due to his girlfriend's mood swings, most notably her angry outbursts and jealous accusations. Their relationship lasted 4 months. Mr. Everett continued to be plagued by the negative memories of these relationships whenever he met anyone new. These experiences contributed to his belief that he is unworthy of love. He was diagnosed with depression in his early 20s but managed it successfully through a balanced lifestyle and cognitive behavioral therapy (CBT) counseling. However, the ending of the relationship with his most recent partner triggered depressive episodes for him. Mr. Everett had been exploring his spirituality over the last year and found some comfort in viewing his struggles through a spiritual lens. Given his openness to different forms of treatment, his therapist referred him to a Reiki practitioner with whom she had successfully worked in the past.

The practitioner explained that Reiki is an energy healing modality that consists of challenging diving energy through the practitioner and into the client, in order to remedy energetic blockages and facilitate healing. Mr. Everett seemed excited and eager as he lay on the treatment table. After a 45-minute session, the practitioner explained where in his body she found his energy to be blocked. She asked Mr. Everett what he had experienced. Mr. Everett reported perceiving temperature changes, specifically heat radiating from the practitioner's hands. Additionally, he reported feeling very relaxed. He briefly fell asleep during the session. He felt that all his anxiety had vanished at the end of the session, and he left feeling hopeful. He scheduled a second appointment for the following week. After the first session, the practitioner decided that six sessions would be sufficient to help Mr. Everett resolve his issues. At the beginning of the second session, Mr. Everett reported that after 3 days his anxiety came back, though the symptoms were not as intense as before. He was also able to sleep better at night, and his appetite increased. The second session was similar to the first, but the practitioner's hands focused more on the area near his heart rather than the whole body. After the end of the second session, Mr. Everett reported feeling relaxed and hopeful. During the next four sessions, treatment changed slightly. As the energy blockages began to be released, the practitioner increasingly focused on specific places and eventually localized treatment to the area near the upper heart. Mr. Everett's symptoms of anxiety and depression slowly dissipated, and he began to go on dates. After the sixth session, he commented, "I never really believed in any of this, but the difference after that first session was so striking, I just had to believe."

This client followed through with a treatment of Reiki therapy as he did not benefit from the mainstream treatment of medication and psychotherapy. The Reiki practitioner was able to identify a pattern of energy blockage in the client's subtle body field. This energy blockage was understood to be fueling the client's maladaptive behavior, thoughts, and emotions. The blockage around his heart corresponded with his thoughts of not being worthy of love. The Reiki treatment dissipated this belief by channeling universal life force to the places in Mr. Everett that were grief stricken, shamed, and fractured. By nourishing these places with Reiki energy, the blockage naturally fell away along with the thoughts and beliefs of being unworthy of love. The treatment served as an experiential reminder of Mr. Everett's worth and capacity to love and be loved. As the number of sessions increased, asymptomatic recovery time increased and reversal time decreased and eventually disappeared. Once Mr. Everett was feeling reliably better, he stopped going to treatments every week. He returned for a "tune-up" once a year. Following Reiki therapy, it was reported that Mr. Everett continued to be successful in his professional life and is now happily engaged.

DISCUSSION QUESTIONS

1. Western medicine methods had been accepted as the primary source of knowledge for health and well-being despite the potential for negative side effects and the failure of some of the treatments. Reflect upon biases, stereotypes, and assumptions you may have toward a healing modality such as Reiki. How are these beliefs limiting your professional practice?
2. Research on Reiki indicates that the modality has potential for improving certain mental health conditions with no side effects. Based on this knowledge, how have your beliefs changed in regards to this modality?
3. Mental health professionals are bound by ethical standards to provide the best care possible without endangering the client. Since Reiki does not have professional standards established, the responsibility falls on the mental health professional. Reflect and discuss what qualities you would look for in a Reiki practitioner.
4. Based on existing research, what criteria would be necessary for you to refer a client to a Reiki practitioner? What would be your expectations of the outcome?

REFERENCES

1. Lubeck, W., Petter, A. F., & Rand, W. L. (2002). The spirit of Reiki. *The complete handbook of the Reiki system.* Twin Lakes, WI: Lotus Press; Yamaguchi, T. (2007). Light on the origins of Reiki. *A handbook for practicing the original Reiki of Usui and Hayashi.* Twin Lakes, WI: Lotus Press.
2. Miles, P., & True, G. (2003). Reiki—Review of a biofield therapy history, theory, practice, and research. *Alternative Therapies in Health & Medicine*, *9*(1), 62–72.
3. Natale, G. W. (2010). Reconnecting to nursing through Reiki. *Creative Nursing*, *16*(4), 171–176; Novoa, M. P., & Cain, D. S. (2014). The effects of Reiki treatment on mental health professionals at risk for secondary traumatic stress: A placebo control study. *Best Practice in Mental Health*, *10*(1), 29–46.
4. Miles & True, Reiki; Natale, Reconnecting to nursing.
5. Novoa & Cain, The effects of Reiki treatment.
6. Natale, Reconnecting to nursing; Novoa & Cain, The effects of Reiki treatment.
7. Kryak, E., & Vitale, A. (2011). Reiki and its journey into hospital setting. *Holistic Nursing Practice*, *25*(5), 236–245.
8. Lubeck et al., The spirit of Reiki; Yamaguchi, Light on the origins.
9. Ibid.
10. Yamaguchi, Light on the origins.
11. Lubeck et al., The spirit of Reiki; Yamaguchi, Light on the origins.
12. Lubeck et al., The spirit of Reiki.
13. Ibid.
14. Ibid.
15. Ibid.
16. Ibid.

17. Lubeck et al., The spirit of Reiki; Yamaguchi, Light on the origins.
18. Ibid.
19. Ibid.
20. Lubeck et al., The spirit of Reiki.
21. Ibid.
22. Ibid.
23. Novoa & Cain, The effects of Reiki treatment.
24. Wardell, D. W., & Engebretson, J. (2001). Biological correlates of Reiki touch healing. *Journal of Advanced Nursing*, *22*(4), 439–445; Shore, A. G. (2004). Long term effects of energetic healing on symptoms of psychological depression and self perceived stress. *Alternative Therapies in Health & Medicine*, *10*(3), 42–48; Richeson, N. E., Spross, J. A., Lutz, K., & Peng, C. (2010). Effects of Reiki on anxiety, depression, pain, and physiological factors in community-dwelling older adults. *Research in Gerontological Nursing. Abstracts in Social Gerontology*, *3*(3), 187–199; Crawford, S., Leaver, E., Mahoney, V. W., & Sandra, D. (2006). Using Reiki to decrease memory and behavior problems in mild cognitive impairment and mild Alzheimer's disease. *Journal of Alternative and Complementary Medicine*, *12*(9), 911–913.
25. Shore, Long term effects; Richeson et al., Effects of Reiki on anxiety; Tsang K., Carlson L. E., Olson K. (2007). Pilot crossover trial of Reiki versus rest for treating cancer-related fatigue. Integrative Cancer Therapy, 6(1), 25–35; Mackay, N., Hansen, S., & McFarlane, O. (2004). Autonomic nervous system changes during Reiki treatment: A preliminary study. *Journal of Alternative and Complementary Medicine*, *10*(6), 1077–1081.
26. Novoa & Cain, The effects of Reiki treatment; Potter, P. J. (2007). Breast biopsy and distress: Feasibility of testing a Reiki intervention. *Journal of Holistic Nursing: Official Journal of the American Holistic Nurses' Association*, *23*(4), 238–248; Bowden, D., Goddard, L., & Gruzelier, J. (2011). A randomized controlled single-blind trial of the efficacy of Reiki at benefitting mood and well-being. *Evidence-Based Complementary & Alternative Medicine*, *8*(1), 1–8; Beard, C., Stason, W. B., Wang, Q., Manola, J., Dean-Clower, E., Dusek, J. A., . . . Benson, H. (2011). Effects of complementary therapies on clinical outcomes in patients being treated with radiation therapy for prostate cancer. *Cancer*, *117*(1), 96–102; Richeson et al., Effects of Reiki on anxiety.
27. Novoa & Cain, The effects of Reiki treatment.
28. Ibid.

SUGGESTED READINGS

Rand, W. L. (2005). *The Reiki touch: Complete home learning system*. Boulder, CO: Sounds True, Incorporated.

This kit contains an instructional workbook, a CD containing three guided meditations, a CD, a DVD, and 30 illustrated Reiki cards. The instructions are easy to follow, and the information is valuable for beginners as well as more experienced practitioners.

Stein, D. (1995). *Essential Reiki: A complete guide to an ancient healing art* (4th printing). Freedom, CA: The Crossing Press.

This is the most comprehensive book on Reiki. It includes all three degrees and explains everything that a healer, apprentice, practitioner, and teacher will like to know. It is very well illustrated.

Usui, M., & Grimm, C. M. (1999). *The original Reiki handbook of Dr. Mikao Usui*. Twin Lakes, WI: Lotus Press.

Usui developed the Reiki system and founded the original Japanese Usui Reiki Ryoho Gakkai organization. This book contains the written materials that Usui passed on to his students. It includes exercises and explanations of the origin of Reiki and pictures of the hand positions. Furthermore, it contains hand positions for specific illnesses recommended by Dr. Usui.

Yamaguchi, T. (2007). *Light on the origins of Reiki: A handbook for practicing the original Reiki of Usui and Hayashi.* Twin Lakes, WI: Lotus Press.

This book addresses the origin and evolution of Reiki in Japan. It describes how it was traditionally taught in Japan and includes cultural background and how world events hindered the development of Reiki in Japan. It also includes Dr. Hayashi's lectures on Reiki and natural body cleansing and the Byosen technique.

PART D

Asian Healing Traditions Inspire Creative Therapies

15 Tai Chi and Meditation

Paul Posadzki and Samantha Jacques

From the Western sciences perspective, the ancient Chinese martial art of Tai Chi (TC) can be classified as mind–body technique that is used to increase an individual's health and well-being. TC consists of gentle, slow movements that can be readily used by the elderly and medically compromised individuals.[1] The training is low impact and involves the coordination of diaphragmatic breathing with graceful motions to achieve tranquility of mind.[2] TC is a popular form of exercise throughout the world and has drawn increasing research interest from international scientists. In addition, more attention is being paid to TC in clinical settings for its health benefits. As a therapeutic intervention, it may provide benefits to patients through its characteristic of combining aspects of meditation with exercise.[3] From the Western scientific paradigms perspective, meditation is a healing discipline that can lead to a deep awareness of the present moment through a quieting of the mind, leading to positive physical and emotional effects.[4] These effects may include happiness, satisfaction, serenity, joy, and freedom, which are achieved via self-realization and self-development. From the Eastern perspective, both TC and meditation are grounded in centuries of experience and are deeply embedded in Asian culture, religion, and philosophy. The essence of these approaches—including the wisdom about life; knowledge about holistic health; ways of self-exploring, self-discovering, self-understanding, and self-development; and deep insight into understanding nature and its mechanisms—was translated from generation to generation.

The purpose of this chapter is to present and discuss research highlighting the beneficial features of TC and meditation and to indicate mutual similarities between them. Consequently, an attempt to illustrate how they may be combined into a coherent construct within the context of psychotherapy and counseling will be performed. The conceptual congruence and implications for practitioners and patients will also be presented.

Introduction to Tai Chi

TC is a time-honored and lifetime exercise, handed down from generation to generation for more than 1,200 years.[5] These movements have their roots in Taoism (a branch of Chinese philosophy). The central doctrine of Taoism is focused on longevity that can be achieved through mind balance and tranquility.[6] TC differentiated into many schools in the process of development, such as Chen, Yang, Sun, and Wu.[7] Each school has its own distinctive features, but the basic concepts of the TC exercise are the same.[8] Similarly, in this chapter, the authors have decided to focus on the mutual features of all TC practices—that is, the essence of these exercises. TC provides an alternative to outdoor and group exercise and, therefore, can be practiced almost everywhere.[9] Moreover, TC is safe, with no evidence of adverse, exercise-related problems for those practicing the form.[10] The practice of TC can lead to significant improvements in physical, mental, and spiritual health, which are discussed in this chapter.

TC as a mind–body technique also serves to integrate physiological improvements with psychological ones, including improved confidence, quality of life (QOL), and motivation. Significant improvements have been detected for QOL dimensions, such as general health perception, social functioning, vitality, and mental health or psychological well-being.[11] The health-related QOL of the people who practiced TC has also been found to improve.[12] In another study, TC participants reported significant improvements in body care and health behaviors due to improved motivation.[13] Significant psychosocial benefits were also observed, such as better-perceived social support and mood state and superior relaxation among TC practitioners.[14] TC has also been associated with significant decreases in sadness, confusion, anger, tension, and fear and with increases in energy and happiness, self-esteem, and self-efficacy.[15] Participant statements in these studies indicated that individuals experienced enhanced well-being and calmness as well as less reactivity, increased self-care and self-awareness, and a sense of interconnection with or interdependence on nature.[16] Participants also reported improved quality of sleep due to combined TC and mindfulness-based stress reduction (MBSR).[17] Knowledge about benefits that TC may bring combined with TC interventions as a part of educational programs or cognitive behavioral approaches could be particularly helpful for individuals intending to improve their mental capacities (i.e., strengthen coping stress strategies or resources) and to prevent mental health disorders (i.e., reduce anxiety, depression, or phobias).

Introduction to Meditation

Meditation opens human's mind to the sacred misterium,

That is taking place every day and every hour; Expands heart in the way that with it every beat, Time's eternity and space's infinity can be felt—Meditation causes that our life is heaven on earth . . .

—Suzuki Roshi

Meditation refers to a family of mental training practices that are designed to familiarize the practitioner with specific types of spiritual and mental processes.[18] These processes may include self-actualization, self-realization, and self-development through self-consciousness. Meditation aims to help the subject achieve serenity and alertness in the present moment, instead of the constant struggle to change or to become.[19] It is an art of efficient management of intentional energy with either total engagement (presence, mindfulness) or disengagement (silence, emptiness).[20] In both states, there is an experience of spontaneous unity with no sense of situational interactive self or personal time. It is a simultaneous, participatory consciousness state with a natural sense of well-being with self-understanding, spontaneous joy, serenity, freedom, and self-fulfillment.[21] It is where the ultimate pursuit of happiness and the search for meaning of life meet and coalesce with each other and one realizes the truth of one's harmonious being in nature and with nature itself. It is being alive at its fullest, when each conscious moment becomes a dynamic process of discovery and continuous learning of the ever-new unfolding reality.[22]

Levey and Levey have claimed that thousands of meditation techniques can be distinguished—that is, breathing and walking as well as loving compassion, mindfulness, and Transcendental or Vipassana Meditation.[23] They also argued that all of these meditation practices might have a similar denominator in reflexive meditation. This kind of meditation can be regarded as the combination of concentrating meditation (aims to concentrate on breath or movements) and receptive meditation (aims to tune brain with everything that appears in consciousness). Reflexive meditation aims to discover deeper levels of the human soul. Analogically, within the scope of this chapter, the authors have assumed that the essence of these "various" meditation practices can be similar because of their "parallel" philosophical roots in Hindu and Buddhism philosophy. Furthermore, the main aim and the essence of these practices are "designed" to facilitate personal–spiritual development of the individuals. Therefore, some of the benefits with regard to the mutual essence of meditation practices will be discussed next.

Benefits of Meditation: Psychological and Wellness

From psychological, neuropsychological, or psychoneuroimmunological perspectives, there is evidence that meditation can reduce anxiety, improve memory and cognitive function, and help individuals retain a balanced pattern of baseline emotion.[24] Meditation may also allow subjects to better moderate the intensity of emotional arousal—as manifested by larger power values in theta-1 (4–6 Hz), theta-2 (6–8 Hz), and alpha-1 (8–10 Hz) frequency bands—and facilitate better integration of brain hemispheres.[25] Meditation improves positive mood states and reduces distractive and ruminative thoughts and behaviors.[26] Orme-Johnson stated that the serotonin increases that may occur through meditation have been associated with increased sense of well-being and better mood.[27]

As the reader might have noticed, meditation practice brings benefits to mind control. This could allow patients to have more sense of freedom and control over their own lives simultaneously. Consequently, the sense of control would imply a further path of hierarchic and continuous development, fulfillment, and growth toward more mature personality (becoming a person) through ecstatic experiencing of God, unity with the universe, and unity within the sea of consciousness. These practices should constantly be developed.

Meditation has been shown to influence spiritual QOL.[28] Patients have been shown to develop the state of love, to transform anger into compassion, and to foster spiritual growth through meditation.[29] Spirituality issues related to meditation are especially worth emphasizing among adolescents, where meditation can facilitate growth toward autonomy by helping them connect to their inner voice.[30] This technique may be especially useful in the adolescent search for self-awareness, meaning, and life purpose and to facilitate expansion of self-perception and individuality.[31] Meditation also increases the state of restful alertness, yields a greater capacity for self-reflection and emotional intelligence (self-control, self-reflection or awareness, and flexibility in emotional response), and may improve academic performance.[32] The state of restful alertness induced by meditation may facilitate the growth of social–emotional capacities necessary for regulating the emotional arousal and interpersonal stress of adolescence.[33] The results also support the hypothesis that meditation and spiritual practices could promote significant social benefits, such as empathy and improved academic performance.[34]

The essence of meditation could be regarded as effectiveness in controlling the brain's features such as cognitive or emotional reactions, behavioral patterns that may bring benefit to numerous life spheres such as social interactions via interpersonal relationships, and spiritual transformation that may facilitate overall QOL through more compassionate attitude. Discovery of life's most important values and essence of truth during **self-actualization** or **self-realization** are also the core components of this kind of practice. Meditation's inevitable role as a therapeutic modality should be broadly acknowledged. Nurses, complementary and alternative medicine (CAM) practitioners, and physiotherapists should implement its essence on a daily basis for patients to obtain the best benefits.

Tai Chi and Meditation: A Conceptual Synthesis

Both meditation and TC have healing potential that can reflect on humans' psychophysiological health and widely understood well-being. Both approaches can be considered as a combination of valuable and vital effects of mindfulness and breathing. As a result of both approaches, an individual is able to achieve a better health state via direct influence on mind–body as a whole. Both can be used interchangeably in the sense of results they offer (i.e., bliss and harmony), fulfillment and life satisfaction, serenity and tranquility, joyfulness, or freedom. TC and/or meditation may be employed as a way of personal and spiritual development toward growing compassion and empathy. Yet another reason why these techniques should be conceived as a conceptual unity is that such amalgamation may bring further health benefits to TC practitioners as they could identify that this mind–body practice holds the quintessence of meditation. Moreover, it can be stated that by combining the essence of these two methods of approaching health into unity a practitioner can benefit "twice," as he or she may incorporate meditative states into TC movements. Therefore, conceptual synthesis of TC and meditation and potential benefits of this synthesis will be performed.

The meditation in motion (MIM) may be regarded as a state of attentive presence with enhanced sense of position in space during the movements along with intentional use of breathing patterns that leads to developed self-cognition.

It is suggested that MIM is undifferentiated reality–consciousness, an essential being state, spontaneous intuition, and unity of mind–body with and within the universe, which can be experienced and expressed by the person, which leads to deeper understanding of the ultimate nature of things and phenomenon as they exist in the reality.[35] An individual should be concentrated on perfectly performed, precise soft movements and natural breath, emotionally serene and tranquil, positively approached with a sense of esthetical beauty. A fully receptive mind ought to be tuned to the experience of self-fulfillment with positive thoughts and emotions, energetic balance, presence in time and space, love and empathy, compassion, creativeness, serenity, and bless-consciousness (Nirvana or Samandi). Therefore, it is being argued that awareness of movement, state of unity with movement, breath, and nature are integral parts and core components of the MIM concept. TC as MIM could refer to a mental training practice that is designed to familiarize the practitioner with specific types of mental processes such as the efficient management of intentional energy with total engagement in its flow. During MIM practices, mind and body should be essentially interrelated and balanced in relaxing harmony.[36]

Potential Benefits of Such Synthesis for Individuals' Health

Within the context of counseling and psychotherapy, MIM may bring potential benefits to numerous life spheres of individuals' health, namely social, spiritual, physical, or psychological. For instance, a reciprocal relationship among individuals' cognitive processes (information encoding, learning), emotional experience, and the bodily physiology might improve, resulting in better interpersonal relationships and spiritual development, enhanced structural and functional homeostasis, and facilitated psychological well-being. The authors have assumed that self-development; more intuitive perception;

and reception of one's own integrity, calmness, and harmony or clear mind—that is, self-awareness—could be an open door to better mental health and ultimately enlightenment during MIM practice.[37] Enlightenment is a self-absorptive, adaptive state with realization of one's being in harmony with (and within) reality and one's own movements, which can have a variety of psychotherapeutic applications.[38]

During MIM, the deepest truth and its simplicity, with full acceptance of natural flow of movements, and continuous emptiness can occur leading to reduced symptoms and improved mental function. MIM may also imply individual continuous transformation of thoughts, feelings, emotions, and behaviors toward the discipline of awareness and development of consciousness, penetrating insight, and awakening.[39] During the consciously performed movements, a discovery of the most important values such as the truth and the essence of life as a part of self-actualization (self-discovery) or self-realization may occur.[40] Furthermore, the essence of MIM could be regarded as effectiveness in controlling positive life attitude—that is, optimism, happiness, and healthy behaviors simultaneously within the here and now.

Spiritual transformation during MIM practices would imply further personal growth as a human being and existential fulfillment through ecstatic experiencing of God, or the higher intelligence.[41] This could lead to further positive development during the cycle of awareness and fuller integration of one's own self. During the course of hierarchic and continuous development, one may become a more mature person through the sense of unity with the universe and the mind, the body, and the soul itself when performing MIM. This practice should constantly be enhanced and developed leading to perfection in the movements' performance and continuous development of self-consciousness. This could allow psychotherapeutic patients to have more sense of freedom and control over their own lives simultaneously.

However, a discussion should be opened, and further explorations may bring some insights into the relationships between TC and meditation in light of their therapeutic values. Psychotherapists or counselors may take inspiration from such synthesis of these concepts for patients' best benefit. Researchers can obtain valuable and additional arguments through such cross-fertilization of ideas across presented studies that may be united by shared assumptions.

Conclusion

Both TC and meditation as a part of Eastern tradition can be regarded as a mind–body medicine or therapies. From the cross-cultural perspective, this chapter describes beneficial features of TC and meditation; indicates mutual similarities between them; and presents values and methods of combination of slow movements, breathing techniques as essential parts of TC, and self-consciousness as an integral part of meditation practices into one unity that can be used in counseling or psychotherapy. This chapter should be regarded as a conceptual synthesis of studies that promotes movements and mindfulness and offers an outlook on this fusion from a counseling or psychotherapy standpoint. Such conceptual combination would be inspiring to each individual who is interested in the health debate and may bring "additional" benefits to TC practitioners as they could recognize that this mind–body technique holds the essence of meditation. It also can be argued that the resulting construct would facilitate greater cognitive understanding of TC from the perspective of meditation and incorporate psychological and physiological benefits—that is, improved structure and function into these movements. MIM should bring happiness, satisfaction, and enjoyment to the practitioner and intentions to continue. MIM may produce beneficial effects (physical, social, psychological); therefore, it can be considered as a wider public health strategy of health promotion and development, plus mental health diseases prevention. In addition, MIM can influence an individual's holistic health and should be regarded as a way of spiritual growth and development. Greater awareness of movements may bring self-realization, self-understanding, and self-control to MIM practitioners. A simultaneous unity of one's own self and movements may promote a fuller perception of coherence with the universe and of a total well-being state.

Various branches of science can be used to explain the beneficial effects of MIM. However, more simplistically, these improvements can be considered as a result of optimized energy within the body. MIM can facilitate the body's "internal intelligence" (adaptation mechanisms) and lead to homeostasis. In this chapter, it has also been suggested that MIM practice can bring measurable changes in structure and function of cells, tissues, organs, systems, body as a whole (i.e., epigenetics of holistic health), total well-being, and overall QOL.

DISCUSSION QUESTIONS

1. Tai Chi (TC) originates from traditional Chinese medicine (TCM), and meditation is deeply ingrained in the Hindu tradition. Are there any philosophical implications of such a combination?

2. This chapter argues that meditation is the essential part of TC. Could the opposite hold true—that is, effortless flow of thoughts (instead of movements) during the practice of meditation?

3. As maintaining mental health is an ongoing challenge, how can meditation in motion (MIM) be more effectively incorporated into mental health promotion campaigns, and to what extent can mental health problems such as depression be prevented?

4. Do we really need more research into MIM? Do you think that more positive research results would encourage people to practice more? Or perhaps more practice of MIM is needed? If so, why?

REFERENCES

1. Irwin, M., Pike, J., & Oxman, M. (2004). Shingles immunity and health functioning in the elderly: Tai Chi Chih as a behavioral treatment. *Evidence-Based Complementary and Alternative Medicine*, *1*(3), 223–232.
2. Richerson, S., & Rosendale, K. (2007). Does Tai Chi improve plantar sensory ability? A pilot study. *Diabetes Technology & Therapeutics*, *9*(3), 276–286.
3. Mansky, P., Sannes, T., Wallerstedt, D., Ge, A., Ryan, M., Johnson, L. L., . . . Gerber, L. (2006). Tai Chi Chuan: Mind–body practice or exercise intervention? Studying the benefit for cancer survivors. *Integrative Cancer Therapies*, *5*(3), 192–201.
4. Wright, S. (2007). Meditation matters. *Nursing Standard*, *21*(39), 18–19.
5. Li, J. X., Hong, Y., & Chan, K. M. (2001). Tai Chi: Physiological characteristics and beneficial effects on health. *British Journal of Sports Medicine*, *35*, 148–156.
6. Ibid.
7. Hong, Y., & Li, J. X. (2007). Biomechanics of Tai Chi: A review. *Sports Biomechanics*, *6*(3), 453–464.
8. Koh, T. C. (1981). Tai Chi Chuan. *American Journal of Chinese Medicine*, *9*, 15–22.
9. Ling, K.-W., Wong, F. S. Y., Chan, W.-K., Chan, S.-Y., Chan, E. P. Y., Cheng, Y.-L., & Yu, W.-Y. (2003). Effect of a home exercise program based on Tai Chi in patients with end-stage renal disease. *Peritoneal Dialysis International*, *23*(Suppl. 2), S99–S103.
10. Barrow, D. E., Bedford, A., Ives, G., O'Toole, L., & Channer, K. S. (2007). An evaluation of the effects of Tai Chi Chuan and Chi Kung training in patients with symptomatic heart failure: A randomised controlled pilot study. *Postgraduate Medical Journal*, *83*(985), 717–721.
11. Abbott, R. B., Hui, K. K., Hays, R. D., Li, M. D., & Pan, T. (2007). A randomized controlled trial of Tai Chi for tension headaches. *Evidence-Based Complementary and Alternative Medicine*, *4*(1), 107–113.
12. Kin, S., Toba, K., & Orimo, H. (2007). Health-related quality of life (HRQOL) in older people practicing Tai Chi—Comparison of the HRQOL with the national standards for age-matched controls. *Nippon Ronen Igakkai Zasshi*, *44*(3), 339–344.
13. Greenspan, A. I., Wolf, S. L., Kelley, M. E., & O'Grady, M. (2007). Tai Chi and perceived health status in older adults who are transitionally frail: A randomized control led trial. *Physical Therapy*, *87*(5), 525–535.
14. Taylor-Piliae, R. E, Haskell, W. L., Waters, C. M., & Froelicher, E. S. (2006). Change in perceived psychosocial status following a 12-week Tai Chi exercise programme. *Journal of Advanced Nursing*, *54*(3), 313–329.
15. Taylor-Piliae et al., Change in perceived psychosocial status; Gemmell, C., & Leathem, J. M. (2006). A study investigating the effects of Tai Chi Chuan: Individuals with traumatic brain injury compared to controls. *Brain Injury*, *20*(2), 151–156; Mustian, K. M., Katula, J. A., Gill, D. L., Roscoe, J. A., Lang, D., & Murphy, K. (2004). Tai Chi Chuan, health-related quality of life and self-esteem: A randomized trial with breast cancer survivors. *Support Care Cancer*, *12*(12), 871–876.
16. Wall, R. B. (2005). Tai Chi and mindfulness-based stress reduction in a Boston Public Middle School. *Journal of Pediatric Health Care*, *19*(4), 230–237.
17. Chen, K. M., Li, C. H., Lin, J. N., Chen, W. T., Lin, H. S., & Wu, H. C. (2007). A feasible method to enhance and maintain the health of elderly living in long-term care facilities through long-term, simplified Tai Chi exercises. *Journal of Nursing Research*, *15*(2), 156–164.
18. Levey, J., & Levey, M. (2005). *The fine arts of relaxation, concentration and meditation*. Boston, MA: Wisdom.
19. Deshmukh, V. D. (2006). Neuroscience of meditation. *Scientific World Journal*, *16*(6), 2239–2253.

20. Venkatesh, S., Raju, T. R., Shivani, Y., Tompkins, G., & Meti, B. L. (1997). A study of structure of phenomenology of consciousness in meditative and non-meditative states. *Indian Journal of Physiology & Pharmacology, 41*(2), 149–153.
21. Travis, F., & Pearson, C. (2000). Pure consciousness: Distinct phenomenological and physiological correlates of "consciousness itself." *International Journal of Neuroscience, 100*(1–4), 77–89.
22. Venkatesh et al., A study of structure.
23. Levey & Levey, *The fine arts of relaxation.*
24. Lee, S. H., Ahn, S. C., Lee, Y. J., Choi, T. K., Yook, K. H., & Suh, S. Y. (2007). Effectiveness of a meditation-based stress management program as an adjunct to pharmaco-therapy in patients with anxiety disorder. *Journal of Psychosomatic Research, 62*(2), 189–195; Wagstaff, G. F., Brunas-Wagstaff, J., Cole, J., Knapton, L., Winterbottom, J., Crean, V., & Wheatcroft, J. (2004). Facilitating memory with hypnosis, focused meditation, and eye closure. *International Journal of Clinical and Experimental Hypnosis, 52*(4), 434–455; Pagnoni, G., & Cekic, M. (2007). Age effects on gray matter volume and attentional performance in Zen meditation. *Neurobiology of Aging, 28*(10), 1623–1627; Barnhofer, T., Duggan, D., Crane, C., Hepburn, S., Fennell, M. J., & Williams, J. M. (2007). Effects of meditation on frontal alpha-asymmetry in previously suicidal individuals. *Neuroreport, 18*(7), 709–712.
25. Aftanas, L., & Golosheykin, S. (2005). Impact of regular meditation practice on EEG activity at rest and during evoked negative emotions. *International Journal of Neuroscience, 115*(6), 893–909.
26. Lane, J. D., Seskevich, J. E., & Pieper, C. F. (2007). Brief meditation training can improve perceived stress and negative mood. *Alternative Therapies in Health and Medicine, 13*(1), 38–44.
27. Orme-Johnson, D. (2006). Evidence that the Transcendental Meditation program prevents or decreases diseases of the nervous system and is specifically beneficial for epilepsy. *Medical Hypotheses, 67*(2), 240–246.
28. Jayadevappa, R., Johnson, J. C., Bloom, B. S., Nidich, S., Desai, S., Chhatre, S., . . . Schneider, R. (2007). Effectiveness of Transcendental Meditation on functional capacity and quality of life of African Americans with congestive heart failure: A randomized control study. *Ethnicity and Disease, 17*(1), 72–77.
29. Carson, J. W., Keefe, F. J., Lynch, T. R., Carson, K. M., Goli, V., Fras, A. M., & Thorp, S. R. (2005). Loving-kindness meditation for chronic low back pain: Results from a pilot trial. *Journal of Holistic Nursing, 23*(3), 287–304.
30. Birnbaum, L. (2005). Adolescent aggression and differentiation of self: Guided mindfulness meditation in the service of individuation. *Scientific World Journal, 23*(5), 478–489.
31. Ibid.
32. Paul, G., Elam, B., & Verhulst, S. J. (2007). A longitudinal study of students' perceptions of using deep breathing meditation to reduce testing stresses. *Teaching and Learning in Medicine, 19*(3), 287–292.
33. Rosaen, C., & Benn, R. (2006). The experience of Transcendental Meditation in middle school students: A qualitative report. *Explore, 2*(5), 422–425.
34. Wang, Y. T., Taylor, L., Pearl, M., & Chang, L. S. (2004). Effects of Tai Chi exercise on physical and mental health of college students. *American Journal of Chinese Medicine, 32*(3), 453–459.
35. Mulamadhyamakakarika, N. (1995). *The fundamental wisdom of the Middle Way.* New York, NY: Oxford University Press.
36. Kulmatycki, L. (1997). *Yoga for health.* Warsaw, Poland: Book and Knowledge.
37. Sangharakshita, B. S. (1996). *In the sign of the golden wheel.* Birmingham, England: Windhorse.
38. Kulmatycki, L. (1997). *Yoga relaxation training and its reception.* Breslau, Poland: Academy of Physical Education.
39. Abe, M. (1985). *Zen and Western thought.* Hong Kong: Macmillan.

40. Sangharakshita, *In the sign of the golden wheel.*
41. Brown, K. (Ed.). (1988). *The essential teachings of Hinduism.* London, England: Century Hutchinson.

SUGGESTED READINGS

Brown, K. (Ed.). (1988). *The essential teachings of Hinduism.* London, England: Century Hutchinson.
This is an extremely resourceful, easy-to-read, and inspiring book on Hinduism.

Hsu, E. (1999). *The transmission of Chinese medicine.* Cambridge, England: Cambridge University Press.
This book is a fascinating account of TCM practices from the perspective of medical anthropology.

Levey, J., & Levey, M. (2005). *The fine arts of relaxation, concentration and meditation.* Boston, MA: Wisdom.
This is an excellent introduction to the fine arts of "mind-enhancing techniques," including meditation. It is also an essential practical guide to beginners offering "simple" solutions for complex life problems.

Mulamadhyamakakarika, N. (1995). *The fundamental wisdom of the Middle Way.* New York, NY: Oxford University Press.
This is a must-read for all those interested in Buddhism as it deeply reflects on the relationship between the ultimate and the relative.

NOTE

1. A full version of this chapter was published in 2009, in the *Journal of Holistic Nursing, 27*(2), 103–114.

16 Hakoniwa: Japanese Sandplay Therapy

Carolyn Zerbe Enns and Makiko Kasai

Hakoniwa, known as Sandplay therapy in North America and Europe, is an important method of counseling children and adults in Japan. The literal English translation of the Japanese word *Hakoniwa* is "box garden" or "miniature garden." Clients work with sand and a variety of figurines and objects within the dimensions of a large, shallow sand tray to construct gardens that reflect their personal worlds.

Japanese gardens convey significant artistic and spiritual values and are often used to depict the beauty of the larger world within a symbolic microcosm. Building on this foundation, the Hakoniwa therapy sandbox resembles some aspects of the Zen dry landscape garden, or ***karesansui***. The dry landscape garden consists of raked sand and gravel patterns, rock formations, and occasional vegetation that depict images from nature.[1] Zen temple visitors view the enigmatic scenes from surrounding verandas and experience the essence of the garden and renewal by engaging in quiet meditation and contemplation. Beyond the temple experience, the act of gardening is also an important Japanese leisure activity that fosters emotional health and allows one to navigate between "the threatening, fearful aspects of the 'outside' nature in the raw, and the safety and security of the 'inside' worlds of social and cultural life" (p. 84).[2] Gardening can also represent human efforts to form an enclosed and protected space in which individuals work through dilemmas as well as cultivate growth and build an orderly, productive world.[3]

Long before its adaptation as a form of psychotherapy in Japan, Hakoniwa involved the creation of miniature gardens within boxes or other small enclosures. Along with other Zen-inspired artistic activities such as flower arranging, calligraphy, painting, and the tea ceremony, Hakoniwa supports mindfulness characterized by absorption in the present moment and can also be conceptualized as a mirror of the mind.[4] In general, these Japanese artways promote health by encouraging participants to (a) communicate important feelings and concepts through nonverbal, symbolic means; (b) develop concentrated attention that facilitates here and now experiencing, and mind–body unity; and (c) experience a restoration of the self through self-discipline, relaxation, and mindfulness of the body and breathing. As can be seen by this brief discussion of the functions of many Japanese gardens and the health-promoting role of many Japanese arts, Hakoniwa was inspired by and is compatible with a long tradition of rich indigenous practices.

Sue and Sue noted that most Western psychotherapies include an emphasis on the individual in isolation, verbal communication, the direct expression of emotion, a linear or direct cause–effect orientation to the world, and a distinction between physical and mental well-being.[5] Hakoniwa facilitates the expression of the individual in context, supports nonverbal and verbal communication, and relies on a whole-body activity that allows for a wider range of emotional expression than abstract emotion words alone. Hakoniwa is also embedded in values that emphasize nonlinear holism and the belief that well-being is enhanced through the integration of physical and mental well-being. Through Hakoniwa, clients create three-dimensional, concrete sand pictures that allow them to express their imagination and depict symbols that hold significant personal meaning. By using this hands-on method, body and psyche as well as matter and spirit can be integrated.[6] When clients have difficulty expressing their dilemmas in words, communicating through images and symbols can provide an alternative language that supports awareness and expression of material about which clients may have limited understanding.[7] Blocked feelings may be released, greater self-trust and self-insight may be facilitated, and spontaneous problem solving and behavior change can occur.[8]

Although Hakoniwa is a distinctive therapy embedded in Eastern traditions, many of the art, drama, play, and music therapies practiced within Western psychotherapy traditions have similar features. The Western therapies that correspond most closely to Hakoniwa are the play therapies, including Sandplay therapy. Although in Western traditions these therapies have been practiced primarily with children, they are now being used more frequently with adults.[9] Throughout its history, Hakoniwa has been an important foundation for psychotherapy with adults and children in Japan, perhaps because of its connection to the arts and spiritual expression and the greater valuing of nonverbal and symbolic communication across life stages in Japan.

The International Roots of Therapeutic Hakoniwa

Although Hakoniwa and dry landscape gardens have historically been associated with art and religious expression in Japan, the use of sand as a therapeutic tool has been influenced by Jungian therapists who used sandplay to integrate Eastern and Western values. Some of the assumptions shared by Jungian and many Asian traditions include (a) a belief in a fundamental internal drive for wholeness and healing and a human capacity to transcend current circumstances; (b) an appreciation of symbols, metaphors, and mythology as important forms of communication; (c) an emphasis on mind–body and person–environment connections; and (d) the importance of balancing apparently opposing psychic forces such as rationality and irrationality.[10] Since the middle of the 20th century, Western and Eastern versions of Sandplay therapy, or Hakoniwa, have evolved along parallel, intersecting tracks, and there has been much cross-fertilization between Western and Japanese practitioners.

Swiss analyst Kalff, who is the founder of therapeutic Jungian Sandplay, viewed the sand tray as a location for clients to express their intrapersonal worlds in symbolic form.[11] She believed that when given the opportunity to construct concrete images of themselves in a safe environment, clients would reconcile disconnected aspects of their inner and outer selves and achieve a new wholeness marked by balance, congruence, and integration of the conscious and unconscious. In her efforts to integrate Western and Eastern traditions, Kalff was inspired by Tibetan Buddhism, which included rituals involving the creation of sand mandalas that were seen as restoring harmony, peace, and balance to the self and the world.[12] She also collaborated with Japanese Zen Buddhist scholar Suzuki and concluded that the sandplayer resembles the Zen pupil who seeks wisdom and is not provided with direct answers to questions but is encouraged to draw on his or her inner resources and imagination to resolve issues.[13] Hayao Kawai, a Japanese Jungian analyst with whom Kalff worked, was instrumental in introducing Hakoniwa to Japan as a formal therapeutic medium and integrating Sandplay therapy principles with Japanese cultural practices and Buddhist philosophy. From the 1960s until his death in 2007, Kawai published prolifically about Hakoniwa (primarily in Japanese language journals and books) and Buddhist perspectives on psychotherapy and Japanese personality, symbolism, and mythology.[14] In 1985, the International Society for Sandplay Therapy was established by practitioners from Japan, the United States, and Europe. The Japan Association of Sandplay Therapy was founded in 1987, publishes the *Archives of Sandplay Therapy*, and sponsors an annual professional conference to support the ongoing development of Hakoniwa.

The Practice of Hakoniwa

The typical Hakoniwa counseling room includes comfortable chairs that allow for face-to-face verbal interaction, as well as a sand tray and shelves displaying miniature figurines and objects. This organization of physical space allows the therapist and client to move naturally between more verbal and nonverbal as well as abstract and concrete modes of expression. The sand tray, which most typically measures 19.5 in. × 28.5 in. × 3 in., is located at table or waist-high level in the center of the counseling room, allowing the sandplayer to work with sand and objects from the various sides of the box. The interior of the sand tray is usually painted blue; the client may work with the half-filled tray of sand to create scenes that depict water or sky, represented by the blue surface, and various qualities of the earth (e.g., hills, snow, movement) represented by sand. Shelves containing miniature objects line the walls of the room, and the client chooses from these objects to construct a living scene.[15] Numerous examples of completed sand trays can also be found in Carey, Morena, Pearson and Wilson, and Steinhardt.[16]

The miniature figures used in Hakoniwa are diverse. Many therapists build their personal collections by gathering potentially meaningful objects from the natural environment and purchasing small figures that represent people, animals, plants, machines, and utensils, or structures used in daily living.[17] These tools may come from a variety of sources, including toy stores, souvenir shops, and nature expeditions. Therapists seek to build collections that will allow clients to express their worlds as completely and imaginatively as possible. Pearson and Wilson proposed that "when the sandplay figurines become symbols they begin to express the language of our unconscious" (p. 1).[18]

When initiating Hakoniwa, or Sandplay, therapy, the therapist introduces the client to the sandbox, tools, and miniatures and provides open-ended instructions such as "You may build any world, make any picture or scene, or create any story in the sand that you wish. You don't have to think about it or understand it. Just do whatever comes. . . . No matter what you do, there is not right or wrong way of doing sandplay" (p. 58).[19] The therapist usually sits quietly and watches, sometimes drawing a sketch or taking notes to maintain records of the client's creation.[20] During the production of the three-dimensional picture, the therapist acts as a supportive participant who observes the energy level of the client, the manner in which he or she shapes the sand, how the person chooses miniatures, the order in which figurines and objects are added, and whether the person makes significant scene changes during the session.[21] The therapist is attentive to (a) how the client creates the sand tray (e.g., where the client stands, variations in the client's mood and body posture) and (b) the content of the sand tray (e.g., shapes created by the client, organization of the tray, spatial relationships, use of elements such as fire and wind, use of space and balance, and potential themes).[22]

The silent building of the sand world may be therapeutic in and of itself. However, most therapists follow the nonverbal construction phase with verbal exploration, which allows the client to gain more conscious awareness of important nonconscious themes, emotions, or beliefs that are expressed in the sand. The therapist typically asks the client to describe the scene or tell the story of the sand picture, using open-ended clarifying questions to help the client describe the creation and elaborate on the meaning he or she attaches to specific images or clusters of items. During this initial discussion, the therapist generally avoids making interpretive remarks, adding commentary only when it supports the client's unfolding self-exploration and understanding of his or her world, concerns, dreams, or approach to living.[23] Depending on time available, the awareness level and needs of the client, and the theoretical orientation of the therapist, the therapist may take on a more active role as a session evolves. For example, to facilitate the working through of a conflict, the therapist might ask the client to imagine and verbalize a dialogue between two figures or objects. The therapist might also encourage the client to consider how the scene reflects current personal issues or to imagine how his or her world might be different if objects, figures, or sand were placed differently or took on different proportions. At the conclusion of a Hakoniwa session, the therapist usually takes a photographic picture to preserve the scene for future discussion.

Hakoniwa may be used as a form of phenomenological assessment, as a single session activity to enhance self-awareness of one's world or a specific issue, or as a major therapeutic intervention during a series of sessions.[24] The process just described focuses primarily on the use of spontaneous sand trays in counseling. However, some therapists also use directed sandplay for purposes such as giving concrete expression to a traumatic event, negotiating a specific internal or interpersonal conflict, expressing grief, or creating an ideal world.[25] When Hakoniwa is used as the primary therapeutic intervention during successive sessions, the therapist and client are able to observe the evolution of changes across sessions with regard to the client's use of themes, creativity, and energy levels.[26] Clients also have opportunities to discuss and integrate images that emerge over time.[27] It is important to note that although the preceding descriptions are indicative of typical Hakoniwa practices, therapists' conceptual frameworks and therapeutic styles may vary, leading to some diversity of practice. Although the practices described in this section are consistent with most procedures that are seen in Western Sandplay therapy, the philosophical underpinnings, goals, applications, and psychotherapy relationship of Hakoniwa are influenced substantially by Asian values and Buddhist concepts.

The Psychotherapy Relationship

The primary roles of the Hakoniwa therapist are to provide a "free and protected space," develop a "wordless rapport" with the client, and bear witness to the sandplayer's act of creation.[28] When the therapist is present without being intrusive and fully appreciates the self-discovery process of the client, the client experiences trust, is open to becoming acquainted with his or her own feelings and life patterns, and learns to access inner capacities that facilitate healing.[29]

The sandplay process often facilitates the therapeutic alliance and, compared to many verbal therapies, may decrease the time needed to unlock nonconscious or blocked themes and issues.[30] Hayao Kawai conceptualized the alliance and curative factors as direct, continuous forms of nonverbal communication between the center, or *hara,* of one person and the center of another person.[31] Building on Buddhist thought, Hakoniwa therapist Kawai described the therapeutic relationship as one in which the therapist waits for the client's "inner possibilities to show themselves" (p. 14).[32]

He added, "I wait for something to happen, without knowing exactly what it will be. . . . Patients are cured by their creative activities, which are fostered by the relationship between them and me (p. 14)."[33] Hakoniwa and Sandplay share many assumptions about healing with humanistic therapies and therapies that are associated with projective techniques; however, nonverbal aspects of connection and healing receive greater emphasis in Hakoniwa.

The therapist's role is also consistent with *muishizen*, an important concept in Taoist philosophy. This attitude, which is attributed to the sage Laozi (or Lao-Tzu), refers to a sharpened intuition that eschews artificiality and supports the spontaneous growth of others. Laozi is quoted as saying, "I take no action and the people of themselves are transformed" and "The way to do is to be" (pp. 104, 107).[34] In keeping with this attitude, the counselor who uses Hakoniwa respects the autonomy and spontaneity of the client by creating an atmosphere in which the client is open to his or her own experiences. The Japanese philosophical ideal that "all things are supposed to evolve and develop by nature without needing rectification" is consistent with the therapist's role (p. 110). [35]

Yet another relevant construct is ***amae***, a central indigenous personality construct for understanding therapeutic and other close relationships in Japan.

Japanese psychiatrist Takeo Doi, who wrote for more than 40 years about the centrality of *amae* to Japanese personality and emotional experience, indicated that *amae* represents the capacity to depend on another person's love and benevolence that is first experienced through the oneness and intimacy of parent–child relationships but that also extends to close friendships and intimate relationships in adulthood.[36] Related to the **Zen** principle that seeks to erase boundaries between subject and object or self and other, *amae* emphasizes being a recipient rather than an actor and being able to "bask in another's indulgence" and experience unconditional acceptance (p. 349).[37] Although similar to concepts such as empathy and unconditional positive regard, actions associated with *amae* emphasize sensitivity to nonverbal rather than verbal cues of acceptance and emotional closeness and are connected to goals of interdependence rather than independence. For the client, the therapist's nonverbal communication of caring and benevolence, provision of a "protected space" and secure holding environment, and emphasis on mutuality and growth-in-relation often represent important therapeutic extensions of *amae*.[38] Issues that emerge when the positive values of *amae* become distorted will be discussed later in this chapter.

Theoretical Foundations: The Integration of Jungian Concepts and Asian Values

As mentioned earlier, the therapeutic practice of Hakoniwa in Japan has been influenced primarily by Jungian psychology and Asian values. In this section, we address Jungian concepts of the collective unconscious, the self, and transcendence; we also discuss the parallels and compatibility between Jungian concepts, Asian philosophies, and indigenous Japanese values. The awareness and change that a client acquires during Hakoniwa therapy are often conceptualized in terms of these Jungian and Asian concepts. According to Jungian analytical psychology, the collective unconscious represents a transpersonal "ancestral heritage of possibilities" that supports the most creative and powerful urges of the individual. Archetypes, the contents of the collective unconscious, are elaborated in mythic tales and symbols that mirror personal dilemmas and provide glimpses of truth that may inspire personal creativity.[39] Symbolism and archetypal themes are also of great importance within Japanese culture and are reflected in images associated with Japanese mythology, art, and religious imagery as well as through Japan's written language, which consists of *kanji* or pictorial characters.[40] From a Jungian perspective, Hakoniwa facilitates nonverbal, symbolic communication and the expression of archetypal themes. Through Sandplay therapy, the client is able to bring unconscious and archetypal themes to a conscious level. This new conscious awareness facilitates client growth and spurs client creativity and wholeness.

Jungian and Buddhist concepts of the self and transcendence are also relevant to Hakoniwa practice. The sand structures individuals build often take the form of a circle, which Jung viewed as a symbol for the self and self-realization. The circular formation, present in many Eastern cultures and often revealed through clients' sand creations, depicts the concept of balance, the union of the conscious and unconscious, and the balancing of competing elements of the psyche.[41] Through transcendence, the guiding force that facilitates the realization of one's full potential, persons are able to integrate unconscious and conscious experiences as well as aspects of self that have been disowned or have acted in opposition to each other.[42] One of the interesting parallels between Buddhist and Jungian concepts is the Buddhist distinction between the lesser self and the greater, boundless self. The lesser or interactional self, which is similar to Jung's descriptions of the persona and conscious ego, is the face-sensitive self that is concerned with one's self-presentation to others. This self is variable and allows one to adapt to various interpersonal demands and situations.[43] In contrast to the lesser self, the greater self resembles the Jungian construct of the self, which allows one to integrate conscious and unconscious material and allows one to develop a sense of unity with nature and other beings.[44]

The boundless or greater self, which is rooted in a Buddhist version of transcendentalism, is able to free itself of the boundaries of the lesser self and transcend dichotomies such as the inner and outer, good and bad, life and death, and subject and object. The boundless self achieves a fundamental self-reorientation by becoming part of the natural world and absorbing the natural world into itself.[45] From a Jungian perspective, the sandplayer literally becomes part of the natural world by engaging in free expression and play, becomes aware of new possibilities for himself or herself, and becomes a more unified person by transcending the limits of the persona or face-sensitive self.

An indigenous Japanese view of transcendence is also reflected in the concept of *arugamama*, which can be defined as a type of acceptance of fate or reality that allows one to achieve harmony with one's circumstances.[46] Members of many Western cultures gain a sense of control and efficacy by "standing out" and attempting to directly influence the people and realities around them. Consistent with the value of *arugamama*, some members of Asian cultures gain a sense of personal control and transcendence by "standing in," which involves making internal adjustments to reality by modifying personal goals, expectations, and attributions so that they facilitate acceptance of one's circumstances.[47] Hakoniwa, which facilitates the expression of self in context, may also support *arugamama*, self-acceptance, and positive coping.

Hakoniwa therapist Kawai proposed that Western ideology often posits a clear distinction between good and evil, and the battle between the two is often intense.[48] In contrast, the distinction between good and evil is not a central characteristic of Japanese mythologies and ideologies, and many Japanese myths explore the "mutual existence of reciprocal elements that maintain a delicate balance among themselves" (p. 74).[49] This ideology reveals interesting parallels to a Jungian approach to personal growth, which proposes that coming to terms with the shadow, or the disowned, negative aspects of the person, is not accomplished through suppressing or disavowing the shadow but rather through recognizing the reality of the shadow within oneself. When one faces and accepts the shadow, one is able to achieve balance and wholeness.[50] The Hakoniwa client develops self-awareness about internal polarities and learns to integrate these facets of the self through the nonverbal and nonconscious expression of important themes in the sand.

From a Jungian conceptual framework, Hakoniwa allows clients to use a vocabulary of symbols to express their imagination, emotion, and thinking. Through the act of shaping sand and placing miniatures in a scene, individuals communicate through personally relevant myths and feelings. This whole body, kinesthetic therapy allows clients to act out internal reality, experience transcendence through experimentation, and prepare themselves for productive action that emerges out of acceptance.

Although Jungian psychology is the primary psychological theory held by Japanese Hakoniwa practitioners, Sandplay practice has also been integrated with a wide range of other theoretical perspectives. From a person-centered perspective, Hakoniwa may be viewed as a method for increasing the range and depth of the client's emotional experience and present awareness. From an Adlerian perspective, creations of sand and miniature objects can be viewed as manifestations of a client's lifestyle, and clients can also use sand expression to reconstruct and reorient their lifestyle statements. From a Gestalt perspective, Hakoniwa can be viewed as a method for increasing the depth and range of self-awareness and for helping clients become aware of and integrate polarities or splits within themselves. Exercises that simulate Gestalt two-chair dialogues between miniature objects can facilitate the resolution of polarities between parts of the self that are depicted in sand trays. Family therapists have also used sand and figurines to encourage families to create family sculptures or pictures of family activity—for examples, see Carey as well as Pearson and Wilson.[51] Sandplay may also be integrated with other expressive therapies, such as drama, music, and art therapy.[52]

The Role of Hakoniwa in Addressing Psychotherapy Challenges

Hakoniwa practice is consistent with many of the values that promote psychological health and offers unique methods for personal growth. In this section, we provide examples of problems and issues for which Hakoniwa may be especially well suited.

Issues Regarding *Amae*

As noted in the previous section on the psychotherapy relationship, the indigenous concept of *amae* involves a type of healthy other-centeredness that promotes the ability to be sensitive to the needs of others and rely on others for unconditional acceptance. This positive form of other-centeredness can become exaggerated or unbalanced, which may lead individuals to become so mindful of minor nuances related to the nonverbal and verbal behavior of others that they experience personal paralysis or a loss of self.[53] Clients who experience an absence or breakdown of healthy *amae* may become overly sensitive to the verbal and nonverbal cues of others, may have limited words for describing personal feelings, or may have difficulty expressing feelings for fear of displeasing others. An exaggerated attentiveness to the cues of others may also affect the client's in-session behavior: He or she may be fearful of inadvertently offending the counselor rather than devoting energy to self-exploration.[54] The very act of sitting face-to-face with a counselor and experiencing direct eye contact may trigger discomfort in some clients. In these situations, Hakoniwa may represent an ideal form of psychotherapy. Because the therapist observes unobtrusively, the client may be less conscious of the presence of another person in the room and may be less likely to spend energy "reading" the counselor's reactions. Furthermore, the client does not need a rich vocabulary of emotional words to describe her or his experience but can create images and emotional scenes that express the client's concerns.

Matsuyuki noted that "*amae* creates attachment and connections to others but often does so along with a sense of obligation to others" (p. 68).[55] The sense of obligation associated with *amae* can be especially problematic for adult caregiving women who bear the burden of fulfilling others' emotional *amae* needs but may only infrequently become the recipients of the benevolence and care of others. Unspoken rules often call on Japanese women to be completely devoted to those around them, anticipate and respond to the needs of others, and avoid expressing any emotions that convey dissatisfaction.[56] As a result, women may experience difficulty expressing their own needs or even giving themselves permission to have personal needs. These women often experience high levels of stress but often have a limited sense of their own desires and acquire a very limited vocabulary for expressing emotions and personal needs.[57] Hakoniwa and other nonverbal techniques may be used in conjunction with verbal, supportive therapy to help clients explore their worlds on their own terms and to gradually develop a language for expressing themselves while also maintaining their ability to stay connected to others and maintain *amae* relationships.

Problems of Internalization

In societies that convey powerful messages about the importance of other-centeredness and interdependence, psychological symptoms are often characterized by internalization of distress. The internalization of distress does not challenge the basic values of a collectivistic culture and allows one to maintain interdependence. Examples of internalization issues found in Japan follow. Student apathy, or ***ryunen***, refers to the experience of students who lack energy and are unable to complete school-related work and/or other everyday life events.[58] A second, closely related problem of withdrawal involves the avoidance of interpersonal relationships, apathy, and flat affect and may be related to a person's belief that it is unacceptable to express one's thoughts or feelings as an individual. A third significant problem, depression, may be associated with the ease with which interdependent individuals, whose self–others boundaries are often fluid or diffuse, identify with significant others and absorb their pain.[59] A fourth problem of internalization is reflected in the relatively common anxiety disorder ***taijin kyofusho***, which manifests itself as a phobia of interpersonal relationships such as having fears of personal inadequacy in social situations, offending others, or causing displeasure to others. Unlike Western anxieties, which tend to involve fears about embarrassing oneself because of failures in voluntary activity (e.g., public speaking or eating out), *taijin kyofusho* tends to involve fears about "involuntary leakage of the self" such as fears of blushing, maintaining eye contact, emitting offensive body odors, or having physical features that may offend others (p. 79).[60]

Each of these problems is marked by difficulties verbalizing problems and behavioral deficits. Hakoniwa's limited face-to-face contact and its emphasis on activity may allow the client to decatastrophize interpersonal fears and act in spite of his or her hypersensitivity to interpersonal cues. Hakoniwa may facilitate "getting unstuck" by providing an environment in which the client experiences freedom to "be" and freedom from the external pressures associated with each of these problems. As an action-oriented approach, Hakoniwa may also help break cycles of inaction that are often associated with internalization.

Hakoniwa Training, Research, and Future Directions

Although Hakoniwa is well-established as a form of therapy, it has only recently become standardized as a component of Japanese counseling psychology and counselor education programs in Japan. Hakoniwa training is integrated with general counseling skills training that resembles microskills training in North America. Training usually begins with an introduction to Jungian psychology and the Sandplay theory of Dora Kalff. The educational process incorporates videotapes of Kalff's work, the study of Jungian symbolism, the significance of sand and miniature placement, various meanings clients attach to sandplay creations, typical stages of Hakoniwa counseling, and problems for which Hakoniwa is considered appropriate. Skill training also focuses on methods of introducing Hakoniwa to the client, developing observational and recording skills, acquiring nondirective support roles, and learning tools for helping clients identify the meaning and implications of their work. Trainees are often asked to create their own sandbox scenes to understand Hakoniwa from an experiential perspective and enhance their personal growth. Trainees also learn by reading case studies, examining Hakoniwa creations depicted in photographs, and participating in practicum assignments.

Limited research has been conducted on Hakoniwa and Sandplay therapy. The absence of research may be related, at least in part, to the difficulty conducting empirical research on Jungian and Asian philosophical concepts and the valued outcomes of Hakoniwa (e.g., *arugamama* or being at peace with oneself), which are difficult to define in concrete, operational terms. One might argue that the objective, linear, and cause–effect language and values of science are inconsistent with the values of Hakoniwa, which focus on artistic, holistic, nonrational, spiritual, and nonverbal aspects of knowing.[61] Research on Hakoniwa should be compatible with the values and assumptions that provide a foundation for this therapy. Much of the research published in Japan consists of case studies of Hakoniwa practice with diverse problems such as dream walking, anorexia, trichotillomania, school refusal, schizophrenia, depression, alcoholism, adolescent crises, obsessive–compulsive disorder, elective mutism, and human relations disorder. Hiramatsu and Yamaguchi's summary of Japanese research since 1969 identified the following categories of research on Hakoniwa: (a) the developmental features of sandplay and the evaluation of sandplay expressions, (b) sandplay manifestations of symptoms and problems, (c) spatial arrangements of sandplay,

(d) infant sandplay expressions, (e) the use of sandplay in assessment and as a projective method, and (f) interview processes in Sandplay therapy.[62] This review noted that most studies had focused only on initial sandplay creations, and authors recommended that psychotherapy process variables needed to be studied to understand therapeutic change.

As training programs in counseling psychology departments in Japan become well established, it is important to build on this initial research base. At a descriptive level, additional studies that focus on the content analysis of clients' sand constructions (e.g., what objects are used, their placement) and clients' descriptions of their created worlds will provide insight about the nature of self-awareness that emerges during Hakoniwa sessions. For clients who construct a sequence of scenes, the content analysis of multiple sand constructions will provide insight about how Hakoniwa creations reveal clients' changing levels of self-awareness, coping strategies, and worldviews. Given the fact that therapeutic change is hypothesized to emerge from clients' self-healing capacities, qualitative research that reveals clients' perceptions of the value, impact, and healing aspects of Hakoniwa will be crucial. One method of exploring perceptions of curative factors may be to ask therapists and clients to identify critical incidents and reconstruct how these events were influential.

Research that examines the types of therapist interventions that facilitate clients' in-depth experiencing and self-understanding during the verbal processing of sand tray pictures will also be useful. The Experiencing Scales, which include a client self-report version and a therapist rating form, hold significant promise for assessing how clients' emotional experience during therapy is related to psychotherapy process and outcomes.[63] Initial research has revealed that Sandplay therapy clients who experienced positive therapeutic progress had significantly higher ratings on these experiencing scales than did clients who did not show therapeutic movement.

This chapter has proposed that Hakoniwa may be especially helpful for clients who experience problems with internalization features. In the future, our understanding of Hakoniwa will be enriched by comparing the therapy outcomes of Hakoniwa clients who have problems marked by internalization (e.g., depression or withdrawal) and externalization (e.g., aggression or bullying). In addition, examining the therapeutic outcomes of Hakoniwa clients at different ages, life stages, or developmental stages will add to knowledge of the relative strengths of this therapy with different populations. Cross-cultural comparisons of Hakoniwa practice will be beneficial for clarifying how the content of clients' sandplay, descriptions of their constructions, and perceptions of Sandplay therapy's curative factors are similar and different across cultures. In addition, it will be useful to study whether Asian and North American clients tend to use concepts that are more collectivistic or individualistic to conceptualize their experiences.

One of Hakoniwa's most notable features is its use of nonverbal communication to support self-awareness and change. Research that examines the therapeutic experiences and outcomes of those who receive Hakoniwa counseling, verbal traditional talk therapy alone, or a combination of Hakoniwa and talk therapy will facilitate knowledge about whether and when nonverbal and verbal methods facilitate different types of awareness and outcomes. Comparisons of the effect and outcomes of Hakoniwa interventions with other expressive therapy interventions such as art therapy or psychodrama will also enhance understanding of the similarities and differences between Sandplay and other whole-body approaches.

Conclusion

Gaining knowledge about the practice of Hakoniwa in Japan can also enrich our understanding of Western Sandplay and the value and uses of a variety of expressive therapies such as psychodrama, art therapy, and drama therapy. Although rooted in a Jungian analytical tradition, Sandplay can be used as a specific, short-term intervention and can be integrated with a variety of theoretical perspectives, such as existential, Adlerian, behavioral, or humanistic approaches.[64]

Japanese perspectives on Hakoniwa may be especially useful for helping clients who prefer to work through issues in holistic, expressive ways, and those who have difficulty expressing deep feelings in words and thus may prefer an active approach to counseling.[65] Indigenous Japanese perspectives on therapy, which tend to emphasize finding internal peace and adapting to one's circumstances in productive ways, may also be especially helpful for working with clients who are coping with situations and "givens" that cannot be changed. By increasing our knowledge of approaches such as Hakoniwa, counseling psychologists can gain additional insight about the boundaries and limitations of Western theories and develop a foundation for integrating Eastern and Western perspectives on psychotherapy. Sandplay and Hakoniwa can help us develop greater appreciation for cultural similarities and differences as well as transcend the tendencies for us to portray cultures and their inhabitants in either–or terms: as individualistic or collectivistic, as high context or low context, or as object focused or contextually focused.

DISCUSSION QUESTIONS

1. Based on this chapter's descriptions of Hakoniwa practice, what types of clients are likely to find this form of psychotherapy to be especially helpful? For what types of problems is this approach most likely to be useful? Why? For what types of clients and life problems might this form of therapy be less beneficial? Why?
2. In what ways are Zen Buddhist and Jungian approaches compatible and incompatible? What are the similarities and differences between Zen and Jungian/Analytical concepts? How are they relevant to Hakoniwa practice?

3. This chapter emphasizes how Hakoniwa is related to Zen Buddhist and Jungian approaches. How might this approach be integrated with other approaches to psychotherapy?

4. Imagine that you are creating a Hakoniwa or sand tray that depicts themes that are important in your life. What types of miniature objects would you choose? How might you arrange or mold the sand? What themes or story would likely emerge from your sand tray?

REFERENCES

1. Berthier, F. (2000). *Reading Zen in the rocks: The Japanese dry landscape garden* (G. W. Parkes, Trans.). Chicago, IL: University of Chicago Press.
2. Hendry, J. (1997). Nature tamed: Gardens as a microcosm of Japan's view of the world. In P. J. Asquith & A. Kalland (Eds.), *Japanese images of nature* (pp. 83–105). Surrey, England: Curzon.
3. Ammann, R. (1994). The sandtray as a garden of the soul. *Journal of Sandplay Therapy*, *4*(1), 46–65.
4. Mizushima, K. (1971–1972). Art therapies in Japan. *Interpersonal Development*, 2, 213–221.
5. Sue, D. W., & Sue, D. (2013). *Counseling the culturally diverse: Theory and practice* (6th ed.). New York, NY: Wiley.
6. Ammann, R. (1991). *Healing and transformation in sandplay.* La Salle, IL: Open Court; Turner, B. A. (2005). *Handbook of sandplay therapy.* Cloverdale, CA: Temenos Press.
7. Morena, G. D. (2001). *The wisdom of Oz: Reflections of a Jungian Sandplay therapist.* Berkeley, CA: Frog.
8. Pearson, M., & Wilson, H. (2001). *Sandplay and symbol work: Emotional healing and personal development with children, adolescents and adults.* Melbourne: Australian Council for Educational Research.
9. Pearson & Wilson, *Sandplay and symbol work*; Garrett, M. (2014). Beyond play therapy: Using the sandtray as an expressive arts intervention in counselling adult clients. *Asia Pacific Journal of Counselling and Psychotherapy*, *5*, 99–105.
10. Morena, *The wisdom of Oz*; Pearson & Wilson, *Sandplay and symbol work*.
11. Kalff, D. M. (1980). *Sandplay: A psychotherapeutic approach to the psyche.* Boston, MA: Sigo Press; Garrett, Beyond play therapy; Steinhardt, L. (2000). *Foundation and form in Jungian sandplay: An art therapy approach.* Philadelphia, PA: Jessica Kingsley.
12. Turner, *Handbook of sandplay therapy*.
13. Mitchell, R. R., & Friedman, H. S. (1994). *Sandplay: Past, present, and future.* New York, NY: Routledge.
14. Kawai, H. (1985). The Japanese mind as reflected in their mythology. *Psychologia*, *28*(2), 71–76; Kawai, H. (1996). *Buddhism and the art of psychotherapy.* College Station: Texas A&M University Press; Uemura, K. (2015). Pioneer of clinical psychology in Japan: The broad achievement of Hayao Kawai. *Kyoto University Research Activities*, *53*, 8–11.
15. Steinhardt, *Foundation and form in Jungian sandplay*; Carey, L. J. (1999). *Sandplay therapy with children and families.* Northvale, NJ: Jason Aronson.
16. Morena, *The wisdom of Oz*; Pearson & Wilson, *Sandplay and symbol work*; Steinhardt, *Foundation and form in Jungian sandplay*; Carey, *Sandplay therapy*.
17. Steinhardt, *Foundation and form in Jungian sandplay*.
18. Pearson & Wilson, *Sandplay and symbol work*.

19. Garrett, Beyond play therapy.
20. Weinrib, E. (1983). *Images of the self: The Sandplay therapy process.* Boston, MA: Sigo Press.
21. Garrett, Beyond play therapy.
22. Pearson & Wilson, *Sandplay and symbol work.*
23. Pearson & Wilson, *Sandplay and symbol work*; Garrett; Beyond play therapy.
24. Vaz, K. M. (2000). When is a sandplay psychotherapy process completed? *International Journal of Action Methods, 53*(2), 66–85.
25. Pearson & Wilson, *Sandplay and symbol work.*
26. Itoh, Y. (1991). Hakoniwa rhohoh (Sand play therapy). In Y. Yamanaka & K. Yamashita (Eds.), *Rinsho shinri test nyumon (Introduction to clinical psychology assessment)* (pp. 244–267). Kyoto, Japan: Higashiyama.
27. Ammann, *Healing and transformation*; Pearson & Wilson, *Sandplay and symbol work*; Weinrib, *Images of the self.*
28. Pearson & Wilson, *Sandplay and symbol work*; Kalff, *Sandplay.*
29. Pearson & Wilson, *Sandplay and symbol work.*
30. Garrett, Beyond play therapy; Carey, *Sandplay therapy.*
31. Kawai, The Japanese mind.
32. Kawai, H. (1998). A Buddhist remedy. *Unesco Courier, 51*(2), 12–14.
33. Ibid.
34. Hayashi, S., Kuno, T., Morotomi, Y., Osawa, M., Shimzu, M., & Suetake, Y. (1998). Client-centered therapy in Japan: Fugio Tomoda and Taoism. *Journal of Humanistic Psychology, 38*(2), 103–124.
35. Ibid.
36. Doi, T. (1989). The concept of *amae* and its psychoanalytic implications. *International Review of Psycho-Analysis, 16*, 349–354.
37. Ibid.
38. Kalff, *Sandplay.*
39. Jung, C. G. (1961). *Memories, dreams, reflections* (A. Jaffe, Ed.). New York, NY: Random House.
40. Kawai, The Japanese mind.
41. Turner, *Handbook of sandplay therapy*; Morena, *The wisdom of Oz*; Vaz, When is a sandplay psychotherapy process completed?
42. Jung, C. G. (1960). The transcendent function. In H. Read, M. Fordham, G. Adler (Eds.), & R. F. C. Hull (Trans.), *The collected works of C. G. Jung* (Vol. 8). New York, NY: Pantheon Books. (Original work published 1916)
43. Lebra, T. S. (1993). Culture, self, and communication in Japan and the United States. In W. B. Gudykunst (Ed.), *Communication in Japan and the United* States (pp. 51–87). Albany: State University of New York Press.
44. Jung, The transcendent function.
45. Lebra, Culture, self, and communication.
46. Bankart, C. P. (1997). *Talking cures: A history of Western and Eastern psychotherapies.* Pacific Grove, CA: Brooks/Cole.
47. Matsuyuki, M. (1998). Japanese feminist counseling as a political act. *Women and Therapy, 21*(2), 65–77.
48. Kawai, The Japanese mind; Uemera, Pioneer of clinical psychology.
49. Ibid.
50. Morena, *The wisdom of Oz*; Vaz, When is a sandplay psychotherapy process completed?
51. Pearson & Wilson, *Sandplay and symbol work*; Carey, *Sandplay therapy.*
52. Garrett, Beyond play therapy; Steinhardt, *Foundation and form.*

53. Doi, The concept of *amae*.
54. Ibid.
55. Matsuyuki, Japanese feminist counseling.
56. Borovoy, A. (2001). Recovering from codependence in Japan. *American Ethnologist, 28*(1), 94–118.
57. Matsuyuki, Japanese feminist counseling.
58. Kasai, M. (1997). *Self-construal, narcissistic vulnerability, and symptoms of psychological distress among Japanese college students* (Unpublished doctoral dissertation). University of Missouri, Columbia.
59. Ibid.
60. Lebra, Culture, self, and communication.
61. Kawai, *Buddhism and the art of psychotherapy.*
62. Hiramatsu, K., & Yamaguchi, S. (1998). A review of fundamental studies of Sandplay Therapy in Japan. *Bulletin of Educational Sciences of Okayama University, 109*, 39–51.
63. Ibid.
64. Pearson & Wilson, *Sandplay and symbol work*; Garrett, Beyond play therapy; Carey, *Sandplay therapy*.
65. Carey, *Sandplay therapy*.

SUGGESTED READINGS

Boik, B. L., & Goodwin, E. A. (2000). *Sandplay therapy: A step-by-step manual for psychotherapists of diverse orientations*. New York, NY: Norton.

This book, written primarily for a Western audience, provides an overview of history and benefits of sandplay and practical information for making use of sandplay techniques with a variety of client populations and for personal growth.

Harding, C., Iwata, F., & Yoshinaga, S. (Eds.). (2015). *Religion and psychotherapy in modern Japan*. New York, NY: Routledge.

This book includes a variety of readings about how religious traditions of Japan have been integrated with psychotherapy traditions of the West. Of particular relevance to this chapter are selections on *amae* theory (Takeo Doi) and information and perspective about the work of Hayao Kawai.

Homeyer, L. E., & Sweeney, D. S. (2011). *Sandtray therapy: A practical manual* (2nd ed.). New York, NY: Routledge.

This volume provides practical and "how-to" information about implementing Sandplay therapy techniques. The book is written primarily for Western practitioners but has been translated into other languages.

Kawai, H. (1996). *Buddhism and the art of psychotherapy*. College Station: Texas A&M University Press.

Hayao Kawai, known for his introduction of Hakoniwa to Japan, was a prolific writer who authored 50 books, written primarily in Japanese. This book is one of only a few of his books that were written in English. This volume provides insight about the profound impact of Buddhism on Kawai's work as a psychotherapist.

NOTE

1. A full version of this chapter was published in 2003, in *The Counseling Psychologist, 33*(1), 93–112.

17 *Oishii:* Japanese Delicious Moment Therapy

Mami Ishii and Ted Lo

Counseling and psychotherapy have evolved over time to address many concerns of people from various cultural settings. That has led to interesting integrations and innovations. In contemporary society, they have become a place for many to find answers about life and living, which used to be guided in traditional cultures by indigenous healers, such as shamans and elders.[1] In such traditional healing, the focus was often on transcending the fragmentations of life toward a meaningful whole, fulfilling the innate desire toward an integral collective oneness.[2] In the postmodern age, many of us are seeking ultimate soul healing in the traditional sense, the intimate remembering and realization of authentic wholesomeness through finding meaning, expanding our consciousness, and living harmoniously with nature. Although psychology, psychotherapy, and even medicine have evolved from such shamanistic practice, its spiritual essence seems to have been forgotten in modern scientific discourse and the current research-based practices of psychology.[3]

The inclusion and integration of traditional healing methods into mainstream counseling and psychotherapy is a creative paradigm shift, which not only makes a difference to multicultural counseling but may also introduce a new lease of life to psychotherapy and counseling generally.[4] Many philosophical and psychological ideas from Asian history and culture are being explored in this integration process because of its relative openness and acceptance of human potential.[5] For example, we see this in the new Japanese psychotherapies of Morita, Naikan, and Hakoniwa, which share the common focus on observing and appreciating one's own life rather than just a cognitive understanding or resolving of tensions and problems.

This unconditional "aesthetic appreciation" of one's life and the world is often layered underneath an active meditative practice that leads to a transformative moment when radical acceptance and healing occur.[6] One way of applying this process of aesthetic appreciation in a contemporary context is an integrative approach that embraces "deliciousness," or ***oishii*** (美味しい), meaning "savoring" in Japanese; with its culinary roots firmly establishing its meaning related to taste and appreciation of food and nutrition, it is nevertheless a symbolic representation of an aesthetic appreciation of the body.

Establishing an aesthetic appreciation of the body, the mind, and the lived experience in Japanese culture is about accepting that the human experience is not a stable state of vanity or perfection but rather a transient cycle of harmony, imperfection, and transcendence of what is. Examples include one witnessing blossoming spring flowers after a long cold winter or a child learning to stand on his feet after countless falls as well as even the resilient recovery of people after a natural disaster. Influenced by Buddhism and Confucianism, it encompasses the values of *monono aware* (transiency of things) and *wabi-sabi* (impermanence, incompletion, and imperfection).[7] Traditional healing rituals are filled with highly aesthetic moments through multimodal experiences where the holistic integration and transcendental harmony are induced. This state of spiritual union is highly regarded as an aesthetic appreciation of human life and indeed in the practice of traditional healing and medicine in Japan.[8]

In this respect, we have employed savoring, deliciousness, and aesthetic appreciation as descriptors or therapeutic constructs to articulate a meditative and transient therapeutic healing process. It engages a person's cognitive, intuitive, and affective self.

Savoring is a process in traditional healing and is also well described in positive psychology. It is a diverse set of processes underlying the regulation of positive feelings including one's emotions, perceptions, thoughts, behaviors, and feelings when mindfully attending to and appreciating positive experiences from the past, present, or future.[9]

Engaging the whole person also means that the concept of *oishii* takes on a larger meaning that incorporates the body (sensation), the mind, and the spirit—a personification of the Eastern idea where the body, mind, and spirit is a single unity and not a Cartesian divide.

While much gets lost in translation in any movement of knowledge across the globe, particularly from cultural texts that are historically seen through a colonial lens, the language and terminology used in this particular therapy can be appreciated if understood through a positive psychology paradigm. Thus, if the concept of *oishii* is employed in counseling and psychotherapy within a positive psychology frame, within which the narratives of clients are listened to, interpreted, and deciphered through the lenses of an aesthetic, deliciousness, and wholeness of a "savoring self," therapy can come to be experienced and understood as a moment of deliciousness. This is experienced through a meditative process using the vital energy, *ki* (氣), manipulated through active guided visualization and vibration via words, aroma, and instruments. This then is an experience of a Japanese Delicious Moment therapy, evolved to integrate a holistic meditative experience of a wholeness of a here and now (gestalt) life.

This chapter first explores the history and philosophy underlying Japanese Delicious Moment therapy, followed by a discussion on the process and practice of Japanese Delicious Moment therapy. The discussion also illustrates how the fulfillment of the innate desire for unconditional love, acceptance, and belonging is achieved.

Theoretical Foundation of Japanese Delicious Moment Therapy

Every society has its own system of health care that reflects its history and culture. In Japan, the Edo period was significant for the beginning of various aspects of its culture. ***Yojokun*** (養生訓) is a holistic health manual written in 1712 by Kaibara Ekken, a samurai physician, Zen master, and neo-Confucianism philosopher. It described the "**art of living**," to cultivate well-lived life, or "*ajiwai-no-aru-jinsei*" (味わいのある人生), meaning "a flavorful or delicious life" and "a fulfilled life with healthy longevity, joy, and meaning."[10] Several important concepts are discussed in the *Yojokun* (養生訓) manual, such as Jin (仁), the human-heartedness or compassion, and *ki*, vital energy. These concepts are discussed next.

Jin (仁), the human-heartedness or compassion, is the key concept in Japanese traditional medicine and the main point of *Yojokun*.[11] It is the expression of benevolence and virtue that enables people to effectively communicate love and nurture harmonious relationships. Individuals possess this innate desire for connection to each other, and to the original source. The ensuing emotion is called *amae* (甘え) in Japanese psychology.[12] It literally means sweetness, coming from the very first sensory experience through tasting the breast milk from the mother, signifying unconditional acceptance and love.[13] The fulfillment of this emotion is aesthetically pleasing and essential not only to the child–mother relationship but also in the realization of *satori* (悟り), a Zen Buddhist idea of reflecting a spiritual state of being that leads to a oneness with the universe.[14] At the heart of traditional Japanese culture is the value of "harmony in all things."[15] This is also the central value of Asian traditional healing practices that recognizes health as a harmonious existence and honors the idea that the whole is greater than the sum of the parts.[16] The traditional (Japanese) rituals and ceremonies tend to engage the wholeness of being with an integration of multisensory experiences that includes music, dance, incense, and herbs. These connect the mind with body, spirit, and society. This holistic and integrative approach toward **flourishing** the authentic self motivates and guides people's attitude and awareness of their own sacred triad (mind–body–spirit), and ultimately to *satori*.

The flow of *ki*, on the other hand, has an essential role in our wellness as it connects, maintains, and promotes the integration of our wholesomeness and harmonious nature. Based on the principle of *ki*, which is the foundation of our being and everything that exists in this world, *Yojokun* presents ways to nourish the vital energy via various *kata* (形).[17] *Kata* are specific forms and designs that were developed and utilized in almost every aspect of daily life to be expressed as an art with functional purpose and spiritual simplicity in living.[18] They inspire people to practice mindful observation and radical acceptance of a constantly changing life from a greater collective perspective, which eventually leads to an experience of transcendence. *Kata* also provides a social and conceptual paradigm for the resolution of the social or personal chaos and ambiguity that emerge as problems in understanding how our worlds are organized and how we identify ourselves within those worlds.[19]

Religious and spiritual concerns, including Shintoism, are critical in Japanese culture. Shintoism is loosely based on Asian traditional values and philosophy, and a central attitude of its healing practice has emphasized individual responsibilities to acquire a power of self-regulation, preservation, and evolution.[20] This motivates and guides people to cultivate a certain attitude toward the fulfillment of life while perceiving oneself as a responsible part of nature. Integration of spirituality into a person's life promotes the states of resilience characterized with coherence, purpose, gratitude, and joy; advocacy for whole-person; a commitment to an ethic of compassion; and a relationship with the sacred. They are both a subjective and an objective reality.[21]

The Process of Japanese Delicious Moment Therapy

Japanese Delicious Moment therapy is a contemporary experiential therapy inspired by Japanese traditional healing and philosophy as described earlier. It is not so much a distinct therapy but an approach, which integrates Eastern philosophy with Western Eurocentric psychological methods. While the goals of this therapy are the same as cognitive behavioral therapy (CBT), person-centered therapy, or the psychodynamic approaches, Japanese Delicious Moment therapy uses Japanese traditional knowledge of the mind, body, and spirit to engage with the therapeutic and healing process.

Some of the four key concepts are (1) flourishing the self, (2) self-cultivation, (3) collective shared experience, and (4) transcendence of the self. These will be discussed next:

Flourishing the self—A person constructs and enjoys a well-lived, delicious life with health, longevity, happiness, and meaning.[22] This is also described in positive psychology as a state of wellness, which is characterized by positive emotions, engagement, relationships, meaning, and accomplishment.[23] In contrast, a languishing life is filled with a sense of emptiness and hollowness.[24] The process of recovery is seen as a personal journey rather than a set of outcomes, and it comprises connectedness, hope, and optimism about the future as well as one's identity and meaning in life.[25] In Kaibara's view, good health is what you owe to yourself but even more so to the world around you so that the gratitude is also to our parents, society, and the heaven and earth, which makes all life possible.[26]

Self-cultivation—Individual responsibility is needed to acquire a power of self-regulation, preservation, and evolution. Kaibara taught and treated people with his nourishing life, "*Yojo* （養生）" principle. Taking a holistic view of health, Kaibara outlined practical methods for the regulation and balance of *ki* as well as a detailed account of the appropriate mental and spiritual attitudes in people's daily life. With the goal of nourishing delicious life with joy, longevity, and meaning, the practice of a health promoting lifestyle and mind-set toward one's harmonious wholesomeness was encouraged.

Collective shared experience—With the focus of Asian culture on the collective, another feature is the idea of healing through a shared experience with the family and community. That requires a responsibility and compassion from each individual. Genuine compassion comes from learning to accept suffering of self as well as others with a sense of the equality and interconnectedness of life. It empowers the person and helps them unlock their strength and courage from within. This is the basis of embracing compassion—nonjudgmental and unconditional acceptance to fulfill *amae*.[27]

Transcendence of the self—This is to find, recognize, and take pleasure in personal goodness but also to strengthen one's character and go beyond connecting with others to a connection to the larger universe.[28] Beyond self-actualization, Maslow's last amended hierarchy of needs indicated self-transcendence as the highest level to understand altruism, social progress, wisdom, religious violence, and the integration of religion and spirituality into psychology and multiculturality.[29]

Japanese Delicious Moment therapy also engages the four domains that are all interconnected: (1) the body (biological), (2) the mind (psychological), (3) the spiritual (metaphysical), and (4) the social (society). Each will be discussed next:

The body (biological)—In traditional healing, a healthy body is seen as an aid in the development of insight toward *satori* and actions pursuing a "delicious life." It is seen as the sacred representative site for the wholesome body–mind–soul sacred triad rather than a separate entity by itself.[30] There are several ways to nourish the body—stimulating the senses, taking in substance (nutrition or medicines), applying substance on the body, working on the body, and using the body. Healing rituals are often accompanied by multiple sensorial stimulation including music, dance, chanting, incense, water, and fire that can set the scene for the healing experience. Since the foundation of life is considered an energy, or *ki*, the manipulation of energy could also be conducted by physical means, such as acupuncture, Qigong (QG), and Reiki healing. The appropriate individualized combination of such interventions leads to the development of a trusting relationship with one's own body by shifting the perception of it from a source of suffering to an ally in healing and comfort. Focusing on these physical sensations also enhances the process of savoring, enabling the person to process thoughts and emotions in the present moment and to develop a heightened self-awareness and a deeper understanding of one's own being in a harmonious way.

The mind (psychological)—While Western psychotherapy works with a vertical dynamic to understand and resolve the emotional conflict that may be deeply repressed, traditional healing works indirectly with the surface dynamic to experience and release such conflict symbolically, energetically, and aesthetically.[31] In this way, the healing process could also be less threatening, more interesting, and often profound—especially when combined with bodywork. Using techniques of meditation and visualization, this process can be reinforced to achieve a state of mindfulness, a natural human mental state of moment-to-moment awareness of the present experience. Often these ritualistic practices are used with the meditative sensorial stimulation to deepen the state into an altered consciousness.

The ritualistic structure of a session with the pleasant physical sensation and hypnotic guidance induces a state of profound relaxation bypassing the conscious mental block of continuous thinking and overwhelmed emotions. Combined with active visualization and often personification of the felt senses, the client is guided to symbolically work with her or his own emotions and memories and connect at a deeper level.[32] This experience eventually builds the foundation for the client to contain the emotional conflicts and challenge the irrational beliefs from the past trauma affecting the present moment. Since flourishing is the ultimate goal of this therapy, traumas and symptoms such as anxiety and sadness are integrated into the heart of savoring to be fully experienced as they are.[33]

The spiritual (metaphysical)—Embedded in the layers of bodily and psychological experiences, the spiritual domain is similarly explored. Based on the cultural relevance, the person is actively encouraged to experience his or her own energy and visualize the spiritual and energetic connection with self, with nature, a higher self, or other applicable spiritual or religious representation. The person's spiritual connection is also gently strengthened through the interactive experience of one's own energy in relation to energy healing and learning of energy systems (e.g., chakra system) and therapeutic power of natural elements such as sun, moon, plants, and stones.

The social (society)—Through an intimate human experience with the therapist, a genuine, accepting, and empathetic relationship, the client seeking help can symbolically fulfill *amae*, promoting self-discovery and personal growth toward an authentic self. This state may also be extended to encourage the development of connections outside the therapeutic dyad, with the family and eventually with the community. The family may be invited to share the savoring experience, or the therapist may go outside with the patient to a park or other community settings to reflect on the process. Clients may also be referred to support groups as well as volunteering or working opportunities so that the person will develop a sense of belonging and recognition in society.

Thus, the Japanese Delicious Moment therapy engages a client with flourishing the self; self-cultivation; collective shared experience; and transcendence of the self through the biological, the psychological, the spiritual, and the social. Indeed, this will eventually lead to what the World Health Organization (WHO) defines as good health: "a dynamic state of complete physical, mental, spiritual and social well-being and not merely the absence of illness or disease."[34]

The Practice of Japanese Delicious Moment Therapy

In Japanese Delicious Moment therapy, the therapist is a guide and cocreator, leading a sequence of actions similar to a traditional healing ritual, such as *misogi* (water cleansing ritual) and *harai* (chanting cleansing ritual), while the client is the other cocreator who is invited to share his or her subjective experience. The client, while receiving the therapist's verbal guidance, verbal questions, and reframing statements toward a self-reflective awareness and consciousness is deeply engaged in the healing process, which focuses on the uniqueness of each person's inner experience and meaning construction.[35]

The sessions usually take place in a quiet, contained room that provides a sense of comfort and security. The use of colors, aromas, lights, and other nature elements such as plants and gemstones can also contribute toward an aesthetic appreciation through the engagement of the five senses, relaxation, and healing. Imbibed at a subconscious level, they can be symbolic representations of the process or the content of therapy (e.g., a picture of a mother and child on a tricycle in the forest at the bifurcation of a road). The length of each session is about 90 to 120 minutes, based on the ultradian neuropsychophysiological profile of the four stages in therapeutic hypnosis.[36] It respects and synchronizes the therapeutic process with the bodily nature of a person. Depending on the individual's needs, goals, and current condition, the treatment period may last from a couple sessions to more than a year. Outside of the office, the clients are also encouraged to re-create, cultivate, and savor their own Japanese Delicious Moment therapy based on what they have experienced in the session.

The four domains (i.e., biological, psychological, spiritual, and social) are experienced in the following way: The biological aspects of treatment are physically engaging experiences through various body work with the use of water, food and herbs as well as the vibrational energy of sound, aroma, and homeopathy. These are part of the repertoire in the practice of naturopathy. Other bodily manipulations are also employed, like bioenergetics.[37] The therapy incorporates visualization and imaginative symbolic work and complements the spiritual dimensions of healing as emphasized in transpersonal psychology. In this symbolic way of exploration, the vague memories and past experience can shift to something more workable, interesting, and non-threatening. The person can allow his own body to express emotions and feelings, release energetically, and gain helpful insights to move on. This aesthetic resolution toward harmony is the main process of healing.[38]

The emotional and practical supports in traditional rituals and ceremonies are well-organized within the community, and the practice of community psychiatry also attempts to make inroads into these areas.[39] They provide an experience of belonging to a group and a view of society as a meaningful and understandable collective possessing potential for growth and acceptance.[40] This healing experience builds a secure foundation for a client to restore integrity through accepting the present moment, cultivating wellness and spiritual abundance through embracing the beauty of an "authentic wholesomeness," which eventually helps to counteract internalized conditions of poor self-worth and negative thoughts.[41] Japanese Delicious Moment therapy can also be an opportunity to explore the relationship between the experiential imagery healing process and induced biomolecular changes such as mirror neurons, gene expression, and brain plasticity.[42] Furthermore, while Japanese Delicious Moment therapy is a highly individualized, ritualized, and experiential process, it can also be conducted with large groups.

Conclusion

As a process-oriented rather than achievement- or goal-directed therapy, its practice can engage a group and inspire hope and meaning in the search of one's own authentic self during one's life journey, while connecting to social, religious, or cultural traditional values that can be extended beyond individual motivations. Moreover, this holistic integrative approach could offer more than a therapeutic option for people to alleviate suffering with mental health issues; it also enhances personal development sought by the nonpatient population at large. Just as our ancestors in traditional cultures strived for cultivation and fulfillment of meaning in daily life by sharing such rituals and ceremonies as a group, Japanese Delicious Moment therapy can provide a collective experience to enhance inner nourishment, spiritual connection, and social cohesiveness. The practice may indeed improve the well-being of the practitioners, reducing burnout and social isolation through realization and practicing own Japanese Delicious Moment therapy and also the aesthetic experience of the therapy, which is encouraging and inspiring for the clients.

DISCUSSION QUESTIONS

1. Symbolic and surface (indirect) processing is one of the characteristics of Japanese aesthetic conceptualization. How can it be useful in the practice of psychotherapy and counseling?

2. Restoring the harmonious relationship with nature is the central value in the traditional Asian healing practices. What are ways to incorporate this point into practice of psychotherapy and counseling?
3. What are some specific characteristics of Japanese traditional healing practices and aesthetic processing that are keys to Delicious Moment therapy? How can they additionally and effectively contribute to the typical Western practice or other multicultural psychotherapy and counseling?
4. How can the concept of Delicious Moment therapy be integrated into psychotherapy and counseling with tools and resources that you have to construct integrative holistic intervention? How would you like to apply this concept into your practice?

REFERENCES

1. Frank, J. D., & Frank, J. B. (1993). *Persuasion and healing: A comparative study of psychotherapy* (3rd ed.). Baltimore, MD: The Johns Hopkins University Press.
2. Moodley, R., & West, W. (Eds.). (2005). *Integrating traditional healing practices into counseling and psychotherapy.* Thousand Oaks, CA: Sage; Tseng, W.-S., Change, S. C., & Nishizono, M. (2005). *Asian culture and psychotherapy: Implications for East and West.* Honolulu: University of Hawai'i Press. Retrieved from http://www.uhpress.hawaii.edu/books/tseng-chap1.pdf
3. Moodley & West, *Integrating traditional healing practices.*
4. Ibid.
5. Tseng et al., *Asian culture and psychotherapy.*
6. Tohata, K. (2012). *Aesthetics and deep conscious psychology.* Kyoto, Japan: Kyoto University Press. [in Japanese]
7. Moodley & West, *Integrating traditional healing practices*; Tohata, *Aesthetics and depth psychology*; Sawada, S. (2011). The art of health maintenance in "Yojokun" by Ekken Kaibara—about selfcare. *Journal of Toho Gakuen, 40*(1), 87–100. [in Japanese]
8. Sawada, The art of health maintenance.
9. Moodley & West, *Integrating traditional healing practices*; Tohata, *Aesthetics and depth psychology.*
10. Sawada, The art of health maintenance.
11. Sawada, The art of health maintenance; Takahashi, H. (2005). *Fundamental research about the Japanese beauty consciousness research on "Aimai" as a concept of the beauty.* Retrieved April 21, 2015, from http://homepage3.nifty.com/naoyuki_oi/Research/biishiki_DRA35.pdf
12. Doi, T. (1986). *The anatomy of dependence* (5th ed.). Tokyo, Japan: Kodansha International.
13. Tohata, *Aesthetics and depth psychology*; Takahashi, *Fundamental research about the Japanese beauty.*
14. Doi, *The anatomy of dependence.*
15. Sawada, The art of health maintenance; Takahashi, *Fundamental research about the Japanese beauty*; Doi, *The anatomy of dependence.*
16. Tseng et al., *Asian culture and psychotherapy.*
17. Takahashi, *Fundamental research about the Japanese beauty.*
18. Griffith, J. L., & Griffith, M. E. (2002). *Encountering The Sacred In Psychotherapy: How To Talk With People About Their Spiritual Lives.* New York: The Guilford Press.
19. Ibid.
20. Tseng et al., *Asian culture and psychotherapy*; Sawada, The art of health maintenance.

21. Griffith, Psychotherapy, religion, and spirituality.
22. Sawada, The art of health maintenance.
23. Peterson, C., & Seligman, M. E. P. (2004). *Character strengths and virtues: A handbook and classification.* Oxford, England: Oxford University Press; Keyes, C. L. M. (2002). The mental health continuum: From languishing to flourishing in life. *Journal of Health and Social Behavior, 43*(2), 207–222.
24. Keyes, The mental health continuum.
25. Leamy, M., Bird, V., Le Boutillier, C., Williams, J., & Slade, M. (2011). Conceptual framework for personal recovery in mental health: Systematic review and narrative synthesis. *British Journal of Psychiatry, 119*(6), 445–452.
26. Sawada, The art of health maintenance.
27. Doi, *The anatomy of dependence.*
28. Griffith, Psychotherapy, religion, and spirituality.
29. Koltko-Rivera, M. E. (2006). Rediscovering the later version of Maslow's hierarchy of needs: Self-transcendence and opportunities for theory, research, and unification. *Review of General Psychology, 10*(4), 302–317.
30. Tseng et al., *Asian culture and psychotherapy.*
31. Frank & Frank, *Persuasion and healing*; Tohata, *Aesthetics and depth psychology.*
32. Gendlin, E. T. (1996). *Focusing-oriented psychotherapy.* New York, NY: Guilford Press.
33. Bryant, F. B., Chadwick, E. D., & Luwe, K. (2011). Understanding the processes that regulate positive emotional experience: Unsolved problems and future directions for theory and research on savouring. *International Journal of Wellbeing, 1*(1), 107–126.
34. World Health Organization. (1998). Review of the constitution of organization: Report of the World Health Organization: Report of the Executive Board special group. Retrieved April 4, 2015, from http://apps.who.int/gb/archive/pdf_files/EB101/pdfangl/angr2.pdf
35. Greenberg, L. S., Rice, L. N., & Elliott, R. (1993). *Facilitating emotional change: The moment-by-moment process.* New York, NY: Guilford Press.
36. Rossi, E. (1982). Hypnosis and ultradian cycles: A new state(s) theory of hypnosis? *The American Journal of Clinical Hypnosis, 25*, 21–32.
37. Frank & Frank, *Persuasion and healing*; Lowen, A. (1994). *Bioenergetics* (Reprint ed.). New York, NY: Penguin Group.
38. Tohata, *Aesthetics and depth psychology.*
39. Moodley & West, *Integrating traditional healing practices*; Tseng et al., *Asian culture and psychotherapy.*
40. Leamy et al., Conceptual framework.
41. Sawada, The art of health maintenance; Greenberg et al., *Facilitating emotional change.*
42. Doidge, N. (2007). *The brain that changes itself: Stories of personal triumph from the frontiers of brain science.* New York, NY: Viking.

SUGGESTED READINGS

Bryant, F., & Veroff, J. (2007). *Savouring: A new model of positive experience.* Mahwah, NJ: Lawrence Erlbaum.

This book describes various aspects of savoring, from the perspective of positive psychology to conceptualize and understand the processing of positive emotion. It is the capacity to attend to the joys, pleasures, and other positive things that we experience in our lives. Related concepts are discussed in terms of human life span, common life concerns and factors, and therapeutic and educational strategies to enhance the experience of savoring.

Doi, T. (1973). *The anatomy of dependence.* Tokyo, Japan: Kodansha International.

This is a classic book for the study of Japanese psyche, defining, analyzing, and exploring *amae,* a foundational emotion in Japanese daily life and behaviors. The word *amae* and its related vocabulary and implication were discussed by the Japanese psychoanalytic psychiatrist Doi to contrast the difference between the East and West cultures as well as their similarities.

Ekken, K. (2008). *Yojokun: Life lessons from a samurai* (W. Wilson, Trans.). Tokyo, Japan: Kodansha International.

This book was originally written by Kaibara, the samurai physician in the 16th century over 6 decades as the collected and compiled experiences, knowledge, and wisdom of holistic health addressing mental, physical, and spiritual matters to daily lifestyles including diet, hygiene, sexual practices, and other healthy habits. Based on the principles of *ki* (*qi,* the essential energy force), *jin* (human-heartedness), spirituality and philosophy (mainly Buddhism and Confucianism), and the art of living, it is a guide that is still applicable today to a traditional way of life and achieving balanced health.

Tohata, K. (2012). *Bi to shinso shinrigaku (Aesthetics and deep conscious psychology).* Kyoto, Japan: Kyoto University Press. (in Japanese)

The role of aesthetics in psychotherapy is explored, analyzed, and discussed from the various perspectives: forms of ailments and disorders, types of therapies and approaches, and levels and directions of its process. It is quite interesting where the author contrasts the difference of aesthetic perception and processing between Japanese and non-Japanese (Westerners) and its implication in psychotherapy.

Conclusion: Integrating Asian Healing Traditions Into Counseling and Psychotherapy

Roy Moodley, Julie Hong, and Na Zhu

Since the 1990s, there has been a tremendous growth in the development, research, and practice of alternative and complementary (medicine) therapies with an increasing number of people engaging in the practices of energy healing, traditional Chinese medicine (TCM), yoga, acupuncture, herbal remedies, Ayurveda, homeopathy, and others. Many professionals in both national and private health care institutions are now sympathetic toward these alternative healing and complementary practices, either practicing some (e.g., mindfulness meditation) themselves or being open to their clients undertaking cultural and indigenous healing. Indeed, Asian and other racialized and marginalized communities have long been engaging in these practices alongside modern medicine, favoring a holistic approach, which seems to be absent in Western health and mental health care. It is not just the new immigrants that appear to be engaging in traditional and cultural healing practices but even second- and third-generation individuals who are now seeking health care practices that reflect their ethnic and cultural traditions of healing.

The current high rate of immigration in North America is not only changing the demography of the ethnic minority populations but is adding to the vociferous call for culturally appropriate health and mental health care. This requires mental health professionals to acquire the knowledge and skills for culturally competent practice. In 35 of the 50 largest U.S. cities, for instance, non-Hispanic Whites are or soon will be the minority, and Asian groups make up a sizable population.[1] In Canada, for example, Asian communities make up the majority of ethnic minority groups.[2] These new racial or ethnic configurations inevitably bring about different worldviews, belief systems, values, customs, lifestyles, etc. In order to meet the health and mental needs of these racialized or marginalized groups, health and mental health clinicians will not only need to integrate their clients' cultural values, attitudes, and ethnic beliefs into diagnosis and treatment but also to seriously consider the inclusion or integration of these groups' cultural, indigenous, and traditional healing practices. Clearly traditional healing integration into Western counseling and psychotherapy will support the diversity and multicultural project, which is now ready for its next stage of development. Indeed, there are of course larger benefits for the counseling and psychotherapy profession if this is to happen—for example, the intersection of Asian healing traditions with Western psychologies will create an opportunity to revisit the conceptualizing and meanings of everyday terminologies in health and mental health; terms such as *healing* and *curing* are understood very differently in traditional Asian healing. Boon-Ooi Lee (see Chapter 7) stated that the focus of Asian traditional healing is about the healing of illness rather than the curing of disease. Lee suggests the following:

> Curing refers to the removal of pathophysiology, which does not recognize the social roots of sickness and social resources for care. By contrast, healing refers to the process of restoring subjective, affective, social, ecological, and spiritual dimensions of illness. Clients may restore their daily functioning, even though they may continuously experience clinical symptoms. Through integration, this holistic approach of traditional healing can broaden the biomedical and psychological model of psychotherapy.

Through the process of both broadening and redefining health and mental health theory and practice, the various chapters in this book explore the possibilities and potentialities of newer forms of health and mental health care. The various chapters in this book explore the many complex facets of Asian healing traditions, such as the mind–body unity, harmony and nature, conduct and the relationship with others, and many others. By juxtaposing the age-old practices of Asian healing with the current lexicon of Western psychotherapies, the chapters attempt to bring to consciousness the ancient art of Asian healing traditions. Beginning with a discussion of the history and philosophy of Buddhism, Confucianism, and Taoism (or Daoism) the chapters develop a rich tapestry of indigenous and cultural traditions of healing; these, in turn, have influenced current Western clinical methods, such as the inclusion of Buddhist mindfulness into cognitive behavioral therapy (CBT) to form mindfulness-based stress reduction (MBSR). Other examples are dialectical behavior therapy (DBT) and acceptance and commitment therapy (ACT). In a more nuanced way, mindfulness can be seen as the foundation of newer forms of cultural healing practice, such as Japanese Morita therapy and Naikan therapy. Both of these chapters (see Chapters 12 and 13) have been interestingly elaborated and described with case studies as did many of the chapters—all illuminating and elucidating the complexity, grace, and sophistication of integrating Asian healing traditions in counseling and psychotherapy. These case studies themselves not only demonstrate how Asian healing traditions can be effectively integrated into Western clinical practices but challenges readers to consider the limitation of Western counseling and psychotherapy. While the clients under discussion (ages ranging from 19 to 50+ years; four men and five women with presenting issues that are typical for counseling and psychotherapy practice, such as depression and anxiety disorders: see Table C.1) are not a representative sample of the population who generally use Asian healing traditions, they do, however, offer an insight into the dual interventions of Western therapy and Asian healing.

Table C.1. Client Characteristics in Case Studies

Chapter	*Ethnicity*	*Age*	*Gender*	*Presenting Issue*	*Traditional Therapy*	*Traditional Philosophy*
6	Caucasian	55	Female	Obsessive–compulsive disorder; anxiety	Acceptance and commitment therapy (ACT); meditation; self-compassion	Buddhism
7	Chinese	46	Female	Major depressive disorder	Taoist rituals; herbal medicine; acupuncture	Taoism
8	Unknown	45	Male	Depression	Tibetan medicine	Tibetan Buddhism
9	Unknown	23	Female	Post-traumatic stress disorder (PTSD)	Mindfulness	Buddhism
10	Chinese	42	Male	Anxiety disorder	Chinese Taoist cognitive psychotherapy (CTCP)	Taoism
11	Chinese	24	Male	Body dysmorphic disorder; panic disorder; social avoidance	Acceptance and commitment therapy (ACT)	Buddhism
12	Unknown	28	Female	Anxiety disorder; conflicting relationship with mother	Naikan therapy	Buddhism
13	Unknown	22	Female	Social anxiety	Morita therapy	Buddhism
14	Caucasian	28	Male	Major depressive episode; generalized anxiety; panic attacks	Reiki therapy	Buddhism

In our brief analysis of the various chapters, two key principles emerge as critical components of Asian healing traditions: (1) the principle of holism and equilibrium and (2) the principle of conduct and ethics. In this conclusion, we explore these principles and their relevance to clinical practice. We also consider the process of integration and discuss its benefits and limitations.

The Principle of Holism and Equilibrium

This concept is understood as a process that explains the mind–body theory. The meaning of the self, selfhood, and the individualized self is very different from the Western Cartesian dualism that informs counseling and psychotherapy. Eastern philosophies offer an alternative knowledge system of the mind–body theory based on a nondualistic (or a monistic) view of the self, within which the body, mind, and spirit are seen as a singular (body–mind–spirit) whole. The Cartesian dialectics in constructing a binary view of the self has been influential in the way that illness and health are conceived, represented, and presented in Western health and mental health care—both structuring diagnosis and mandating clinical governance in counseling and psychotherapy. Indeed, the larger meanings of holism and equilibrium are more than just seeing the client as a unification of the body–mind–spirit concept, or the aggregation of the sum of the (self) parts but is deeply embedded in the relationship of the individual with the environment and vice versa. In other words, the individual is constituted through the reciprocal relationship with the environment and all things universal; this, in turn, influences the evolution and development of the multilayered self in the context of group of seven (race, gender, class, sexual orientation, disability, religion, and age).[3] This idea of the global influence in the makeup of the self is best summarized by Amy L. Ai (see Chapter 4): "The universe, including humans, depends on reciprocal influences and transforms between opposite but interdependent energetic forces in the ever-changing world. As such, parts become meaningful only in relevance to the whole context." The person's wholeness and equilibrium is dependent on the inner and outer contextual and environmental relationships. As Kwang-Kuo Hwang (see Chapter 1) noted, "harmony is constructed on the concepts of *yin* and *yang*, the five primary elements (*wu-hsin*), and the eight trigrams (*ba-gua*)." Harmony with nature and the environment, with oneself, and with others are critical to developing a holistic self. In other words, the principle of holism and harmony establishes a practice within which all aspects of the individual are interconnected and come together under their respective environmental context. The healer considers all of the parts of the person, which includes their physical senses (i.e., sight, sound, smell), physical presentation (i.e., facial expression, body posture, other nonverbal but physical cues), auras, *shen* (soul or spirit), *qi* (life force), life context, as well as nonphysical presentations (i.e., attitudes and emotional states). Mental illness, under the guiding principle of holism, is conceptualized as "destabilization" of the parts; likewise, mental health is defined as achieving a harmonious balance between the parts. Balance and harmony can be understood as a dialectical and interdependent worldview where opposing forces reciprocally influence and transform each other as described by the *yin* and *yang* forces. Asian healing traditions approach diagnosis as first identifying the parts and location of destabilization, followed by specific remedies and rituals that reestablish balance and harmony.

Consistent with the teachings of Taoism and Buddhism, clients are guided to recognize their feelings of dissonance, accept themselves as to who they are, and integrate this new meaning into their identities. This focus on acceptance appears to be present in many of the case studies and therefore becomes an important component in therapy. In fact, the holistic principle of acceptance is one of the underlying tenets of ACT and mindfulness, modalities that are becoming increasingly mainstream in Western counseling and psychotherapy. For example, in the Chapter 10 case study, there is a dissonance between who Mao is and who he wants to be, resulting in feelings of distress. Using the teachings of Taoism, the therapist was able to help Mao to let go of his yearnings and to be at peace and harmony with himself. In the Chapter 6 case study, the client Mia was counseled into integrating Buddhist teachings of acceptance; as a result, Mia was able to accept her inner experiences without forming attachment to it, leading to alleviation of some of her symptoms. It appears that when clients are able to integrate and assimilate their intrinsic and extrinsic self, they are at peace and harmony in the present while letting go of some of their attachments that contributed to psychological distress.

Within many of the case studies, there is a theme of mind–body–spirit interconnection. The unique therapeutic treatments emphasized awareness of the holistic and harmonious self in relation to lived experience; for example, constructive activities and light work (see Chapter 13), universal life force (see Chapter 14), meditation (see Chapters 6 and 9), movement (see Chapter 9), and traditional medicine to treat the body (see Chapters 7 and 8) to alleviate clients' psychological symptoms. Achieving a state of harmony and equilibrium of the body, mind, and spirit is an active engagement between the therapist and the client. Chikaki Ozawa-de Silva and Brendan Richard Ozawa-de-Silva reminded us that self-cultivation practices indicate "that this 'unity' is often understood as a 'potential,' and that mind-body unity is not a natural state, but rather something to be achieved" (p. 96).[4]

A wealth of remedies and special rituals exist to treat the fractured and multiple parts of the individual toward an integrated harmonious whole; for example, herbal medicines to treat imbalances within the body; acupuncture and acupressure to remove obstructions to the flow of *qi* (Chinese) or *ki* (Japanese); food and medicinal cuisine to counteract extreme moods; *taiji* and Qigong (QG) practices to promote physical exercise, as well as balance of the *qi;* and Taoist meditation to facilitate balance as well as promote emotional and physical health by fostering greater self-awareness and self-control. Less invasive remedies consist of art and talk therapies, involving dream interpretation, speaking with a healer or elder, doing music therapy, and painting and doing calligraphy. Many of these remedies have been integrated with Western counseling and therapeutic practice; for example, the use of meditation in pain management such as MBSR or the use of mindfulness in adaptations, addictions, and depression, such as mindfulness-based cognitive therapy (MBCT). And, indeed, newer approaches are also on the horizon—for example, the use of calligraphy, with particular attention to emotion regulation when used as a grounding technique through deliberate and mindful focus of brushstrokes, as suggested by Catherine Tien-Lun Sun (see Chapter 2). Through these and other methods, counselors and psychotherapists can actively engage the principle of holism and equilibrium and make integration a reality. As Ben C. H. Kuo and Beatriz Rodriguez-Rubio (see Chapter 6) discussed, counselors and psychotherapists would need to "expand their therapeutic and conceptual perspectives by giving consideration to the psychological, the medical, and the spiritual well-being of their clients and the mutual connections and implications among these critical dimensions."

The Principle of Conduct and Ethics

The ways in which an individual gains an awareness and understanding of his or her inner world—as well as how he or she relates to the outer world and the people in it—could be understood as the principle of conduct and ethics. Woven into the fabric of Asian healing traditions are the ancient wisdoms of Buddhism, Confucianism, and Taoism and their healing methods. These rich culturally and historically tried and tested teachings have over time evolved and are available as guides to support principled ways of conduct for positive health, fruitful and harmonious relationships, and ethical values and morals. The core principle that underpins the practice of authenticity of self and equitable actions with the other is the principle of conduct and ethics, where a person's thoughts and actions are sincere and congruent and achieved by fostering greater self-awareness through the practice of meditation and self-reflection. In other words, the individual undertakes an inward journey of self-examination—a time of psychological stocktaking. For instance, Tadashi Ogawa and Mama Ishii (see Chapter 5) urged us to practice QG not only for attaining better health but also to enable us to find "our own authentic selves in the answer to the fundamental question of who we are." The history and philosophy of QG and healing is elaborated in great detail by Amy L. Ai in Chapter 4. Furthermore, the Four Noble Truths in Buddhism often serve as the foundations of Asian healing traditions, governing the practice of conduct and ethics of others. According to Tony Toneatto (see Chapter 3), in regard to this process of introspection, "through discipline and discernment (fourth Noble Truth), one can develop a new *experiential* understanding of oneself, our social relationships, and the 'world' based on uncontrived acceptance and equanimity rather than obsessive clinging and fear (third Noble Truth)." Toneatto noted that "the pervasive dissatisfaction, lack of fulfillment, and mental suffering and illness that is part of life (first Noble Truth) is caused by the strong tendency to look for happiness, satisfaction, and reality in the phenomenal world that, by definition, cannot provide such dissatisfaction (second Noble Truth)." In addition, Toneatto argued that the "Buddha demonstrated that phenomenal experience, due to its transience and conditionality, can never provide us with genuine health and happiness but only conditional states of mind." The teachings of Buddha on moral conduct and self-understanding are demonstrated in many of the case studies in various chapters. For example, in the case studies in Chapters 12 and 13, the clinicians were able to integrate these Buddhist ideas into their Western clinical approach by undertaking this through an awareness of the principle of conduct and ethics. Furthermore, as mentioned previously, both mindfulness and ACT (see Chapters 6, 9, and 11) stemmed from Buddhist teachings and have become increasingly practiced in Western counseling and psychotherapy. From analyzing and synthesizing the case studies, it appears that there is value to the integration of clients' values, beliefs, and practices that are consistent with Eastern traditions.

The principle of conduct and ethics can also be applied as a self-disciplinary principle where an individual practices acceptance of self in a nonjudgmental way. In other words, an individual can exercise the choice to engage or not to engage a train of thought, a fleeting feeling, or the drive for action. The Taoist and Buddhist philosophy of being mindful of these thoughts, feelings, and possible actions also infuses an understanding of acceptance and letting go of these attachments (discussed in Chapters 3, 6, and 9). Specifically for the case study in Chapter 11, while in group therapy, Mr. Lee experienced behavioral exposure and disconfirmation of his maladaptive beliefs about himself, which are techniques consistent with CBT. These occurred in combination with learning to let go and connect with others in the present moment, which are teachings of Buddhism. The detachment from thoughts allows the individual to engage in humility and interpersonal harmony as well as compassion toward self and others (see Chapters 6 and 7).

The principle of conduct and ethics can also be extended beyond self-awareness, authenticity, and self-disciplinary principle and be applied in the interpersonal and intersubjective contexts. Asian philosophy defines the ways in which an individual conducts himself or herself with others, which determines the potential as a healer of suffering and a facilitator of harmony and wellness. The principle of conduct tends to inculcate values such as benevolence, propriety, and reciprocity necessary to minimize conflict and promote interpersonal harmony in a collectivistic environment. This is explored in-depth through the lens of "Confucianism and healing" in the first chapter. Of particular importance is the notion of uncovering the socialization process of the client in order to understand their unique ways of conducting their life, which includes lifestyle, coping, conflict resolution, and interpersonal styles and choices. Indeed, these are the objectives of Western counseling and psychotherapy as reiterated by Ben C. H. Kuo and Beatriz Rodriguez-Rubio (see Chapter 6): "Similar to the holistic framework assumed by traditional healers, counselors are challenged to expand their therapeutic and conceptual perspectives by giving consideration to the psychological, the medical, and the spiritual well-being of their clients and the mutual connections and implications among these critical dimensions."

Many chapters focused on interpersonal harmony and interdependence, as well as forbearance as values that are essential for conduct and ethical relationships with the other. To forbear is to restrain one's temper in order to avoid conflict and to refrain from casting judgment on others. This is illustrated in several case studies; clients shared the same kinds of issues where the presenting issues arouse from clients' conflict, or perceived conflict, with the social world. In Chapter 10, for example, Mao's symptoms were partially related to a lack of a romantic relationship, which served as a stressor for him given the cultural and societal expectation of him for his age. In Chapter 12, the client was guided to reevaluate her relationship with her mother, the origins of her distress, by taking a different perspective such that the focus is less "I"-centered and with a better understanding of the interdependent nature of her relationship with her mother. While taking a different perspective is a strategy that is often utilized in Western counseling and psychotherapy, this client was encouraged to explore the new perspective that is aligned with Buddhist teachings. An emphasis on relationships and the social world is consistent with the collectivist worldview of the Eastern cultures in which the focus is on the group rather than on the individual since the self is framed within a collective that emphasizes the values, wants, and needs of the cultural group before those of the individual.[5] Individuals in counseling and psychotherapy in one form or another will have an awareness of this collective self and will in a similar culture or race dyad reflect and share these cultural narratives. This could also be experienced in any clinical setting irrespective of race or culture or ethnic dyad similarity but indeed requires a culturally competent clinician with a strong clinical compatibility to engage such individuals.

Integration: Benefits and Limitations

Given the changing demographics in North America, it is inevitable that traditional or indigenous healing methods will in one form or another become part of the counseling and psychotherapy process in the future. As stated earlier, this process has already begun, with mindfulness meditation integration into CBT. Indeed, there are several ways in which integration of Asian healing traditions into Western counseling and psychotherapy may be understood and accomplished.

First, awareness, acknowledgment, and recognition of the critical importance of Asian healing traditions and its potential healing aspects would need to be a part of counselor education and training. Even if clinicians do not themselves practice these methods personally or professionally, it would be within their remit to refer some patients for appropriate traditional and cultural healing treatments. However, if the recognition of Asian healing traditions is at the professional organizational level, then it may be much easier for state and provincial levels of health and mental health policy and registration bodies to accommodate it. Following government legitimacy, mental health care providers and trainers will implement Asian healing traditions as part of their "culturally competent care" strategy.

Second, at the practitioner level, the counselors and psychotherapists will require critical multicultural competency training to be culturally competent. This includes an experience in deep self-reflection in order (a) to examine their assumptions and beliefs about cultural forms of healing and wellness; (b) to uncover any negative biases they may hold about indigenous, traditional, and cultural healing practices; (c) to acquire knowledge and skills to work in an ethical and non-oppressive way; and (d) to be more accommodating of the principle of holism, engaging in mind–body integration and intervention. An example of this can be found in the case study presented in Chapter 7 where the client entered therapy with a Western-trained psychotherapist to work through her grief after her mother's suicide. The therapist understood that there was a spiritual component underlying the grief. Referring and supporting the client to work with a Buddhist nun ensured a cultural, ethical, and clinical process for this client. Consulting a Buddhist nun assured the client that her mother would not return as a revengeful spirit. Clearly, the traditional teachings that are embedded in the cultural healing methods are an important factor in the treatment process as these likely promote a match between the therapeutic orientation and the client's spiritual beliefs about death and dying. The connection between the client and the Buddhist nun offered a sense of cultural or historical connection within which the client may feel better understood and motivated in her healing journey given the alignment in values and beliefs with the traditional healer. Furthermore, in using a Western psychotherapy technique, the empty-chair technique, the client was able to ask for forgiveness from her deceased mother. A culturally sensitive counselor will make sure that the client is in agreement with the exercise of "talking" to the dead mother. For some clients, talking to someone who is dead is not part of their cultural practice and can be seen as taboo. In circumstances where this is done—for example, in particular religious or spiritual contexts—an elder or priest would need to be present to conduct the ceremony. If this is the case, then the empty chair exercise will not work. In addition, there is the added dimension of language. If clients agree to do the empty chair exercise, they may prefer to speak in the vernacular, which may pose difficulties to a therapist who strongly desires to direct the exercise rather than accept a translation after the exercise.

Third, it may be difficult to envision what an ideal integration might look like in matching client's mental health needs with a particular healing tradition as many clinicians are not trained in Asian healing methods. However, for counselors and psychotherapists to gain an appreciation and understanding of Asian healing methods, certain features have been identified as key to a helpful integrated healing model. Specifically, a thoughtful and sound theoretical rationale forms an important foundation for integrating therapies and healing strategies. The primary rationale should be centered on developing a common framework or shared worldview that connects the counselor and the client, enabling them to work together in the safety of a supportive and respectful space, and one that is culturally sensitive. This means that prior to integration, the counselor should gain an in-depth understanding of the client's worldview in order to determine what kind of Asian healing practice might be of interest and whether they complement or contradict the work that is being done. In other words, it is essential to determine whether the models of healing that are to be integrated complement one another in terms of theoretical framework, paradigmatic methodological approaches, and negotiated clinical outcomes. In this process of integration and cross-fertilization, Linda Barnes argued that we modify and adapt "in our own image" as "a matter of felt need" and that "the transformation which some Chinese practices are undergoing through having been transplanted into American soil has had the effect not only of intensifying certain nuances that were already present, but also of introducing questions that had not even entered the Chinese system as rejected possibilities" (p. 438).[6]

Conclusion

Asian healing traditions may not be of interest or a desire by all counselors and psychotherapists. There may be critiques against the use of Asian healing methods, arguing that these are not grounded in evidence-based research. Even if the methods are supported by research, there continues to be doubts about its utility. For example, even though mindfulness has a huge canon of research that supports its use in various psychological and medical settings, there are still claims about the serious adverse effects to mindfulness meditation. The same arguments could be made for Asian healing traditions, such as acupuncture, TCM, Morita, and others. Even with volumes of research to indicate the positive outcomes, there will be clinicians who will always be anxious, concerned, or afraid for whatever reason to appreciate, accept, and acknowledge the use of traditional and indigenous healing practices. For those practitioners who are interested in integrating Asian healing traditions and acquiring competency in some of the Asian healing methods, the process can be an organic one, depending on interest, motivation, and context within which they practice. For some, becoming skilled at mindfulness meditation or acupuncture can take years of training and education. Likewise, becoming a spiritual healer (shaman, elder, healer) is a journey that requires renouncing one's current way of life and training in specific institutes in Asia. However, a modicum of knowledge and appreciation of Asian healing traditions may be essential if clinicians are working in a multicultural setting, particularly with clients who identify as Asian. For example, the psychotherapist in the case study in Chapter 7, while not trained in any of the Asian healing traditions, was culturally competent enough to refer his client to a Buddhist nun so that she could learn meditation to regulate her moods and thoughts and to undertake a ritual—to make an offering to the "tiger god" at a Taoist temple. Also, in Chapter 7, Lee explored the idea that the Taoist ritual worked because it "symbolically transformed her emotional experiences within a culturally legitimate myth consistent with her Taoist and Buddhist worldviews"; it seems that "her emotional experience was attached to the transactional symbols (ritual) derived from the myth." Consistent with Asian healing traditions, the therapist "reinforced" the clients' beliefs and perceptions of traditional healing through the referral to a Buddhist nun for Taoist healing and at the same time this process engaged in a "reduction" of her anxiety. As Zhang and Chi noted, "Reinforcing (adds something positive into the system) and reducing (remove something negative from the system) are important categories of TCM methodology, which govern innumerable specific treating skills, including psychological interventions" (p. 361).[7]

The significance of referring to indigenous healers and elders is twofold. First, given past colonial appropriation of cultural artifacts and rituals, it avoids the possibility of cultural exploitation of certain cultural practices that appear to be "sacred" to traditional shamans, healers, and elders. Second, inviting indigenous healers and elders to conduct their rituals and remedies legitimizes traditional and cultural healing practices and conveys respect and acceptance of their healing philosophies, values, and "psychologies." In other words, the counselor perceives the ritual and practice to be sacred and special and understands that it ought to be conducted by someone who is respected in that particular cultural community who specializes in that role. This way, the counselor demonstrates that he or she trusts in the traditional healer and in the cultural healing practice. Indeed, consulting with traditional and indigenous healers and elders of the client's community could lead to more substantive collaboration in the future as well as the possibility of gaining deeper and richer knowledge and insights of the unique facets of the particular cultural healing methods which could lead to, in the very least, a genuine collaboration between the Western healing systems and Asian healing traditions.

REFERENCES

1. U.S. Census Bureau. (2006). https://www.census.gov/quickfacts/table/PST045215/00Statistics
2. Statistics Canada. (2006). *2006 census of population.* Retrieved from https://www12.statcan.gc.ca/census-recensement/2006/index-eng.cfm
3. Moodley, R. (2011). *Outside the sentence: Readings in critical multicultural counseling and psychotherapy.* Toronto, Canada: Centre for Diversity in Counselling and Psychotherapy, Ontario Institute for Studies in Education (OISE), University of Toronto.

4. Ozawa-de-Silva, C., & Ozawa-de Silva, B. R. (2011). Mind/body theory and practice in Tibetan medicine and Buddhism. *Body & Society*, *17*(1), 95–119.
5. Moodley, R., & Kinha, B. (2015). Therapy without borders: Bridging counseling and psychotherapy across cultures. In R. Moodley, M. Lengyell, R. Wu, & U. P. Gielen (Eds.), *International counseling: Case studies handbook*. Washington, DC: American Counseling Association.
6. Barnes, L. L. (1998). The psychologizing of Chinese healing practices into the United States. *Culture, Medicine and Psychiatry*, *22*, 413–443.
7. Zhang, P., & Chi, X. (2013). Reinforcing and reducing: Dialogue between traditional Chinese medicine and psychoanalytic psychotherapy. *International Journal of Applied Psychoanalytic Studies*, *10*(4), 361–367.

Glossary

Amae **(甘え):** *Amae* means "sweet" in Japanese, symbolizing the first of experience of love with a mother through the sweetness of breast milk. It refers to the opportunity to depend on the benevolence or indulgence of others with whom one has close relationships (e.g., parents, children, romantic partners). This quality of relatedness is communicated primarily through nonverbal means and involves feelings of warmth, intimacy, and security. It also implies unconditional acceptance within close relationships.

Art of living: This refers to the pragmatic and skillful approaches described in *Yojokun* to take responsibility for one's wholesomeness and to appreciate abundance and savor the fulfillment of one's life with purpose and meaning. Detailed instructions were described over eight volumes about food and drink, hygiene and bathing, illness and preventive treatment, aging and longevity, education, acupuncture, and medicinal herbs. The moral practice also emphasized the respect for parents and the heaven and earth due to the strong influence of neo-Confucianism.

Biomedical psychiatry: This is the dominant conceptual framework within which mental illness is understood, diagnosed, and treated in the context of Western biomedicine. This broad framework is based on contemporary biological models of brain function at the level of neurotransmitters and functional brain circuits.

Buddhism: Considered one of humanity's great religions, Buddhism was founded by Siddhartha Gautama in Nepal approximately 2,500 years ago. Its core belief defines suffering (and its resolution) as a result of our distorted beliefs about the world we experience, specifically about the nature of the self. A goal of Buddhism is to experientially realize the true nature of the self and what it perceives in order to eliminate suffering and attain enlightenment.

Byosen scanning: Byosen is a scanning technique used in Reiki to detect energy blockages on the client's body. The technique uses the sensitivity on the practitioner's hands to perceive disrupted energy. The disrupted energy may present as areas with different density or different temperature. The disrupted areas will need more Reiki healing energy.

Chinese Taoist cognitive psychotherapy (CTCP): This is a form of indigenous psychotherapy developed in China. The process of CTCP resembles cognitive behavioral therapy (CBT), but it is infused with Chinese values. Clients learn to replace their maladaptive beliefs with Taoist doctrines.

Chinese worldview model of equilibrium: This traditional Chinese cosmology is designated to maintain harmony and balance among humans and nature, humans and society, and within any human being.

Common factors model: This model is one of the approaches for psychotherapy integration. It postulates that the effectiveness of the many counseling theories is due to their similarities (common factors) rather than their specific processes. Past research has identified a number of common factors, including shared worldviews, the therapeutic relationship, interventions, client expectations, extra-therapeutic factors, hope, and placebo effects.

Confucian self-cultivation: This is a doctrine for practicing the Confucian core values of "self-exertion" and "putting oneself in the place of others."

Confucianism: This is a system of philosophy developed by Chinese philosopher Confucius (551–479 BC). There is an emphasis on ethics, harmony, and maintenance of social order. At an individual level, people strive to become an upright person, or *junzhi*, who is concerned with justice, morality, and welfare of others while reinforcing social order.

Dao Yin (導引): This is a series of exercises, a practice as a precursor of Qigong (QG). Literally, it means leading and guiding the vital energy, following Dao and sometimes tracing the channel of bodily *qi*—that is, meridians and its key points, in this ancient practice. The Daoist Canon (AD 1145) comprises 1,120 volumes, including 1 dedicated to the classic version of *Dao Yin*, which contains all the principles involved in QG.

Eightfold Path: This describes the Buddha's teachings on how one can attain the end of suffering and realize enlightenment. These can be summarized into three major teachings on ethics (how to behave toward others), wisdom (how to perceive reality as it is), and meditation (how to understand the mind).

***Feng shui*:** It is written as "wind–water (風水) " in Chinese character. It is an ancient Chinese art and the practice of a philosophical system that governs spatial arrangement of objects and things in relation to the flow of energy (*qi*) in a living environment. The purpose of *feng shui* is to enhance the harmonization of the environments to support health and well-being and invite wealth and happiness.

The five elements: This is a foundational concept in Chinese medicine that is also used in other disciplines, including feng shui, martial arts, and philosophy (e.g., *The I Ching*). The elements are metal, wood, water, fire, and earth. This schema is used to describe the interaction between nature and different dimensions of the human being, including internal organs and emotions.

Flourishing: This is a positive psychology concept that is a measure of overall life wellness including positive emotion, engagement, interest, meaning, and purpose. In mental health, flourishing individuals are filled with emotional vitality and functioning positively in their lives rather than merely existing.

Forbearance: This is a psychological mechanism for Chinese people to restrain their tempers and to cope with frustrations or interpersonal conflicts in a harmonious way.

Four Noble Truths: These truths or insights encapsulate the core Buddhist beliefs that life is characterized by emotional suffering, that the cause of suffering is a tendency to project our beliefs onto the outside world (leading to attachment and aversion toward experience), and that such tendencies can be corrected through the pursuit of personality transformation.

***Futei* (wind–body):** It is a term to describe the "atmosphere" around a person and written as "wind–body (風体)." In this case, the atmosphere includes all aspects of the external appearance, including style, shape, complexion, dress, facial expression, demeanor, countenance, and so on. It is often used to describe the impression of a person.

Holistic: This is treatment of the whole person, which takes into account the physical, emotional, psychological, spiritual, and environmental factors of a person's health.

***Huangdi Neijing*:** This is an ancient Chinese medical text, the foundation source of traditional Chinese medicine (TCM). The manuscript is composed of two texts each of 81 chapters in a question-and-answer format.

***The I Ching*:** This is an ancient book on the results of divination. Confucianists' reinterpretation of it had transformed it into a classic of Confucian cosmology and self-cultivation.

Indigenous healing: This is localized helping beliefs, practices, and strategies that originate within a given culture or society that are not imported from other regions and are intended to treat the members of that given cultural groups.

***Karesansui*:** The word *karesansui* can be translated as a dry landscape or rock garden. The garden may include rocks, sand, pruned trees and bushes, water features, and other elements that are used to depict natural scenes. These landscapes, often referred to as Zen gardens, are typically enclosed by a wall and are often integrated within a Zen temple context. A porch-like sitting area allows individuals to view the garden and engage in meditative practices.

***Maha-satipatthana Sutta*:** This is the great aphorism or sermon on the foundation or establishment of mindfulness. These are the Buddha's instructions on the foundations of mindfulness, and it is regarded as the canonical Buddhist text that contains the most comprehensive teachings on mindfulness meditation techniques. The word *satipatthana* is the name for an approach to meditation aimed at establishing *sati*, or mindfulness.

Meditation: This is the primary means by which the mind is transformed. Buddhist meditation practices encourage the development of one-pointed concentration and equanimity as well as a clear insight or understanding of the true nature of phenomena. With discipline, meditation becomes the means by which the personality is transformed and suffering ended.

***Mensetsu-sha*:** Naikan practitioners are called *mensetsu-sha* in Japanese, and the term literally means "a person who interviews." A *mensetsu-sha* is also a *Naikan-sha*.

Metabolic syndrome: This is a disorder caused by abnormal use and storage of the body's metabolic energy and is often associated with abdominal (central) obesity, elevated blood pressure, elevated fasting plasma glucose, high-serum triglycerides, and low high-density lipoprotein (HDL) levels that place individuals at increased risk of developing heart disease and diabetes. Several widely prescribed antipsychotics and other medications are associated with significantly increased risk of developing a metabolic syndrome.

Metacognitive acuity: What various definitions of mindfulness hold in common is the notion of a cultivated meta-cognitive capacity to observe events in awareness (i.e., thoughts, feelings, and sensations) without reacting to them in an automatic, habituated pattern.

Mindfulness: The term is derived from the Pali word *sati* or *smṛti* in Sanskrit and translates as nonforgetfulness or recollection. The term is related to the verb *sarati*—"to remember" or "to keep in mind" and can be used in the context of recall or memory of past events or remembering to do some activity in the future. In the context of mindfulness meditation, it relates to present-focused attention, the "keeping in mind" of arising phenomena—that is, the object of one's meditation, such as the sensations related to breathing (*ānāpānasati*). "Right-mindfulness" is defined in the context of the Buddhist Eightfold Path as being, guided by the right view, grounded by ethics, and motivated by the right intention.

Mindfulness-based stress reduction (MBSR): This is a manualized treatment program developed by Kabat-Zinn for the management of chronic pain. The typical protocol is an 8- to 10-week program for groups of up to 30 participants who commit to meeting for 2 to 3 hours a week. Examples of mindfulness techniques introduced in MBSR training are the body scan (a participant directs their attention through the body, cultivating increased proprioception), walking meditation, hatha yoga, diaphragmatic breathing, and seated meditation.

***Mishirabe*:** This term literally means "self-examination," and this Buddhist meditational practice involves severe and ascetic meditation-like bodily engagement such as fasting and deprivation of sleep until one achieves spiritual awakening. *Mishirabe* forms part of the basis of Naikan, but the founder of Naikan, Yoshimoto Ishin, modified *mishirabe* so that it would be more accessible to a wide range of people regardless of their religion.

Morita therapy: Japanese psychiatrist Shoma Morita developed Morita psychotherapy and counseling. Its primary tenets include accepting reality as it is and taking constructive action in one's life. It works closely with harmonizing oneself to nature and following one's own natural rhythms.

Multicultural counseling competencies: Multicultural counseling competencies refer to three specific domains associated with counselors' cultural competencies: awareness, knowledge, and skills. These competencies enable counselors to work effectively with clients of various cultural and diversity backgrounds.

Multitheoretical psychotherapy (MTP): Multitheoretical psychotherapy is one of the approaches for psychotherapy integration. It aims at integrating different counseling theories at both conceptual and practical levels. It adopts a pragmatic approach whereby theories do not have to be reconciled or synthesized.

Naikan: This is a Japanese indigenous introspective healing practice that has been derived from Japanese Mahayana Buddhism and established as a secular form of therapeutic self-cultivation. Naikan lies at the border of psychotherapy and spirituality. *Nai* means "inside," and *kan* means "looking," so Naikan literally means "introspection" or "inner-looking." When Naikan is offered at Naikan centers, it is usually simply called Naikan. Naikan is referred to as Naikan therapy when it is offered in the clinical setting with the necessary medication and supervision by medical professionals.

Naikan's three themes or questions: These are the three themes or questions: (1) what the client received from the person on whom he or she is reflecting, (2) what he or she gave back to that person, and (3) what trouble he or she caused that person. These three themes are the essence of Naikan. They are simple and yet complex, as they require interpretation by the client. How clients respond to these questions reflects the level of their introspection. Naikan clients engage with their past in accordance with these three questions.

***Naikan-sha*:** The term literally means "a person who does Naikan." Both Naikan clients and Naikan practitioners are *Naikan-sha*. In this book, the convention of using the terms *client* and *practitioner* will be retained for clarity, but these terms could be misleading if they are not understood within this context.

Reiki symbols: The Reiki symbols are the essence of the technique. The symbols are the vehicle in which the Reiki teacher transfers the energy to the practitioner during the attunements. During a session, they are better described as keys to different healing energies to address specific issues on the recipient.

***rlung*:** *rlung* (wind) is one of the "humors" in Tibetan medicine (Sowa-Rigpa) and is generally associated with the mind and heart. Imbalances in *rlung* may result from or cause imbalances in the other humors and manifest as complex symptom patterns of emotional and somatic symptoms that resemble psychosomatic disorders described in Western medicine.

***Ryunen*:** *Ryunen* refers to a sense of apathy seen in some Japanese young people. It is often related to a lack of clarity, sense of purpose, or personal goals and may be related to feeling alienated or disenchanted about opportunities available to young people. *Ryunen* may be reflected in lack of work aspirations, apathy about or feeling disconnected in intimate relationships, or disengagement from one's community.

Savoring: It is a positive psychology concept and refers to the action to increase the intensity, duration, and appreciation of positive experiences and emotions while coping and dealing with negative emotions. It is a way to optimize the potential benefits of positivity on people's lives through mindful engagement and conscious awareness to the experience of pleasure in various time frames.

Self: This is a central tenet of Buddhism that concerns the nature of the self, which is considered to be "empty." The self is composed of a number of psychophysical processes (i.e., consciousness, feeling, perception, volition, materiality)—the nature of which is without inherent substance or essence.

Self-actualization: This is a concept of the integrity of a person's nature in which the organism spontaneously reorganizes its capacities to actualize its potential through whichever avenues are available.

Self-realization: It brings a value of richness of the human existence that expands horizons and maximizes potential.

***Shinkeishitsu*:** This is a Japanese term describing a nervous predisposition and feelings of anxiety. The original Morita therapy was designed to treat clients with *shinkeishitsu*-related symptoms, such as excessive introspective tendencies, perfectionistic obsession, hypersensitivity, and a highly anxious character.

Shinpiden: The term *Reiki master* was created by Hawayo Takata to refer to the Reiki teacher's level or Shinpiden as it is known in Japan. The term *master* is traditionally used in the East to denote a person who has achieved spiritual enlightenment or in the West to denote experience and knowledge on a subject. So what is referred to in the West as "Reiki master level" following Japanese Reiki tradition is actually Reiki teacher level.

Social anxiety: This is a persistent fear of one or more social or performance situations in which a person has an excessive and unreasonable fear. Anxiety (intense nervousness) and self-consciousness arise from a fear of being closely watched, judged, and criticized by others. The feared situations are avoided or else are endured with intense anxiety and distress.

Somatization: A tendency for clients to express their psychological disturbances in terms of physical complaints.

Sowa-Rigpa: "The science of healing" is being used more increasingly instead of "traditional Tibetan medicine." However, scholars of Tibetan medicine claim that Sowa-Rigpa incorporates principles and clinical methods from both Ayurvedic medicine used in India and indigenous medical practices used in Tibet.

Subtle body: The subtle body can be defined as an extension of the physical body. Any solid object has an energetic field. The subtle body pertains to the energetic field of living beings. Within this field lies the blueprint of our thoughts, feelings, and spirit. This blueprint can manifest in the physical body as a particular behavior, emotional state, or illness. The Reiki practitioner channels universal life force into the subtle body of the client in order to remove and rectify blockages and rebalance the client's energetic constitution.

***Taijin kyofusho*:** This disorder can be translated as fear (*kyofusho*) of interpersonal relationships (*taijin*). This culture-specific syndrome is related to social anxieties and involves concerns about offending others. Symptoms may include fear of eye contact, fear of showing improper facial expressions, or fear of emitting body odors that may embarrass others. *Taijin kyofusho* may be accompanied by *hikikomori*, which involves a pattern of social isolation and shutting oneself away from others for a period of at least six months.

Taoism: A philosophical doctrine of Chinese origin that emphasizes living in harmony with nature (macrocosmos) and own self (microcosmos); based on writings attributed to Laozi (or Lao-tzu), Zhuangzi (or Chuang-Tzu), and others and advocates conforming one's behavior and thought to the Tao. Taoism is based on the founder Laozi, a philosopher and sage in China in the 6th–5th century BC and his work *Tao Te Ching* (or *Dao De Jing*). There is an emphasis on nonaction, naturalness, spontaneity, simplicity, and purification of the heart through nonstriving and being in harmony with the Tao. Tao, which means "way," "path," or "principle," is thought to be the natural source or force behind everything: the basic, eternal principle of the universe that transcends reality and is the source of being, nonbeing, and change. Taoist philosophy is distinguished from Taoism practiced as a religion.

Third-wave behavioral psychotherapies: This is a term based on a behavioralist perspective. The origin of psychotherapy is considered psychoanalysis. The first wave began with behavioral therapy when there was an attempt to move toward empiricism and principles governing observable behaviors. The second wave refers to cognitive behavioral therapy (CBT) when there was a shift to focus on one's thoughts. The third-wave interventions have in common the incorporation of mindfulness and acceptance.

Three higher trainings: The Buddha's Eightfold Path was subdivided into three divisions, often referred to as the three higher trainings—wisdom (*paññakkhandha*), ethical conduct (*silakkhandha*), and mental development (*samadhikkhandha*). Mental development was further subdivided into right effort, right mindfulness, and right concentration.

Traditional and conventional therapy integration: These are systematic efforts to generate counseling or therapy approaches that incorporate the assumptions, the principles, and the practices of both traditional cultural healing and Western counseling and psychotherapy.

Traditional healing practices: These are helping beliefs and methods originating in a particular cultural group. There are many forms of traditional healing practices, such as traditional and complementary medicine, shamanism, spirit mediumship, and religious healing.

Universal life force: Universal life force can be defined as the energy that permeates, creates, and connects all things. It has held different names across cultural contexts such as *chi* (China), *ki* (Japan), *ni* (Lakota), *nilch'i* (Navajo), *prana* (India, Yogic tradition), and even the Force (Star Wars). No matter what name it is given, or what culture it appears in, universal life force holds the same characteristics and can be harnessed for use in healing. Universal life force is ever present and available to all beings. It is said to hold its own consciousness and awareness.

Worldviews: are beliefs, assumptions, and values that describe reality, human nature, the meanings of life, and one's relationships with the world.

***Wu wei*:** Idea evolving from Confucianism and tenet of Taoism philosophically describing the right way of being still as a life attitude.

***Wu-chin-his* (Five Animal Dances):** This is an ancient Qigong (QG) exercise practiced by the legendary traditional Chinese medicine (TCM) physician Hua Tua (c. 140–208). The practitioner mimics dancing movements, sounds, and breathing of the five animals (i.e., monkey, bear, deer, bird, and tiger) to bring the energy system back to the free human nature. Symbolically, the animals are related to the five elements in colors, seasons, internal organs, sensory organs, and emotions.

***Yamai wa ki kara* (病は気から):** It is a Japanese proverb, literally saying that sickness arises from one's spirit (*qi*), meaning that one's illness starts with the mind. It implies the causational relationship between one's mind and body and mental stress can lead to physical health.

***Yin* and *yang*:** This presents a core philosophical idea in Daoism and other Chinese philosophy. The pair symbolically describe how opposite or contrary forces are actually complementary, interconnected, and interdependent in the natural world and how they give rise to or control over each other as they interrelate to one another. It indicates complementary (but sometime contradictive) forces that interact to form a dynamic system in which the whole is greater than the assembled parts. *Yin* is associated with the properties of darkness, softness, and passivity, and *yang* with the properties of brightness, hardness, and activity. *Yin* and *yang* are constantly in a dynamic interplay from which change becomes a constant in the universe. *Yin* and *yang* generate and attenuate each other.

***Yojokun*:** This is a concept, written as 養生 and literally meaning "nourishing life." It is the basic philosophy in *Yojokun*, the teaching manual written by Kaibara Ekken for holistic health to fulfill longevity, self-responsibility for taking care of one's own body as well as mind and spirit. It was widely read and practiced by people of the Edo period, the final period of traditional Japan characterized by unified political stability and rise of agriculture, economy, and industrial development.

Zen: This is a school of Mahayana Buddhism originating from China as Chán and became known as Zen in Japan. It is a branch of Buddhism that emphasizes meditative practice, insight into Buddha–nature, and its application for the benefit of others. Its development has been influenced by Taoism.

Zi-Wu-Liu-Zhu: This indicates the movement of *qi* in the mind–body system involving its flowing and ebbing in paired organ systems and corresponding meridians. Of this system, each energetic organ–emotional pair has its own peak time around a circadian system covering a 24-hour cycle. This system can be used as a guiding principle in practicing Qigong (QG) and acupuncture.

Index

About the Editors

Roy Moodley, PhD, is associate professor of counseling psychology at the Ontario Institute for Studies in Education, University of Toronto. He is also the director of the Centre for Diversity in Counselling and Psychotherapy. Roy's research interests include critical multicultural counseling and psychotherapy, race and culture in psychotherapy, traditional healing practices, and gender and identity.

Ted (Hung-Tat) Lo, MBBS, MRCPsych, FRCPC, is a cultural psychiatrist in Toronto. He was assistant professor in the Department of Psychiatry at the University of Toronto, consulting to the Culture, Community and Health Studies Program. Ted has developed many programs in culturally competent practice and has written and lectured widely on the topic. He also founded the Friends of Alternative and Complementary Therapies Society and organized workshops and conferences on traditional healing. With Mami Ishii, he established the Integrative Mental Health Centre of Toronto.

Na Zhu, MEd, is currently pursuing a PhD in clinical psychology at the University of Windsor in Canada. She has a master's degree in counseling psychology from the Ontario Institute for Studies in Education, University of Toronto. Na has many years of experience in the mental health field, integrating culturally sensitive practices. Her current research interests are in developmental psychopathology and emotional competence.

About the Contributors

Amy L. Ai, PhD, is a professor at Florida State University. She has practiced Qigong (QG) since her teenage years. Amy has led many funded projects and published 120+ academic papers. She is a Fellow of the American Psychological Association (APA), Association for Psychological Sciences (APS), and the Gerontological Society of America (GSA); a Hartford scholar, a Fulbright specialist, and a delegate to the 2005 White House Conference on Aging.

Yu-ping Cao, MD, PhD, is a professor at the Mental Health Institute of Second Xiangya Hospital, Central South University in China. She is the vice chairman of the young member committee of the division of Psychiatry of the Chinese Medical Association, and a committee member of the China Association of Psychological Counseling and Psychotherapy.

Charles P. Chen, PhD, is a professor of counseling psychology and is the Canada Research Chair at the University of Toronto. His book *Career Endeavour* received the 2008 Canadian Best Counselling Book Award. Charles is a prominent social scientist featured in Canadian Who's Who and Who's Who in the World.

Carolyn Zerbe Enns, PhD, is a professor of psychology at Cornell College. She was born and raised in Japan, which shaped her lifelong interests. Carolyn served as resident director of the Japan Study program (study abroad). Carolyn has explored and written about Japanese indigenous psychotherapies, Japanese feminisms, and contemporary gender issues.

Kenneth Fung, MD, FRCPC, MSc, is staff psychiatrist and clinical director of the Asian Initiative in Mental Health program, Toronto Western Hospital, University Health Network, and associate professor with Equity, Gender and Population Division, Department of Psychiatry at the University of Toronto. Kenneth's interests include both cultural psychiatry and psychotherapy.

Julie Hong, MEd, is currently pursuing her doctorate in counseling psychology at the University of Toronto. Her clinical practice involves working with adult community populations, with special interest in trauma-related sequelae. Julie's current research area focuses on career and life transitions of new immigrants in Canada.

Kwang-Kuo Hwang, PhD, is the National Chair Professor at National Taiwan University, awarded by Taiwan's Ministry of Education. He has endeavored to promote the indigenization movement of psychology in Chinese society since the early 1980s and has published eight books and more than 100 articles on related issues.

Mami Ishii, ND, MT-BC, Lac, is the project coordinator for Clinical Cultural Competence Consultants, consultant for the Asian Initiative in Mental Health at Toronto Western Hospital, and a lecturer at the Canadian School of Natural Nutrition. With Ted Lo, she established the Integrative Mental Health Centre of Toronto.

Samantha Jacques, PhD, FACHE, is director of Clinical Engineering at Penn State Health Milton S. Hershey Medical Center. Prior to Penn State Hershey, Jacques was director of Biomedical Engineering at Texas Children's Hospital. She has a PhD in biomedical engineering and is a Fellow of the American College of Healthcare Executives.

Makiko Kasai, PhD, is a professor at Naruto University of Education in Japan. She is a member of the American Psychological Association (APA) and on the board of directors of the Association of Japanese Clinical Psychology and the Japanese Society of Certified Clinical Psychologists. Her research includes diversity and sensitivity training for counselors.

Emily Kedar, BA, MEd (candidate), is studying psychotherapy at the University of Toronto. She is a published poet, Reiki practitioner, and professional tarot reader. She currently works at distress centers doing grief support for survivors of suicide loss. Emily plans to establish Kanaka Village, a wellness retreat center in British Columbia, Canada.

Ben C. H. Kuo, PhD, is Full Professor of Clinical Psychology at the University of Windsor. His main research and teaching are cross-cultural psychology and multicultural counseling. Ben is actively involved in international teaching and has lectured in countries such as Taiwan, China, Thailand, the United States, Australia, and New Zealand.

James H. Lake, MD, is a psychiatrist in the San Francisco Bay Area. He was previously assistant professor in the Department of Psychiatry and Behavioral Medicine at Stanford. James founded and chaired the American Psychiatric Association Caucus on Integrative Medicine. He is a founding member and former chair of the International Network of Integrative Mental Health.

Boon-Ooi Lee, PhD, is the senior lecturer in counseling psychology at the National Institute of Education, Nanyang Technological University in Singapore. His research focuses on culture and mental health. Boon-Ooi's research is interdisciplinary, combining the knowledge and methods from psychology, cultural psychiatry, and medical anthropology.

Tenzin Lhundup, MD, is staff physician in the Department of Internal Medicine and full-time faculty at Men Tse Kang, Lhasa. He served as a staff physician in Tibetan medicine at the Qu Su County Nyi thng Village hospital, Lhasa Taktse County Bonthu Village Hospital, and Lhasa Tak tse County Hospital.

Marco Mascarin, PhD, RP, is codirector of the Institute of Traditional Medicine and Buddhist chaplain at the University of Toronto Multi-Faith Centre. He is facilitator of the Nalanda Institute's Contemplative Psychotherapy program (Toronto) and clinical associate at the Mindfulness Clinic. Marco also served as codirector of University of Toronto's Inter-Professional Mindfulness Program.

Yoshihiko Miki, is professor emeritus at Osaka University in Japan, a clinical psychologist, and an author of many publications. He established Nara Training Center of Naikan Therapy with his wife, Junko, and continues research on the clinical application of Naikan therapy.

Martha P. Novoa, PhD, Reiki Master, has over 15 years of experience in Reiki therapy, practicing and teaching Reiki therapy as an intervention for physical and emotional illnesses on an international level. Her interests are integration of energy therapies and quantum realities as a tool for transformation in everyday life.

Tadashi Ogawa, PhD, is professor emeritus at Kyoto University and was president of Koshien University, Japan. Ogawa's research interest is phenomenology of *qi*, mood, and atmosphere. He is the editor of nine journals, including the *Monist*, and the author of 15 books. He has presented at many conferences in Japan, Germany, and Italy.

Chikako Ozawa-de Silva, PhD, is associate professor in the Department of Anthropology at Emory University. Her research focuses on cross-cultural understandings of health and illness, especially mental illness, by bringing together Western and Asian (particularly Japanese and Tibetan) perspectives on the mind-body, religion, medicine, and therapy.

Paul Posadzki, PhD, is Research Fellow in Health Services and Outcomes Research Programme at Lee Kong Chian School of Medicine, Singapore. His interests are evidence-based medicine and health care, safety, and effectiveness of complementary and alternative medicine, psychosocial health, preventive medicine, physical activity and sport, physiotherapy and rehabilitation, research and practice of pain, and public health.

Beatriz Rodriguez-Rubio, PhD, received her doctoral degree in clinical psychology at the University of Windsor in 2015. Beatriz specializes in qualitative research. Her doctoral dissertation qualitatively examined therapist–trainees' experiences while providing therapy to first-generation refugee clients in Canada. Beatriz is currently practicing in St. John's, Newfoundland.

Catherine Tien-Lun Sun, PhD, is academic vice president and professor of the Department of Counseling and Psychology at Hong Kong Shue Yan University. She has an abiding interest in developing a body of knowledge in psychology and psychotherapy, which bears cultural relevance and is useful to people in Asia, particularly those of Chinese descent.

Tony Toneatto, PhD, is associate professor in the Department of Psychiatry and director of the Buddhism, Psychology and Mental Health program at the University of Toronto. He has published on substance and behavioral addictions, especially pathological gambling. Tony is a registered clinical psychologist and a psychoanalyst.

Jie Zeng, MD, PhD, received her master's degree in neurology at Shanghai Jiao Tong University and PhD in psychiatry at Central South University. She has a special interest in the integration of Chinese traditional culture and psychotherapy. Jie Zeng is currently completing her psychiatry residency at Shanghai Mental Health Center.

Ya-lin Zhang, MD, PhD, is a professor at the Mental Health Institute of Second Xiangya Hospital, Central South University in China. He is the vice chairman of the China Association on Psychological Counseling and Psychotherapy, and one of the founders of Chinese Taoist cognitive psychotherapy (CTCP).

Zhuo-Hong Zhu, PhD, is a professor at the Institute of Psychology at the Chinese Academy of Sciences. He is also the president of the China Chapter of the Association for Contextual Behavioral Science (ACBS) and director of the Central State Organs and Staff Mental Health Counseling Center.